Serono Symposia USA
Norwell, Massachusetts

W0050578

Springer Science+Business Media, LLC

PROCEEDINGS IN THE SERONO SYMPOSIA USA SERIES

Continued after Index

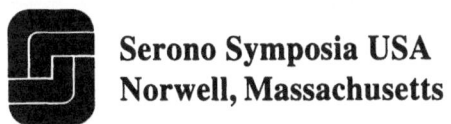

Serono Symposia USA
Norwell, Massachusetts

Eli Y. Adashi

Editor

Ovulation

Evolving Scientific and
Clinical Concepts

With 89 Figures

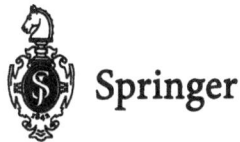

Springer

Eli Y. Adashi, M.D.
Department of Obstetrics and Gynecology
University of Utah Health Sciences Center
Salt Lake City, UT 84132
USA

Proceedings of the International Symposium on Ovulation: Evolving Scientific and Clinical Concepts, sponsored by Serono Symposia USA, Inc., held September 24 to 27, 1998, in Salt Lake City, Utah.

For information on previous volumes, contact Serono Symposia USA, Inc.

Library of Congress Cataloging-in-Publication Data
Ovulation: evolving scientific and clinical concepts/Eli Y. Adashi, editor.
    p. cm.
    "Proceedings of the International Symposium on Ovulation: Evolving Scientific and
Clinical Concepts, sponsored by Serono Symposia USA, held September 24 to 27, 1998,
in Salt Lake City, Utah"—T.p. verso.
    Includes bibliographical references and index.
    ISBN 978-1-4899-0521-5
        1. Ovulation—Congresses. I. Adashi, E.Y. II. Serono Symposia, USA.
III. International Symposium on Ovulation: Evolving Scientific and Clinical Concepts (1998:
Salt Lake City, Utah)
    [DNLM: 1. Ovulation—Congresses. 2. Gonadotropins, Pituitary—Congresses.
3. Ovary—physiology—Congresses. WP 540 O949 2000]
QP261 .O93 2000
612.6'2—dc21   00–059480

Printed on acid-free paper.

© 2000 Springer Science+Business Media New York
Originally published by Springer-Verlag New York, Inc. in 2000
Softcover reprint of the hardcover 1st edition 2000

Production coordinated by Chernow Editorial Services, Inc., and managed by Francine McNeill; manufacturing supervised by Jacqui Ashri.
Typeset by KP Company, Brooklyn, NY.

9 8 7 6 5 4 3 2 1   SPIN 10778215

ISBN 978-1-4899-0521-5   ISBN 978-0-387-21508-2 (eBook)
DOI 10.1007/978-0-387-21508-2

SYMPOSIUM ON OVULATION: EVOLVING SCIENTIFIC AND CLINICAL CONCEPTS

Scientific Committee

Eli Y. Adashi, M.D., Chair
University of Utah Health Sciences Center
Salt Lake City, Utah

Organizing Secretary

Leslie Nies
Serono Symposia USA, Inc.
100 Longwater Circle
Norwell, Massachusetts

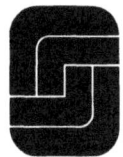

Preface

One can think of few more fundamental biological processes than ovulation. There is little doubt that the extrusion of the mature, fertilizable oocyte, surrounded by a layer of somatic cumulus cells, subserves a single purpose: the preservation of the species. Although much has transpired in the understanding of follicular rupture, many gaps remain in our knowledge with respect to this fundamental biological process. It has become clear that ovulation, in the final analysis, constitutes a series of highly synchronized and exquisitely timed transcriptional events. In other words, a cascade of gene activation is inevitably launched to a point of no return such that transformation into a corpus luteum is all but inevitable. One cannot help but reflect on the sad irony that a process so central to the creation of life is also the one responsible for the genesis of one of the most virulent forms of human cancer; namely, epithelial ovarian cancer. If for no other reason than to conquer this major scourge, understanding ovulation is a must so as to shed light on the genesis of this disease.

This volume, by some of the best minds in the discipline of ovarian physiology, is unique. The authors spent 3 days together dedicating the discussion exclusively to the process of ovulation and its mechanistic underpinnings. These thoughts and more are contained in this volume, which to the best of my knowledge represents a first. It is my sincere hope that you, the reader, will enjoy reading this book as much as I did. It is by far the next best thing to being there.

ELI Y. ADASHI

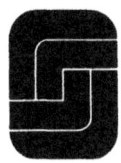

Contents

Part VI.   Clinical Frontiers

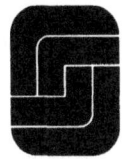

Contributors

JUDITH M. ADAMS, Reproductive Endocrine Unit and National Center for Infertility Research, Massachusetts General Hospital, Boston, Massachusetts, USA.

KARA J. ALLEN, Prince Henry's Institute of Medical Research, Clayton, Victoria, Australia.

MARTINE ANTAYA, Center of Research in Animal Reproduction, Faculty of Veterinary Medicine, University of Montreal, Saint-Hyacinthe, Quebec, Canada.

ANNA J. BAILLIE, Prince Henry's Institute of Medical Research, Clayton, Victoria, Australia.

HAROLD R. BEHRMAN, Department of Obstetrics and Gynecology, Yale University School of Medicine, New Haven, Connecticut, USA.

ANGELINE N. BELTSOS, Department of Obstetrics and Gynecology, Washington University School of Medicine, St. Louis, Missouri, USA.

DEREK BOERBOOM, Center of Research in Animal Reproduction, Faculty of Veterinary Medicine, University of Montreal, Saint-Hyacinthe, Quebec, Canada.

PATRICIA BOLAND, Regeneron Pharmaceuticals, Inc., Tarrytown, New York, USA.

MATS BRÄNNSTRÖM, Department of Obstetrics and Gynecology, Göteborg University, Göteborg, Sweden.

KARA L. BRITT, Prince Henry's Institute of Medical Research, Clayton, Victoria, Australia.

PATRICK D. BURNS, Department of Animal Science, University of Kentucky, Lexington, Kentucky, USA.

ANTONELLA CAMAIONI, Department of Public Health and Cell Biology, University of Rome Tor Vergata, Rome, Italy.

CHARLES L. CHAFFIN, Division of Reproductive Sciences, Oregon Regional Primate Research Center, Beaverton, Oregon, USA.

YASMIN A. CHANDRASEKHER, Division of Reproductive Sciences, Oregon Regional Primate Research Center, Beaverton, Oregon, USA.

VICTORIA A. COX, Prince Henry's Institute of Medical Research, Clayton, Victoria, Australia.

WILLIAM F. CROWLEY, JR., Reproductive Endocrine Unit and National Center for Infertility Research, Massachusetts General Hospital, Boston, Massachusetts, USA.

THOMAS E. CURRY, JR., Department of Obstetrics and Gynecology, University of Kentucky, Lexington, Kentucky, USA.

ANITA DHAR, Prince Henry's Institute of Medical Research, Clayton, Victoria, Australia.

MONICA DI GIACOMO, Department of Public Health and Cell Biology, University of Rome Tor Vergata, Rome, Italy.

GREGORY A. DISSEN, Division of Neuroscience, Oregon Regional Primate Research Center, Oregon Health Sciences University, Beaverton, Oregon, USA.

ANN E. DRUMMOND, Prince Henry's Institute of Medical Research, Clayton, Victoria, Australia.

DIANE M. DUFFY, Division of Reproductive Sciences, Oregon Regional Primate Research Center, Beaverton, Oregon, USA.

MITZILEE DYSON, Prince Henry's Institute of Medical Research, Clayton, Victoria, Australia.

JOHN J. EPPIG, The Jackson Laboratory, Bar Harbor, Maine, USA.

GREGORY F. ERICKSON, Department of Reproductive Medicine, University of California, San Diego, La Jolla, California, USA.

LAWRENCE L. ESPEY, Department of Biology, Trinity University, San Antonio, Texas, USA.

JOCK K. FINDLAY, Prince Henry's Institute of Medical Research, Clayton, Victoria, Australia.

JOANNE E. FORTUNE, Department of Biomedical Sciences, Cornell University, Ithaca, New York, USA.

CSABA FULOP, Department of Biomedical Engineering, The Lerner Research Institute of the Cleveland Clinic Foundation, Cleveland, Ohio, USA.

ALAIN GOUGEON, INSERM U-407, Faculty of Medicine Lyon-Sud, Oullins Cedex, France.

GILBERT S. GREENWALD, Department of Molecular and Integrative Physiology, University of Kansas Medical Center, Kansas City, Kansas, USA.

JANET E. HALL, Reproductive Endocrine Unit and National Center for Infertility Research, Massachusetts General Hospital, Boston, Massachusetts, USA.

ALES HAMPL, Institute of Animal Physiology and Genetics, Academy of Sciences of the Czech Republic and Mendel University of Agriculture and Forestry, Brno, Czech Republic.

VINCENT C. HASCALL, Department of Biomedical Engineering, The Lerner Research Institute of the Cleveland Clinic Foundation, Cleveland, Ohio, USA.

TIMOTHY M. HAZZARD, Division of Reproductive Sciences, Oregon Regional Primate Research Center, Beaverton, Oregon, USA.

YUJI HIRAO, Faculty of Agriculture, Kobe University, Kobe, Japan.

AARON J.W. HSUEH, Department of Gynecology and Obstetrics, Stanford University School of Medicine, Stanford, California, USA.

JOSEPH ITSKOVITZ-ELDOR, Department of Obstetrics and Gynecology, Rambam Medical Center, and Faculty of Medicine, Technion-Israel Institute of Technology, Haifa, Israel.

ALBINA JABLONKA-SHARIFF, Department of Obstetrics and Gynecology, Washington University School of Medicine, St. Louis, Missouri, USA.

PETER F. JOHNSON, Eukaryotic Transcriptional Regulation Section, Molecular Basis of Carcinogenesis Laboratory, ABL-Basic Research Program, National Cancer Institute, Frederick Cancer Research and Development Center, Frederick, Maryland, USA.

ERVIN E. JONES, Department of Obstetrics and Gynecology, Yale University School of Medicine, New Haven, Connecticut, USA.

MARGARET E.E. JONES, Prince Henry's Institute of Medical Research, Clayton, Victoria, Australia.

PINAR H. KODAMAN, Department of Obstetrics and Gynecology, Yale University School of Medicine, New Haven, Connecticut, USA.

SHAHAR KOL, Department of Obstetrics and Gynecology, Rambam Medical Center, Haifa, Israel.

CAROLYN M. KOMAR, Department of Obstetrics and Gynecology, University of Kentucky, Lexington, Kentucky, USA.

JIANMIN LIU, Center of Research in Animal Reproduction, Faculty of Veterinary Medicine, University of Montreal, Saint-Hyacinthe, Quebec, Canada.

KATHRYN A. MARTIN, Reproductive Endocrine Unit and National Center for Infertility Research, Massachusetts General Hospital, Boston, Massachusetts, USA.

ARTUR MAYERHOFER, Molecular Anatomy, Anatomical Institute, Technical University, Munich, Germany.

MASATO M. MIKUNI, Department of Obstetrics and Gynecology, Hokkaido University School of Medicine, Kita-ku, Sapporo, Japan.

THEODORE A. MOLSKNESS, Division of Reproductive Sciences, Oregon Regional Primate Research Center, Beaverton, Oregon, USA.

PREMA NARAYAN, Department of Biochemistry and Molecular Biology, University of Georgia, Athens, Georgia, USA.

WARREN B. NOTHNICK, Department of Obstetrics and Gynecology, University of Kentucky, Lexington, Kentucky, USA.

SERGIO R. OJEDA, Division of Neuroscience, Oregon Regional Primate Research Center, Oregon Health Sciences University, Beaverton, Oregon, USA.

LISA M. OLSON, Department of Obstetrics and Gynecology, Washington University School of Medicine, St. Louis, Missouri, USA.

C. MATTHEW PETERSON, Division of Reproductive Endocrinology and Infertility, Department of Obstetrics and Gynecology, University of Utah Health Sciences Center, Salt Lake City, Utah, USA.

SANDRA L. PRESTON, Department of Obstetrics and Gynecology, Yale University School of Medicine, New Haven, Connecticut, USA.

DAVID PUETT, Department of Biochemistry and Molecular Biology, University of Georgia, Athens, Georgia, USA.

JOANNE S. RICHARDS, Department of Cell Biology, Baylor College of Medicine, Houston, Texas, USA.

REBECCA L. ROBKER, Department of Cell Biology, Baylor College of Medicine, Houston, Texas, USA.

MICHAEL J. ROSSI, Department of Biology and Environmental Science, University of New Haven, New Haven, Connecticut, USA.

EVA RUNESSON, Department of Obstetrics and Gynecology, Göteborg University, Göteborg, Sweden.

ANTONIETTA SALUSTRI, Department of Public Health and Cell Biology, University of Rome Tor Vergata, Rome, Italy.

EVAN R. SIMPSON, Prince Henry's Institute of Medical Research, Clayton, Victoria, Australia.

JEAN SIROIS, Center of Research in Animal Reproduction, Faculty of Veterinary Medicine, University of Montreal, Saint-Hyacinthe, Quebec, Canada.

ESTA STERNECK, Molecular Mechanisms in Development Group, Regulation of Cell Growth Laboratory, National Cancer Institute, Frederick Cancer Research and Development Center, Frederick, Maryland, USA.

RICHARD L. STOUFFER, Division of Reproductive Sciences, Oregon Regional Primate Research Center, Beaverton, Oregon, USA.

JOEL S. TABB, Department of Biomedical Sciences, Cornell University, Ithaca, New York, USA.

MASASHI TAKAMI, Department of Obstetrics and Gynecology, Yale University School of Medicine, New Haven, Connecticut, USA.

ANN E. TAYLOR, Reproductive Endocrine Unit and National Center for Infertility Research, Massachusetts General Hospital, Boston, Massachusetts, USA.

ANNE K. VOSS, Department of Biomedical Sciences, Cornell University, Ithaca, New York, USA.

CORRINE K. WELT, Reproductive Endocrine Unit and National Center for Infertility Research, Massachusetts General Hospital, Boston, Massachusetts, USA.

STANLEY J. WIEGAND, Neural and Endocrine Biology, Regeneron Pharmaceuticals, Inc., Tarrytown, New York, USA.

GEORGE D. YANCOPOULOS, Regeneron Pharmaceuticals, Inc., Tarrytown, New York, USA.

ULF J. ZACKRISSON, Department of Obstetrics and Gynecology, Göteborg University, Göteborg, Sweden.

MARY B. ZELINSKI-WOOTEN, Division of Reproductive Sciences, Oregon Regional Primate Research Center, Beaverton, Oregon, USA.

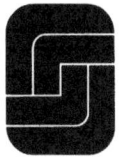

1

An Overview of 37 Years
of Research on Ovulation

LAWRENCE L. ESPEY

Introductory Remarks

Thirty-seven years ago, the first major publication that I read on the same topic as this volume was a book entitled, *Control of Ovulation* (1). That text consisted of the proceedings of a conference held in Dedham, Massachusetts, in 1960. The conference was organized by Professors Claude Villee, Roy Greep, and Duncan Reid and co-sponsored by Harvard University and the Association for the Aid of Crippled Children. In reviewing this reference several months ago, I was struck by three notable realizations. First, the insights from that conference have influenced the direction of my own research on ovulation more than I heretofore appreciated. Second, the participants in that conference demonstrated an inspiring determination to decipher the mechanism of ovulation and give clinical relevance to the existing knowledge of the process. Third, the discussions that were published as part of the proceedings disclose an impressive attitude of cooperation among the investigators who participated in the conference. As we commence this study, therefore, I cannot help but think of the groundwork we are laying for the next century of research on ovulation.

Thirty-seven years ago, I could only dream of what it must be like to participate in a conference such as this. To be sure, I never imagined that someday I might have the privilege of being the initial speaker at such a gathering. Faced with this reality, it has been difficult to select the most befitting subject matter. My first thought was to prepare an overview of the significance of the work of the other authors, but I then realized that should be the privilege of each of the other participants themselves. Next, I considered summarizing the current status of the hypothesis that the ovulatory process is comparable to an inflammatory reaction, but that topic has been reviewed adequately elsewhere (2). Finally, realizing that I might never again have the opportunity to interact with such an assembly of scientists with a mutual interest in ovulation, I have concluded that a more fitting approach might be to categorize those observations over the years that have had the greatest influence on my current conception of the ovulatory process. This presentation, therefore starts with a brief review of the principal changes in the ultrastructure of a mammalian follicle that is approaching rupture. It then highlights 10 different factors that must be considered in formulating any hypothesis on the mechanism of ovulation. Next, it itemizes 10 experimental procedures that can cause confusion for investigators working on ovulation. It subsequently lists 10 topics that are worthy of further investigation and/or represent novel approaches to the study of ovulation. Finally, it summarizes the value of the molecular method known as "differential display" in isolating and identifying unique gene expression in ovarian tissue during ovulation, and it provides a synopsis of the information that has been gained to date by this procedure.

Brief Comments on the Ultrastructure of Ovulatory Follicles

These brief observations on the most conspicuous changes that occur at the apex of ovulatory follicles are based primarily on electron micrographs of rabbit follicles (3–6). In a mature rabbit follicle, the theca interna appears to be the most metabolically active layer of the follicular wall. This deduction is based on the evidence that most of the ovarian vascular supply is distributed to this layer, and on the incidence of steroidogenic components in the secretory cells that comprise this layer.

After a follicle has been stimulated by an ovulatory surge in gonadotropin(s), there is no conspicuous change in the ultrastructure for several hours. Then, near the time of rupture, four major modifications become discernible. First, the thecal capillaries expand, and there appears to be exudation of their serous contents into the extracellular matrix of the thecal layers of the follicular wall. Second, lipid droplets begin to form in the cytoplasm of the granulosa cells, and this layer becomes steroidogenically active. Third, and most notable, the numerous fibroblasts in the theca externa and tunica albuginea at the follicular apex become very elongated and manifest attributes of proliferation. Fourth, the epithelial cells on the apical surface of the follicle appear to be necrotic, and these cells are less firmly attached to the surface of the ovary.

In the minutes preceding rupture, a thin stigma of tenacious connective tissue balloons above the normal curvature of the follicle, and this bulging tissue is an indication that rupture is eminent. At this final stage of the ovulatory process, the cells of the surface epithelium are usually completely absent from the apex, and the stratum granulosum retracts laterally along the inner surface of the follicular wall. The theca interna sometimes also retracts with the granulosa cells. The collagenous tissue of the tunica albuginea and theca externa eventually begin to disintegrate.

Seven Impressionable Characteristics of the Ovulatory Process

This section itemizes seven different sorts of data that I have found to be particularly useful in formulating a comprehensive image of the ovulatory process. Selection of these seven items is not intended to imply that other colleagues have not arrived at additional insights that are of equal, or greater, value in understanding the mechanism of ovulation. It is instead simply a list of results that have had the most lasting impression on my own perception of the overall process. Most of the items in the list arise from biophysical studies, perhaps because biophysical methods provide more tangible data than the sophisticated molecular and biochemical procedures of today. In any case, they represent some of the more obvious manifestation of the underlying molecular processes.

Importance of Intrafollicular Pressure

The hydrostatic pressure of the fluid inside a mature follicle is in the range of 15–20 mmHg (7). This intrafollicular pressure is directly dependent on the hydrostatic pressure in the matrix of capillaries in the theca interna. Although the earlier hypothesis that follicular rupture is the consequence of a substantial increase in follicular pressure is not true, this pressure nonetheless serves as an essential hydrostatic force to cause dissociation of the connective tissue elements in a weakening follicular wall. The relevant point is that the modest intrafollicular pressure is important for ovulation; therefore, any conditions that disrupt the vascular supply to a follicle, or otherwise reduce the ovarian blood pressure, can impair ovulation.

Loss of Tensile Strength of the Follicular Wall

Measurements of the tensile strength of sow follicles at intervals during the ovulatory process have shown that the collagenous layers of the follicle become significantly less tenacious during the hours preceding rupture (8). Shortly after rupture there is a subsequent re-establishment of the tensile strength of the follicular wall. The important point is that the molecular events of ovulation create a temporal "window" during which the follicular integrity is more vulnerable to the force exerted by the modest intrafollicular pressure. It remains to be determined whether this ephemeral disintegration of the follicle wall is the consequence of some kind of biphasic effect of the biochemical mediators of the ovulatory process.

Induction of Rupture by Proteolytic Enzymes

If one dissolves a collagenolytic enzyme in physiologic saline and carefully injects 1 μL of such a solution in situ into the antrum of a mature rabbit follicle, then the injected follicle will rupture within 7–10 minutes (9). A similar response occurs following the injection of elastin or trypsin into a follicle. The important point is that potent proteolytic enzymes can rapidly induce the rupture of a mature follicle, which implies that such enzymes have a central role in the ovulatory process.

Proliferation of Thecal Fibroblasts

As described earlier, the fibroblasts in the tunica albuginea and theca externa change from a position of quiescence to a state of proliferation during ovulation (5). During this transition, the fibroblasts display unusually long cytoplasmic processes that extend from the cell-body along the tangential plane of the follicular surface. In other words, the fibroblasts exhibit evidence of motility and appear to begin moving within the dense thecal layers of the follicular wall. The important point is that in order for these connective tissue cells to move they must produce agents such as proteolytic enzymes to soften the extracellular matrix of collagen and ground substance that is characteristic of the thecal tissue that provides the tensile strength to the follicular wall.

Progesterone Production and Ovulation

It is well known that luteinizing hormone (and homologous glycoproteins that can induce ovulation) initiate a massive increase in ovarian progesterone synthesis (10). Although there has been speculation about the possible role of this steroid in the mechanism of ovulation, the magnitude of this role was firmly established by experiments that showed that epostane, an inhibitor of progesterone synthesis, can block ovulation, whereas exogenous progesterone can reverse this epostane-induced action (11). Because the synthesis of ovarian progesterone is the principal indicator of the onset of luteinization, the important point from the epostane experiment is that the luteinization process is an integral part of the ovulatory process. In the final analysis, it may turn out that the proliferation of cells during the early stages of the luteinization process degrade the extracellular matrix to the extent that the follicular apex expands and ruptures under the force of a modest, but constant, intrafollicular pressure.

Lipoxygenase Activity and Ovulation

There is ample evidence that ovarian prostanoid synthesis increases substantially during ovulation (although the precise functions of the prostaglandins have yet to be established). The presumed importance of this group of compounds is not based solely on the measurable increase in prostaglandins E_2 and $F_{2\alpha}$; rather, it is also based on the consistent reports that the cyclo-oxygenase inhibitor, indomethacin, suppresses ovulation. There is more recent evidence, however, that indomethacin is not a specific blocker of prostanoid synthesis—it also inhibits the action of lipoxygenases on arachidonic acid, thereby preventing the normal increase in synthesis of products such as 12- and 15-HETE in ovulatory follicles (12). It is noteworthy, therefore, that eicosanoids other than the prostanoids may also contribute to the metabolic events of ovulation.

Ovarian Hyperemia and the Inflammatory Cascade

It is obvious to the eye that ovulatory follicles become progressively redder. This hyperemic condition has been confirmed by experiments that measure the amount of blood in ovaries that have been stimulated with an ovulatory dose of gonadotropin (13). Such hyperemic conditions are the cardinal sign of inflammatory reactions. This fact, along with the evidence that indomethacin and other nonsteroidal anti-inflammatory agents inhibit ovulation, has lead to the idea that the ovulatory process is comparable to an inflammatory reaction (14). The important point, therefore, is that ovulation probably involves a more complex cascade of metabolic events than originally thought. Such complexity may be necessary in order to confine the degradative events to a localized area of the ovarian surface.

Seven Sources of Confusion and/or Inconsistency

Over the course of 37 years of work on the physiology of ovulation, one cannot help but encounter certain problems with different methodologies, or other circumstances that can make it difficult to interpret data. In some instances, such problems arise in the form of biological "booby traps" that lead investigators to take experimental approaches that can be, in the final analysis, misleading. This section arbitrarily selects seven such circumstances. Most of the observations are based on problems with immature rats because this organism has become the most common experimental model in studies on ovulation.

PMSG/hCG Injections in the Immature Rat Model

In the methods sections of many manuscripts, it is commonly reported that immature rats are selected on the basis of their age. The animals are usually weaned at 23 days of age, and they receive the first injection of gonadotropin on day 24 or 25. The problem with this age-related selection procedure, however, is that the litter sizes within a group of 100 gravid rats can range from as low as five pups to as high as 20 pups. This being the case, the competition for maternal milk varies significantly from litter to litter. As a result, at the age of 23 days, pups in a small litter can weigh twice as much as those in large litters. The ovulation rate in response to fixed doses of gonadotropins can consequently vary substantially within and/or between groups of experimental animals. From our experience with tens of thousands of immature rats, more consistent ovulation rates can be obtained by selecting the animals on the basis of their weight, rather than their age. It is preferable to use animals in the body weight range of 42–48 g, although a 40–50 g range can yield reproducible results. In contrast, animals weighing less than 38 g have substantially lower ovulation rates, whereas those above 55 g also have progressively lower ovulation rates.

Induction of ovulation in immature rats is usually carried out by an initial injection of 10 IU of pregnant mare serum gonadotrophin (PMSG) (i.e., eCG) followed two days later by an injection of 10 IU of hCG. It is imperative to administer the dose of hCG during the morning hours on the second day after treatment with PMSG because there are reports that PMSG-primed immature rats often experience an endogenous surge in LH secretion at approximately 7 hours after the animals are exposed to light on the second day following the PMSG injection (15). In addition, the dose of PMSG (but not hCG) is crucial for consistent results. There is an exponential increase in ovulation rate with doses of PMSG ranging from about 4 IU to 10 IU per rat. On the other hand, doses of 20 IU or higher cause a progressively lower ovulation rate (15). Finally, the route of administration of gonadotropin also can affect the results. A subcutaneous injection will provide a more consistent ovulation rate than intraperitoneal and intravenous injections.

Whole Ovaries Versus Cell Cultures

It has become common practice to isolate specific cell types (especially granulosa cells) and study their metabolic responses to gonadotropins and other hormones. Although this kind of in vitro work can provide useful information about the immediate responses of granulosa cells to G-protein-coupled receptor stimulation, there is one certain limitation to this experimental approach. Granulosa cells do not ovulate—only intact follicles ovulate. The ovulatory process also involves secretory cells in the theca interna, connective tissue cells in the theca externa and tunica albuginea, and probably endothelial cells in the follicular capillaries. In essence, rupture requires a synergistic sequence of events involving all of these cells; without the omnium gatherum in their natural setting, it would be impossible to decipher the complete sequence of events.

Glutaraldehyde-Fixed Tissues for Electron Microscopy

At least one major study has reported that rodent follicles do not contain collagen fibrils in the thecal layers (16). In that instance, however, the ovarian tissue was fixed for electron microscopy by using glutaraldehyde, an agent that causes collagen to loose its electron density. In such a preparation, it is necessary to treat the ultrathin sections with a metallic solution such as phosphotungstic acid (17).

Follicular "Smooth Muscle" Cells versus Thecal Fibroblasts

The controversial role of follicular "smooth muscle" in the mechanism of ovulation has been debated for more than a century (18). Common evidence in favor of the smooth muscle theory arises from microscopic studies that report an abundance of "spindle-shaped" cells in the thecal layers and from histochemical studies that show actin filaments in such cells; however, electron micrographs taken at a 90 degree angle to the usual cross-sectional view of the follicle wall reveal that the thecal cells are actually platter-shaped fibroblasts rather than spindle-shaped smooth muscle cells (5). Furthermore, fibroblasts and other motile cells usually contain strands of actin within their cytoplasm (5); therefore, actin is not a reliable indicator of smooth muscle tissue.

Localization of the Rupture Site at the Follicular Apex

Anyone who has observed the actual rupture of a follicle cannot help but wonder whether there is an apical area that is cytologically different from the rest of the spherical surface of a mature follicle. There is no evidence, however to delineate any significant difference in the cellular composition at the apex, versus the base, of follicles from most species of mammals. Furthermore, if one dissects a follicle from the rest of the ovarian mass, or measures the tensile strength of a follicular strip taken lateral to the apex, it becomes obvious that the degradative activity is dispersed throughout the follicle. It seems reasonable, therefore, to deduce that an ovulatory follicle balloons out at the apex simply because this is, morphologically, the weakest link to the outside.

Nonspecificity of Inhibitory Agents

A wide variety of agents that inhibit diverse metabolic reactions have been tested on ovulation. These agents have been selected to block the synthesis of serine proteases, metalloproteases, eicosanoids, steroids, kinins, angiotensin, and many other compounds that have been implicated as mediators of the ovulatory process. It is usually difficult, however, to certify the specificity of such inhibitory agents. A prime example is the antiovulatory agent indomethacin, which has been widely used as "proof" that prostaglandins E_2 and $F_{2\alpha}$ are essential components of the ovulatory process. It is now clear, however, that indomethacin is not specific for the prostanoids. This anti-inflammatory agent also inhibits the formation of products of 12- and 15-lipoxygenase (12). The lesson is that the results from experiments involving inhibitory agents must be interpreted with circumspection.

Simultaneous Decomposition and Recomposition of the Follicular Wall

As mentioned earlier, the ovulatory process has been likened to an acute inflammatory reaction. In such a process, there is evidence that destructive metabolic events are occurring simultaneously with processes that are operating to bring about healing and repair (5,14); unfortunately, there is not a set of criteria to follow to establish whether any newly discovered ovulation-related substance is promoting the degradative events that lead to rupture, or is facilitating the postovulatory healing process. It is important, therefore, to keep this metabolic contradiction in mind when attempting to interpret experimental data on ovulation.

Seven Suggested Areas for Future Studies

It seems worthwhile to use this occasion to suggest several new experimental approaches that might yield useful information about the mechanism of ovulation. A deliberate effort has been made to avoid significant overlap with the various other scientific subjects that will be discussed in this book. The very fact that the other topics are herein serves as affirmation that such projects are worthy of further pursuit.

Determine the Function(s) of Progesterone

It is clear that the ovulatory increase in ovarian progesterone synthesis is important for ovulation; however, the precise function of this steroid is uncertain. Two suggestions follow:

Biphasic Effect of Progesterone

A novel approach to decipher the role of progesterone in ovulation would be to investigate the hypothesis that the acute effects of this steroid contribute to the degradative events of an inflammatory reaction, whereas the chronic effects (exerted during the lutein phase) are anti-inflammatory in nature. In essence, the hypothesis is that progesterone might exert a long-term effect on reproductive tissue that is comparable to the anti-inflammatory action of the glucocorticoids (19).

Effect of Progesterone on Uteroglobin Production

Glucocorticoids express their anti-inflammatory action by promoting the formation of lipocortins (19). These highly charged glycoproteins are especially known for their ability to block the enzyme phospholipase A_2. Progesterone similarly induces the formation of uteroglobin by uterine and other tissues. This homologue is structurally and functionally similar to the lipocortins, and it suppresses inflammatory reactions by inhibiting phospholipase A_2. This agent, therefore, hypothetically might mediate the chronic effect of ovarian progesterone that was suggested in the previous paragraph.

Determine the Function(s) of Prostaglandins

It appears that the ovarian increase in prostaglandins E_2 and $F_{2\alpha}$ are important for ovulation. As with progesterone, however, the precise functions of these eicosanoids have not been established. Although I do not have any specific experiments to suggest that would clearly establish their functions, there are several facts to consider in future studies on ovulation. First, contrary to a number of reports during the 1970s, there is evidence that exogenous prostaglandins cannot reverse the anti-ovulatory action of indomethacin (20). This later observation needs to be confirmed. Second, as mentioned earlier, the literature on inflammation attributes both pro- and anti-inflammatory properties to the prostaglandins (5,14), and it has not yet been established which of these two opposing actions are dominant in ovulatory follicles. Third, any future studies on arachidonate metabolism in ovulation should bear in mind that products of the lipoxygenase pathway (e.g., the lipoxins) might also be contributing to angiogenic activity, or to other metabolic events associated with ovulation.

Compare Ruptured Follicles
with Granuloma Tissue

Ruptured follicles (and, in some instances, unruptured follicles) rapidly transform into functional corpora lutea. Because there is evidence to suggest that the ovulatory process is merely a part of the luteinization process, useful insights might be gained from studies that relate the ovulatory process with luteal function. In particular, it would be interesting to assess the extent to which luteal tissue is comparable to a granuloma. A granuloma is a firm nodular mass that forms in conjunction with angiogenesis and fibroplasia that develops during the wound-healing process in injured and inflamed tissues (14). Thus, in many respects, the later stages of the ovulatory process resemble the early stages of granuloma formation, and this theoretical correlation merits further consideration.

Analyze Electrochemical Activity in the Stratum Granulosum

G-protein-coupled receptors are usually linked through the signal transduction process to ion gates (19). It would be interesting to know, therefore, the extent to which LH and hCG induce changes in the plasma membrane potential of granulosa cells. Application of the patch-clamp technique, the fura-2 method, and similar procedures could provide useful information about the extent to which various ligands influence ion currents across the membranes of these follicular cells. In addition, in view of the extensive network of gap junctions that appear to organize the stratum granulosum into a syncytium, it would be interesting to use an oscilloscope to determine whether this inner layer of the follicle wall can conduct an action potential across its surface. This would serve as a novel approach to analyze the hypothesis that the granulosa is electrically coupled to the oocyte, and vice versa.

Demonstrate the Activation of Thecal Fibroblasts by Blood Serum

It has been suggested that the inflammatory agents in an ovulatory follicle might induce vascular exudation of serum into the follicular connective tissue to activate the thecal fibroblasts (6). Serum is commonly used to convert quiescent fibroblasts into proliferating cells. It is therefore feasible to anticipate that the significant vasodilatation and hyperemia that occurs in ovulatory follicles could result in leakage of serum (and, unspecified serum proteins) into the thecal layers. Preliminary tests of this hypothesis could include the addition of serum proteins to the medium circulating through an in vitro perfusion system. If one or more test proteins happens to increase the ovulation rate in vitro, then the results would provide indirect support for the idea that exudation has a role in ovulation. Positive results from such tests could simultaneously provide clues to help explain the unusually low recovery of ova from in vitro perfusion systems.

Evaluate the Termination of Early Pregnancy by Ovulation

Pregnancy in rats can be terminated by a single dose of menotropin, administered during the first trimester (21). Termination of pregnancy is the result of menotropin-induced ovulation in the gravid animals. The mechanism of this abortifacient action of the ovulatory process has not been determined, yet an analysis of this phenomenon might simultaneously provide useful information about the mechanism of ovulation itself.

Assess the Degradative Action of the Cumulus Mass

The ovulation rate in gonadotropin-primed immature rats is determined by counting the number of ova in the oviducts at 20–24 hours after hCG. The ova (actually the cumuli oopheri) congregate midway along the length of the oviduct at a region known as the ampulloischemic junction. This segment of the oviduct balloons significantly in response to the presence of the ova, and this morphological change appears to be an effect of chemical secretions from the cumulus cells, rather than from the physical volume of the cumulus masses. This deduction is based on preliminary studies in which we have assayed the wall of the ampulloischemic junction for prostaglandin E_2 before and after the arrival of the ova at this segment of the oviduct. The preliminary data indicate a significant increase in prostaglandin synthesis in the wall of the oviduct and suggest that the cumulus masses induce a local inflammatory reaction. Further analysis of this unique experimental model could therefore also provide useful information about the mechanism of mammalian ovulation.

Early Insights from Differential Display

Introductory Remarks

To date, about two dozen bioactive agents have been implicated as components of the ovulatory process. Molecular studies of ovarian tissue have confirmed the transcription and translation of about a dozen of the genes that encode these agents. It is impossible to predict the total number of genes that are uniquely expressed in the different follicular cells during the ovulatory process, but it is likely that many more genes remain to be identified. This deduction is based on evidence that as many as 100 new mRNAs are usually transcribed during cell–tissue responses to various stimuli (22,23).

In simple metaphorical terms, the metabolic events of ovulation can be likened to a 100-piece jigsaw puzzle (i.e., an "ovulation puzzle"). At present, only about 12 fragments of the puzzle have been placed on the table for assembly. Although certain properties of any one of these parts (e.g., of progesterone) are known, the connection of a given piece to any other piece is presently uncertain. For example, the functional association between the ovulatory rise in progesterone and the rise in prostaglandins has not been determined. To gain a better picture of the relationships among the existing fragments, more of the unknown pieces of the puzzle need to be placed on the assembly table. That objective can be achieved by modern molecular methods.

After so many years of research on ovulation, I could not have imagined that an ultramolecular procedure like "differential display" would become available at the end of my career. This novel methodology permits the detection of previously undiscovered mRNA expression (in the form of fragments of cDNA) from genes that are upregulated (or downregulated) during ovulation (24). The cDNA fragments that are isolated by differential display can be sequenced, and this information can be submitted to gene databases to identify the specific regulatory proteins that are translated in the experimental tissue during ovulation. The next section is an overview of the kind of information that can be gained from the differential display procedure.

Preliminary Results from Differential Display

Immature Wistar rats were used in this study. In this experimental model, PMSG-primed animals begin ovulating at approximately 12 hours after hCG administration. In order to gain information about the time-course of gene expression, therefore, mRNA was extracted from ovaries at six periovulatory intervals, including 0, 2, 4, 8, 12, and 24 hours after hCG treatment of the rats. Details of the methods of procedure can be found at the internet address *www.trinity.edu/~lespey* under the hyperlink "Manuscripts."

The cDNA fragments that have been discovered by differential display as being uniquely related to the ovulatory process are presented in chronological order in Table 1.1. Most of the fragments are significantly homologous to a variety of genes that have previously been registered in the database at the National Center for Biotechnology Information, while a number of the transcripts are not homologous to any of the registered genes. To date, the identifiable fragments can be associated with (1) genes that regulate steroid metabolism, (2) genes that have been implicated in tumor growth, and (3) genes with miscellaneous metabolic affiliations.

Potential Significance of the Results

This work with differential display is still very much in the data collection phase. Nevertheless, at this stage, several noteworthy trends are emerging. First, several of the newly discovered, ovulation-specific genes are providing new insights about the nature of ovarian steroid activity during ovulation. In particular, the repetitious discovery by differential display of a carbonyl reductase that has been linked to both steroid and prostanoid metabolism (25,26), may provide a significant connection between the well established, simultaneous increase in progesterone and prostaglandin synthesis during the ovula-

TABLE 1.1. Chronological order of discovery of ovulation-unique cDNA fragments.

cDNA	Description	Signal from northern blot lanes (hours after hCG)					
		0	2	4	8	12	24
G7-8A	carbonyl reductase		-	++	+++++	+++++	-
G3-12B	unknown	-	-	-	++++	++++	-
A3-8A	LINE repeat element	=	=	=	=	=	=
A16-8A	nerve growth factor-induced A		+++	+++	+++	+++	
A15-8E	LINE repeat element	=	=	=	=	=	=
G4-8A	carbonyl reductase		-	++	+++++	+++++	
G21-8A	Niemann Pick C disease protein	-	-	++	+++++	++	-
C22-8A	unknown		-	++	+++++	++	-
C23-0B	c-Ha-ras protooncogene	+++++	+++++	+++++	++	+	+
A24-8A	G-protein-coupled receptor		-	+	+++	+	-
C23-8A	3α-hydroxysteroid dehydrogenase		-	++	+++++	++++	+
C23-12AA	AD1/CD63 (melanoma antigen)	+	+	+	+++	+++	+
G24-8A	unknown	-	-	+	+++	-	-
G75-8A	unknown			-	+++	-	
A72-8A	helix-loop-helix basic phosphoprotein		-	+++++	++++	+++	-
A65-8A	unknown		-	++++	+++++	+++	-
A65-8F	unknown (same as above)		-	++++	+++++	+++	-
G65-8A	unknown (same as above)		-	++++	+++++	+++	-
G72-4A	G-protein signaling regulator	-	-	++++	++++	+++	-
A58-8A	cyclooxygenase-2 isoform			-	++	-	
A58-8B	carbonyl reductase		+	+++	+++++	+++++	
G58-8C	carbonyl reductase		-	+++	+++++	+++++	-
G67-8A	steroidogenic acute regulatory protein	-	+++	++++	+++++	++++	+++
C26-8A	vimentin (rat prostatic tumor protein)		-	+++	+++++	++	-
G62-8C	pancreatitis-associated protein III			-	+++	++	-

"-" = trace; "+" = intensity of hybridization signal; "=" = multiple hybridization sites.

tory process. Second, the discovery of gene expression for antigens associated with melanoma (i.e., the antigen AD1/CD63) (27) and with a highly aggressive prostatic tumor (i.e., the vimentin) (28) indicates that the ovulatory process may have certain similarities with a tumorous growth. Such an analogy, which was originally suggested 25 years ago (29), is worthy of further assessment because ovulation and luteinization involve rapid proliferation of several types of follicular cells. Third, the differential display procedure has thus far yielded five different cDNA fragments that do not share homology with any genes that are registered in the common databases. The further characterization of these "unknown" genes should also provide significant new information about the molecular events of the ovulatory process. In this regard, it is worthy to note that one of these unknown genes has been further characterized (by Dr. Darryl Russell in Dr. Joanne Richards laboratory at Baylor College of Medicine), and this preliminary analysis has revealed that the fragment is homologous to a retroviral sequence that is endogenous to most mammalian species (30). Although such sequences of viral genes may represent little more than evolutionary aberrations of mammalian genomes, additional investigations may be necessary to rule out any possible relationship between such transcripts and the mediation of an inflammatory reaction in ovulatory follicles.

Concluding Remarks

I would like to conclude with a summary of the three principal reasons I believe that further research on ovulation is worthwhile. First, purely on scientific grounds, it is important to understand the metabolic events that coordinate this stage of the procreative process. Second, the ovulatory process is an exceptional experimental model to study the manner in which a distinct target tissue (namely, an ovarian follicle) responds to a glycoprotein hormone such as luteinizing hormore or hCG. Third, and perhaps most important, there is a thoughtful admonition expressed by Dr. Frederick Hisaw during one of the discussion sessions at that earlier conference on ovulation four decades ago (1). He stated:

> The destiny of mankind most certainly depends more on control of the world's population than it does on the curious international competition now raging over such comparatively trivial things as who is to enjoy the dubious distinction of being the first to get a peek at the sea's bottom or the moon's backside. Even so, finding a method for the inhibition of ovulation is in reality a problem in endocrine engineering which relies on basic information.

It is ironic that since that erudite admonition by Dr. Hisaw, we have found the *Titanic* and walked on the Moon, and we now control ovulation at will; however, the world's population continues to expand relentlessly toward global congestion and chaos. Nevertheless, this remorseless situation should not deter us from seeking more effective and efficient means of controlling fertility. It is certain that just as the papers from that earlier conference provided the foundation for the progress on ovulation, the information in this volume will set the stage for the advancement of our knowledge on ovulation in the next millenium.

Ackowledgments. The author expresses appreciation to Dr. Joanne Richards, Baylor College of Medicine, Houston, Texas, for her assistance in learning some of the molecular procedures used in this chapter. Technical assistance in recent years has been provided by postdoctoral associates Drs. Takeshi Ujioka and Shinya Yoshioka, and by undergraduate students Bogdan Vladu, Molly Skelsey, Matt Call, and Linh Tran. The differential display work was supported in the past by NIH AREA Grant HD-21649 and currently by NSF Grant 7890793.

References

1. Villee CA, ed. Control of ovulation. New York: Pergamon Press, 1961.
2. Espey LL. Current status of the hypothesis that mammalian ovulation is comparable to an inflammatory reaction. Biol Reprod 1994;50:233–38.
3. Espey LL. Ultrastructure of the apex of the rabbit Graafian follicle during the ovulatory process. Endocrinology 1967;81:267–76.
4. Espey LL. Ultrastructure of the ovulatory process. In: Familiari GS, Makabe S, Motta P, eds. Ultrastructure of the ovary. Boston: Kluwer Academic Publishers; 1991:143–59.
5. Espey LL. Ovulation. In: Knobil E, Neill JD, eds. The physiology of reproduction. New York: Raven Press; 1994:725–80.
6. Espey LL. Ovulation. In: Knobil E, Neill JD, eds. Encyclopedia of reproduction. Vol. 3. San Diego: Academic Press; 1999:605–14.
7. Espey LL, Lipner H. Measurements of intrafollicular pressure in the rabbit ovary. Am J Physiol 1963;205:1067–72.
8. Espey LL. Tenacity of porcine Graafian follicle as it approaches ovulation. Am J Physiol 1967;212:1397–401.
9. Espey LL. Enzyme-induced rupture of rabbit Graafian follicle. Am J Physiol 1965;208:208–13.
10. Snyder BW, Beecham GD, Schane HP. Inhibition of ovulation in rats with epostane, an inhibitor of 3β-hydroxysteroid dehydrogenase. Proc Soc Exp Biol Med 1984;176:238–42.
11. Espey LL, Adams RF, Tanaka N, Okamura H. Effects of epostane on ovarian levels of progesterone, 17β-estradiol, prostaglandin E_2, and prostaglandin $F_{2\alpha}$ during ovulation in the gonadotropin-primed immature rat. Endocrinology 1990;127:259–63.
12. Espey LL, Tanaka N, Adams RF, Okamura H. Ovarian hydroxyeicosatetraenoic acids compared to prostanoids and steroids during ovulation in the rat. Am J Physiol 1991;260:E163–69.

13. Tanaka N, Espey LL, Okamura H. Increase in ovarian blood volume during ovulation in the gonadotropin-primed immature rat. Biol Reprod 1989;40:762–68.
14. Espey LL. Ovulation as an inflammatory reaction—a hypothesis. Biol Reprod 1980;22:73–106.
15. Espey LL, Shimada H, Okamura H, Mori T. Increase in plasminogen activator in the involuting uterus of the postpartum rat. J Endocrinol 1985;32:1087–94.
16. Parr EL. Histological examination of the rat ovarian follicle wall prior to ovulation. Biol Reprod 1974;11:483–503.
17. Espey LL. The distribution of collagenous connective tissue in rat ovarian follicles. Biol Reprod 1976;14:502–6.
18. Espey LL. Ovarian contractility and its relationship to ovulation: a review. Biol Reprod 1978;19:540–55.
19. Espey LL. A review of factors that could influence membrane potentials of ovarian follicular cells during mammalian ovulation. Acta Endocrinol 1992;126(suppl. 2): 1–32.
20. Espey LL, Tanaka N, Stacy S, Okamura H. Inhibition of ovulation in the gonadotropin-primed immature rat by exogenous prostaglandin E_2. Prostaglandins 1992;43:67–74.
21. Espey LL, Stacy S, Hayter H, Fujii S. Termination of early pregnancy in the rat by a single dose of human menopausal gonadotropin. Early Pregnancy: Biol Med 1997;3: 23–26.
22. Hedrick SM, Cohen DI, Nielsen EA, Davis MM. Isolation of cDNA clones encoding T cell-specific membrane-associated proteins. Nature 1984;308:149–53.
23. Mohn KL, Laz TM, Hsu JC, Melby AE, Bravo R, Taub R. The immediate-early growth response in regenerating liver and insulin-stimulated H-35 cells: comparison with serum-stimulated 3T3 cells and identification of 41 novel immediate-early genes. Mol Cell Biol 1991;11:381–90.
24. Liang P, Pardee AB. Differential display of eukaryotic messenger RNA by means of the polymerase chain reaction. Science 1992;257:1642–50.
25. Wermuth B, Mader-Heinemann G, Ernst E. Cloning and expression of carbonyl reductase from rat testis. Eur J Biochem 1995;228:473–79.
26. Inazu N, Satoh T. Activation by human chorionic gonadotropin of ovarian carbonyl reductase in mature rats exposed in vivo to estrogens. Biochem Pharmacol 1994;47:1489–96.
27. Nishikata H, Oliver C, Mergenhagen SE, Siraganian RP. The rat mast cell antigen AD1 (homologue to human CD63 or melanoma antigen ME491) is expressed in other cells in culture. J Immunol 1992;149:862–70.
28. Dumortier J, Daemi N, Pourreyron C, Anderson W, Bellaton C, Jacquier MF, et al. Loss of epithelial differentiation markers and acquisition of vimentin expression after xenograft with laminin-1 enhance migratory and invasive abilities of human colon cancer cells LoVo C5. Differentiation 1998;63:141–50.
29. Espey LL. Ovarian proteolytic enzymes and ovulation. Biol Reprod 1974;10: 216–35.
30. Godwin AK, Miller PD, Getts LA, Jackson K, Sonoda G, Schray KJ, et al. Retroviral-like sequences specifically expressed in the rat ovary detect genetic differences between normal and transformed rat ovarian surface epithelial cells. Endocrinology 1995;136:4640–49.

Part I

The Follicle

2

Histologic Definition of Ovarian Follicles and Analysis of Folliculogenesis Disruptions Due to Gene Mutations

ALAIN GOUGEON

Introduction

Significant insights in the knowledge of ovarian function have been brought by analysis of fertility potentials in either knockout mice or rodents bearing spontaneous mutations of genes involved in reproduction. When ovarian follicular growth is disrupted in these rodent models, the lacking molecule is expected to play a key role in the control of follicular development. It is therefore tempting to extrapolate this role to other mammals and especially to humans.

On the other hand, in humans, some cases of infertility are due to a gene defect. When ovarian biopsies are performed, the exact time at which follicular growth is impaired is difficult to identify because, among others, of the great confusion existing in the terms used to name follicles at the various stages of their development.

The aim of this chapter is to give some examples of gene mutations that leading disruption of follicular growth in rodent and human models, then to describe the step at which follicular growth is arrested, and finally to analyze the role played by the lacking molecule in the control of ovarian follicle development.

Stock of Nongrowing Follicles and Initiation of Follicular Growth

In the mammalian ovary, three types of very small follicles can be observed in the ovary: primordial follicles in which the oocyte is surrounded only by flattened granulosa cells (Gcs) (Fig. 2.1), intermediary follicles in which the oocyte is surrounded by a mixture of flattened and cuboidal GCs (Fig. 2.2), and primary follicles in which the oocyte is surrounded by a single layer of cuboidal GCs (Fig. 2.3).

One of the reasons for which progress in the knowledge of the precise mechanisms controlling initiation of follicular growth has been slow is perhaps because it is difficult to distinguish resting follicles from early growing follicles. As a result, a first question arises regarding the pool of very small follicles: Which follicles are nongrowing and which are earlygrowing?

The earliest criteria that have been used to distinguish nongrowing from growing follicles are morphological criteria such as oocyte size and GC shape. It has been stated that in mice, entry into the growth phase takes place when 8–20 GCs are present in the largest cross-section (LCS) (1). In humans, active follicular growth starts at the primary stage when the oocyte nucleus reaches critical diameter of 19 μm and when approximately 15 GCs are present in the LCS (2). Physiological criteria have also been used extensively to distinguish nongrowing from growing follicles. The labeling of GCs by tritiated thymidine (3H-TdR) is considered to be the start of follicular growth. By using pulse-labeling with 3H-TdR, Pedersen (3) found that mouse follicles similar to human primordial and intermediary follicles seldom contain labeled GCs and are nongrowing, whereas primary follicles often contain labeled GCs but to a varying degree, and that most of them are growing follicles. By using a different follicular classification in mice, Oakberg (4) estimated that follicles morphologically similar to human primordial intermediary, and small primary follicles are nongrowing follicles.

These conclusions are disputed by Hirshfield, however, who considers that studies that rely on morphometric criteria and pulse-labeling with 3H-TdR are not sufficiently sensitive to discriminate between nongrowing follicles and those that have begun to grow. By using a 7-day continuous infusion of 3H-TdR (5) she observed that both flattened and cuboidal GCs of the smallest follicles were often labeled. She concluded that many follicles that would be classified as nongrowing follicles by their morphological characteristics alone are nonetheless growing and that a substantial proportion of the smallest follicles in adult rats ovaries are growing. This assumption has been reinforced by other studies. The proliferating cell nuclear antigen (PCNA) is absent in cells of primordial follicles, but it begins to appear in intermediary follicles, even in flattened GCs (6). After injection of 5-bromodeoxy uridine, 30% of intermediary and primary follicles are labeled (7).

Thus, in laboratory rodents, morphological and physiological studies have led to a different appreciation of what defines nongrowing and growing follicles. In the early studies (1,3,4), the primary follicle was considered to be the stage at which follicle growth start. In more recent studies (5–7), it has been observed that some GCs, even in primordial follicles, are proliferating cells, and Hirshfield (5) assumed that more than one third of follicles with four or fewer GCs in the LCS, more than two thirds of follicles with 5–8 GCs,

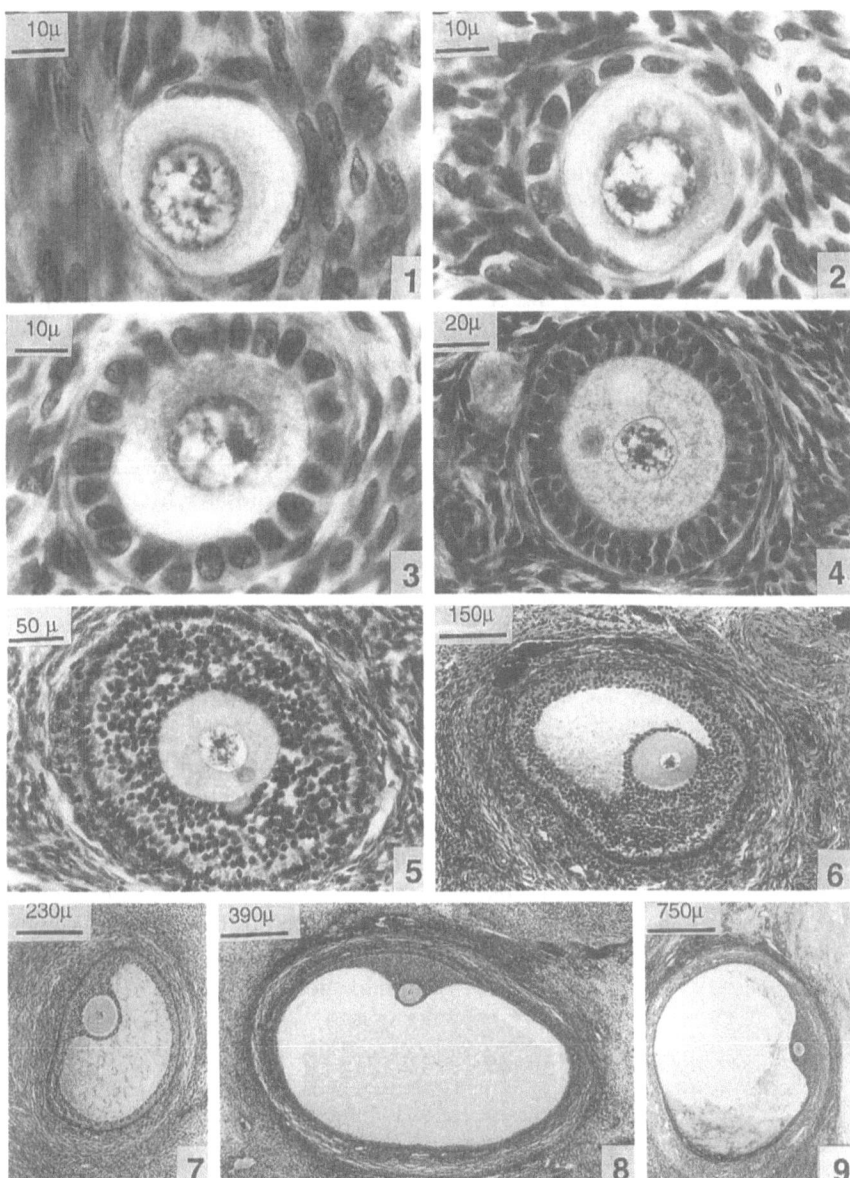

FIGURE 2.1. Primordial follicle in which the oocyte is surrouded by flattened GCs, ×1000. FIGURE 2.2. Intermediary follicle in which the oocyte is surrounded by a mixture of flattened and cuboidal GCs, ×1000. FIGURE 2.3. Primary follicle in which the ooctye is surrounded by a single layer of cuboidal GCs, ×1000. FIGURE 2.4. Secondary follicle, no epithelioid theca cell, ×550. FIGURE 2.5. Preantral follicle, the TI is differentiated (class 1, 0.11–0.22mm), ×200. FIGURE 2.6. Early antral follicle (class 2, 0.2–0.4mm), ×90. FIGURE 2.7. Small antral follicle (class 3, 0.5–0.9mm), ×55. FIGURE 2.8. Small antral follicle (class 4, 1–2mm), ×33. FIGURE 2.9. Selectable follicle (class 5, 2–5mm), ×17.

and more than three quarters of follicles with 9–12 GCs (i.e., more than 40% of the total number of follicles present in the ovaries) are growing follicles.

A second question then arises: Does the presence of proliferating GCs signify that follicles exhibiting such cells are growing follicles (i.e., have entered the process at the term of which they either become atretic or ovulate)? In humans, although primordial, intermediary, and small primary follicles differ in their diameter, they do not differ in the mean diameters of their oocyte and its nucleus (Table 2.1). The oocyte nucleus is about 16 μm in diameter, which is a size is below that of 19 μm observed when active follicular growth start (2). It can therefore be assumed that in human, primordial, intermediary, and small primary follicles are nongrowing follicles, whereas large primary follicles possessing an oocyte nucleus over 19 μm in diameter are early growing follicles. In addition, the number of follicles possessing at least one cuboidal GC is so high (Table 2.2) that, in agreement with van Wezel and Rodgers (8), we can assume that if all these follicles were growing follicles, then the ovary could be expected to be devoid of follicles within a matter of months. Because a similar comment could be made in rats if more than 40% of the follicles present in the ovaries were growing, the findings of early investigators (3,4) that initiation in rodents starts at the primary stage appear to be the most reliable.

In conclusion, studies in both human and rodent models indicate that the morphological events of initiation seem to be similar in humans and rodents.

The mechanisms that underly the initiation of follicular growth are unknown. A role for gonadotropins in this process has been debated for a long time. In rodents, some studies suggest that gonadotropins might be involved in the initiation of follicular growth observed at days 5–7 of life (for a review, see Ref. 9). Nevertheless, this postnatal initiation of follicular growth cannot result in a gonadotropic stimulation because efficient gonadotropin receptors are not present at this age (10), and because initiation of follicular growth can occur in vitro in absence of follicle stimulating hormone (FSH) in mice (11), in cattle (12) and in baboon (13). In mice homozygous for severe com-

TABLE 2.1. Percentages of different types of small follicles from human ovarian samples in various age groups.

	Age groups (years)				
	19–30 (6)	31–35 (10)	36–40 (13)	41–45 (31)	≥46 (26)
Primordial	62.2 ± 1.9	57.8 ± 3.6	54.5 ± 3.0	49.5 ± 1.9	45.1 ± 3.2
Intermediary	29.7 ± 1.7	30.9 ± 2.6	35.4 ± 2.0	36.3 ± 1.0	35.0 ± 1.5
Primary	6.0 ± 1.4	7.5 ± 1.5	7.9 ± 1.1	11.3 ± 1.2	15.3 ± 2.0
Secondary	1.7 ± 0.3	4.1 ± 1.2	2.2 ± 0.4	2.9 ± 0.4	4.5 ± 0.6

Values are mean ± e.m., number of ovaries in the brackets.

TABLE 2.2. Morphometric characteristics of very small follicles in the adult human ovary.

Follicle	Follicular diameter	Oocyte diameter	Oocyte nuclear diameter	Granulosa cells Mean $n°$	Granulosa cells Range
Primordial (408)	35.4 ± 0.3	32.1 ± 0.3	16.1 ± 0.3	13 ± 6	7–23
Intermediary (409)	37.8 ± 0.4	31.7 ± 0.4	16.3 ± 0.2	28 ± 6	9–50
Primary (153)	46.0 ± 0.5	32.6 ± 0.4	16.7 ± 0.2	76 ± 27	23–223
Early growing (30)	77.2 ± 2.0	47.8 ± 2.2	20.9 ± 0.6	360 ± 34	60–990

Diameters in microns expressed as mean ± SEM, and number of granulose cells expressed as mean ± SD for the number of follicles given in the brackets.

bined immunodeficiency (SCID) and hypogonadism (hpg), xenografts of human ovarian tissues exhibit follicles up to the secondary stage (14). Finally, FSH is not mandatory to initiate follicular growth because initiation is abolished neither in FSH knockout mice (15), nor in women presenting a mutation in the FSH-β subunit (16) or bearing mutated FSH-receptors (17,18). Taken together, these data strongly suggest that FSH is not involved in the initiation of follicular growth.

IGF-I is similarly not involved because IGF-I knockout mice (19) and women suffering from the Laron syndrome (20) exhibit a normal follicular growth, at least up to the antral stage for IGF-I knockout mice.

Because in growth differentiation factor-9 (GDF-9) knockout mice, follicular growth is prematurely arrested (21), it has been suggested that GDF-9 may be involved in the initiation of follicular growth. The presence of secondary follicles in ovaries from GDF-9 knockout mice, however, suggests that this molecule is not involved in initiation. A mutation of the *steel* locus encoding the kit ligand (KL) (22) and treatment of mice with an antibody against c-kit (23) result in arrest of follicular growth beyond the primary stage. Thus, it appears that both the KL, produced by GCs, and its c-kit receptor, present on the oocyte membrane, (24) might be involved in initiation.

In conclusion, many molecules have been suggested to be involved in the initiation of follicular growth because they are developmentally regulated and, when absent, lead to impaired follicular growth. When the precise stage of follicular development at which these molecules act and when the stage at which initiation occurs are taken into consideration, however, it appears that the KL/c-kit system is the only known system that might be involved in initiation.

Early Follicular Growth Up to the Preantral Stage

In humans, when primary follicles enter the growth phase, they enlarge, both by GC proliferation and by an increase in size of the oocyte. Follicles progressively become secondary (Fig. 2.4), and the surrounding connective tissue stratifies and differentiates into two parts the theca externa and the theca interna (TI), which contain some steroid-producing cells, also referred to as epithelioid cells. Morphological studies in women have shown that definitive theca layers appear only when follicles contain three to six layers of GCs (follicle diameter: 103-163 μm) (25).

There is a general assumption that early growing follicles are not gonadotropin-dependent despite the presence of functional FSH-R as soon as the primary stage (26). In FSH knockout mice (15), the number of growing follicles does not seem to be reduced and follicle growth can process up to the large preantral stage. In a women bearing mutated FSH-β subunit, ovulation was obtained within 15 days (16). Women bearing mutated FSH-R display various stages of follicular development up to a size of at least several millimeters (17,18). Some data, however, indicate that FSH may play a primary role in early follicular growth. In GDF-9 knockout mice, follicles do not develop beyond the secondary stage. Because signals downstream the FSH-R are altered in these mutant mice, FSH appears to be mandatory for early follicular growth (21). Hypophysectomized rodents (27) and *hpg* mice, which lack pituitary hormones (28), display preantral follicles, but in low number when compared with control animal; however, treatment with gonadotropins restores the normal situation (29). Because available models lead to opposite conclusions, it appears, in conclusion, that the needs of a gonadotropic support for early follicular growth remains unclear.

Problems in the Interpretation of Ovarian Biopsies in Sterility of Ovarian Origin

In humans, some reproductive failures are due to a gene mutation. These pathological situations are exceptional opportunities to understand which factors are or not involved in folliculogenesis, and at which stage of development the presence of these factors is mandatory for further growth. In most cases, examination of an ovarian biopsy has been reported but the exact time at which follicular growth is impaired is often difficult to identify because of the great confusion existing among the terms used to describe the successive stages of follicular development. The lack of experience of pathologists in analyzing human follicular growth has led them to use imprecise term (e.g., small follicles, large, cystic, small antral, large antral, and even Graafian, either used for antral or preovulatory follicles). A correct interpretation of these ovarian biopsies therefore requires a good knowledge of the kinetics of follicular growth in humans.

Basal Follicular Growth

In humans, epithelioid theca cells specifically bind LH as soon as the preantral stage (30,31). Thus, when the TI commences its epithelioid differentiation, the follicle becomes responsive to circulating gonadotropins because LH and FSH receptors (30,31) are present in the TI and GCs, respectively. This does not mean, however, that these follicles are highly responsive to gonadotropic hormones because transduction pathways can be partly inhibited by factors not clearly identified (32).

From the time of appearance of epithelioid cells in the TI, the secondary follicle becomes a preantral follicle (Fig. 2.5), the first class of growing follicles in a classification based on morphological aspect and total number of GCs in each individual follicle (25). These various classes represent the stages of development through which the single ovulatory follicle will pass.

Appearance of an antral cavity starts with the development of small fluid-filled cavities of 40 μm in diameter that aggregate to form the antrum. In humans and monkeys, follicles pass from the preantral (class 1) to the early antral stage (class 2, Fig. 2.6) at a follicular diameter comprised between 180 and 250 μm (25). With the accumulation of fluid in the antral cavity and proliferation of GCs and TI cells, the follicle progresses through subsequent stages of development (class 3, Fig. 2.7, and class 4, Fig. 2.8) until it reaches a size of about 2 mm.

The time required by a follicle to grow from the preantral stage to a size of 2 mm is approximately 70 days (25). This part of folliculogenesis is named basal follicular growth because many observation have shown that the development of these follicles can be sustained by basal levels of FSH up to a size of 2 mm (for a review, see Ref. 25). During basal growth, GCs proliferate at a slow rate and follicular steroidogenesis is low, which suggests that follicular cells are undifferentiated and poorly responsive to gonadotropins. Because the follicle cell content in gonadotropin receptors seems to be unchanged through the successive stages of development, various molecules produced by the follicle itself may be acting in a paracrine–autocrine fashion to maintain follicle cells in an undifferentiated stage (25). Among them, EGF/TGFα, which inhibits androgen synthesis and aromatase activity at TI (33) and granulose (34) cell levels, respectively, and WT1, which inhibits follicle differentiation (35), might be involved.

It has been reported that some patients suffering from a hypergonadotropic ovarian failure, characterized by elevated levels of circulating gonadotropins and unresponsive ovaries to exogenous gonadotropic stimulation, carry mutation(s) of the FSH receptor (FSH-R) gene (17,18). The mutated receptors are either nearly completely (17) or partially (18) inactive. Pelvic ultrasonography of a patient displaying partially inactive FSH-R revealed that follicular growth can proceed up to a size of 5 mm. Ovarian biopsies from this patient, however, indicated that only follicles up to a size of approximately 0.5 mm are healthy, whereas, follicles more than 2 mm are atretic and possess a hypertrophied TI (18). Ovarian biopsies from the patients beating neatly completely inactive FSH-R exhibited healthy follicles only at either primary or secondary stages (17); however, the size of the biopsies was so small that the existence of healthy follicles at further stages of development cannot be excluded.

In six of eight patients of the same age, follicles were detected by transvaginal sonography (17), indicating that these ovaries contained follicles 2 mm or more in diameter and suggesting that although FSH-R were nearly completely inactive, follicular development could occasionally proceed up to a size of several millimeters, but in a lesser extent than in the patient bearing partially inactive FSH-R. Taken together these observations confirm that follicle growth up to a size of several millimeters can be sustained by a very low FSH message and that there is a possible relationship between the level of the FSH message and the size reached by the follicles.

The Selectable Stage

In humans, 2- to 5-mm follicles (Fig. 2.9) are present throughout the cycle. It is during the late luteal phase that the follicles that have entered the preantral stage 70 days earlier become selectable follicles (25). It is among these follicles that the one destined to ovulate in the subsequent cycle will be selected to ovulate approximately 2 week later (36). From a size of 2 mm, there is a body of evidence indicating that follicle development become dependent of high levels of FSH. The percentage of atretic selectable follicles decreases when FSH increases (37). From the mid- to the late luteal phase, GCs of selectable follicles exhibit a significant increase in the rate of proliferation (37), which parallels the increase in circulating levels of FSH. In addition, when stimulated with hMG during both the late luteal and early follicular phase, selectable follicles can grow more quickly than unstimulated selectable follicles (38).

In some women suffering from a Kallman syndrome (39,40), or in the patient with a mutation in the β-subunit of FSH (16), ovulation can be induced within approximately 2 weeks. Because this is the time required for a selectable follicle to reach the ovulatory size during an unstimulated cycle, and because exogenous gonadotropins strongly stimulate GC proliferation (38), it appears that either selectable follicles or follicles slightly smaller may be present in the ovaries of these women.

Preovulatory Maturation

From the early follicular phase to the late follicular phase, the size of the preovulatory follicle passes from 6.9 ± 0.5 to 18.8 ± 0.5 mm by follicle cell multiplication and accumulation of fluid in the antrum (36). The mean number of GCs rises from approximately 2–5 million to 50–100 million at the time of ovulation (25). During the final phase of development, the granulosa layer of the follicles destined to ovulate is subjected to marked morphological transformations resulting from a modulation of the actin cytoskeleton organization, which may be related to the programmed events that lead to GCs differentiation (25). In humans, GCs express aromatase only in healthy follicles larger than 8–10 mm in diameter; consequently, the only follicle to produce significant levels of estradiol in humans is the preovulatory follicle.

During its maturation, the preovulatory follicle produces increasing levels of IGF-II and inhibin, acting, respectively, at the GC level to enhance expression of aromatase, and at the TI level to enhance the LH-induced production of androstenedione leading to an increasing production of estradiol (for a review, see Ref. 25).

After the midcycle LH surge, the preovulatory follicle passes from an estrogen-producing to a progesterone-producing structure. In its GC layer, mitotic figures have disappeared and it picnotic index rises up to 0.3% (25).

Conclusions

When a large resection is examined to assess its follicle content, a classification based on the number of GCs can be used, however, this constitutes a painstaking task. Because there is a strong correlation between the number of GCs and the follicle diameter, the former can be conveniently replaced by the measurement of the latter (36). As a result, terms such as small, large, and cystic follicles must be discarded and replaced by the size of the considered follicle.

In small ovarian biopsies, all follicles up to preantral/early antral stage can be easily observed and measured, especially in young patients. In these biopsies, however, follicles more than 0.5 mm in diameter, it they exist, are observed by chance. When such biopsies are performed in infertile patients it is therefore extremely difficult to appreciate the stage at which follicular growth is disrupted. Given the small size of most biopsies, analysis of their follicular content only allows the investigator to discriminate between the absence of nongrowing follicles, either due to an ovarian dysgenesis or to a premature exhaustion of the follicular stock, and a disruption of follicular growth, either at the initiation level or at the early stages of development. Identification of further stage of development at which follicular growth is disrupted requires additional investigations. For example, transvaginal sonography can indicate the presence of follicles more than 2 mm in diameter (i.e., selectable follicles), which can be either healthy or atretic. Only healthy follicles are stimulable by exogenous gonadotropins and can reach the ovulatory size. In the case of follicular growth disruption at the selectable stage, a successful induction of ovulation with exogenous gonadotropins can be obtained only if these selectable follicles are both healthy and possess functional FSH-R. If induction of ovulation is uncussessful, it can be assumed either that selectable follicles are atretic or that they do not possess functional FSH-R.

Thus, a careful examination of the stages at which follicular growth is disrupted in ovarian biopsies from infertile patients in addition to the analysis of steroids and gonadotropins circulating levels, ovarian sonography and ovarian stimulation with exogenous gonadotropins in the same infertile patient, may provide significant insights in the knowledge of the mechanisms controlling ovarian follicular development.

References

1. Lintern-Moore S, Moore GPM. The initiation of follicle and oocyte growth in the mouse ovary. Biol Reprod 1979;20:773–78.
2. Gougeon A, Chainy GBN. Morphometric studies of small follicles in ovaries of women at different ages. J Reprod Fertil 1987;81:433–42.
3. Pedersen T. Follicle kinetics in the ovary of the cyclic mouse. Acta Endocrinol 1970;64:304–23.
4. Oakberg EF. Follicular growth and atresia in the mouse. In Vitro 1979;15:41–49.
5. Hirshfield AN. Granulosa cell proliferation in very small follicles of cycling rats studied by long-term continuous tritiated-thymidine infusion. Biol Reprod 1989;41:309–16.
6. Oktay K, Schenken RS, Nelson JF. Proliferating cell nuclear antigen marks the initiation of follicular growth in the rat. Biol Reprod 1995;53:295–301.
7. Gaytan F, Morales C, Bellido, Aguilar E, Sanchez-Criado JE. Proliferative activity in the different ovarian compartments in cycling rats estimated by the 5-bromodeoxyuridine technique. Biol Reprod 1996;54:1356–65.
8. van Wezel IL, Rodgers RJ. Morphological characterization of bovine primordial follicles and their environment in vivo. Biol Reprod 1996;55:1003–11.
9. Hirshfield AN, DeSanti AM. Patterns of ovarian cell proliferation in rats during the embryonic period and the first three weeks postpartum. Biol Reprod 1995;53:1208–21.
10. Sokka TA, Huhtaniemi IT. Ontogeny of gonadotrophin receptors and gonadotrophin stimulated cyclic AMP production in the neonatal rat ovary. J Endocrinol 1990;127:297–303.
11. Eppig JJ, O'Brien MJ. Development in vitro of mouse oocytes from primordial follicles. Biol Reprod 1996;54:197–207.
12. Braw -Tal R, Yossefi S. Studies in vivo and in vitro on the initiation of follicle growth in the bovine ovary. J Reprod Fertil 1997;109:165–71.
13. Wandji SA, Srsen V, Nathanielsz PW, Eppig JJ, Fortune JE. Initiation of growth of baboon primordial follicles in vitro. Hum Reprod 1997;12:1993–2001.
14. Oktay K, Newton H, Mullan J, Gosden RG. Development of human primordial follicles to antral srages in SCID/*hpg* mice stimulated with follicle-stimuating hormone. Hum Reprod 1998;13:1133–38.
15. Kumar TR, Wang Y, Lu N, Matzuk MM. Follicle stimulating hormone is required for ovarian follicle maturation but not for male fertility. Nature Gen 1997;15:201–4.
16. Matthews CH, Borgato S, Beck-Peccoz P, Adams M, Tone Y, Gambino G, et al. Primary amenorrhoea and infertility due to a mutation in the β-subunit of follicle-stimulating hormone. Nature Gen 1993;5:83–86.
17. Aittomaki K, Herva R, Stenman U-H, Juntunen K, Ylöstalo P, Hovatta O, et al. Clincal features of primary ovarian failure caused by a point mutation in the follicle-stimulating hormone receptor gene. J Clin Endocrinol Metab 1996;81:3722–26.
18. Beau I, Touraine P, Meduri G, Gougeon A, Desroches A, Matuchansky C, et al. A novel phenotype related to partial loss of function mutations of the follicle-stimulating hormone receptor. J Clin Invest 1998;102:1352–69.
19. Baker J, Hardy MP, Zhou J, Bondy C, Lupu F, Bellvé A, et al. Effect of an *igf1* gene null mutation on mouse reproduction. Mol Endocrinol 1996;10:903–18.
20. Menashe Y, Sack J, Mashiach S. Spontaneous pregnancies in two women with Laron-

type dwarfism: are growth hormone and circulating insulin-like growth farctor mandatory for induction of ovulation? Hum Reprod 1991;5:670–71.

21. Dong J, Albertini DF, Nishimori K, Kumar TR, Lu N, Matzuk MM. Growth differentiation factor-9 is required during ovarian early folliculogenesis. Nature 1996;383:531–35.

22. Huang EJ, Manova K, Packer AI, Sanchez S, Bachvarova RM, Besmer P. The murine steel panda mutation affects kit ligand expression and growth of early ovarian follicles. Dev Biol 1993;157:100–9.

23. Yoshinda H, Takakura N, Kataoka H, Kunisada T, Okamura H, Nishikawa S-I. Stepwise requirement of c-kit tyrosine kinase in mouse ovarian follicle development. Dev Biol 1997;184:122–37.

24. Motro B, Bernstein A. Dynamic changes in ovarian c-kit and Steel expression during the estrous reproductive cycle. Dev Dynamics 1993;197:69–79.

25. Gougeon A. Regulation of ovarian follicular development in primates: facts and hypotheses. Endocrinol Rev 1996;17:121–55.

26. Oktay K, Briggs D, Gosden RG. Ontogeny of follicle-stimulating hormone receptor gene expreesion in isolated human ovarian follicles. J Clin Endocrinol Metab 1997;82:3748–51.

27. Jones EC, Krohn PL. The effect of hypophysectomy on age changes in the ovaries of mice. J Endocrinol 1961;21:497–509.

28. Halpin DMG, Charlton HM, Faddy MJ. Effects of gonadotrophin deficiency on follicular development in hypogonadal (hpg) mice. J Reprod Fertil 1986;78:119–25.

29. Halpin DMG, Charlton HM. Effects of short-trem injection of gonadotrophins on ovarian follicle development in hypogonadal (*hpg*) mice. J Reprod Fertil 1988;82:393–400.

30. Shima K, Kitayama S, Nakano R. Gonadotropin binding sites in human ovarin follicles and corpora lutea during the menstrual cycle. Obstet Gynecol 1987;69:800–6.

31. Kobayashi M, Nakano R, Ooshima A. Immunocytochemical localization of pituitary gonadotrophins and gonadal steroids confirms the "two-cell, two-gonadotrophin" hypothesis of steroidogenesis in the human ovary. J Endocrinol 1990;126:483–88.

32. Jonassen JA, Bose K, Richards JS. Enhancement and desensitization of hormone-responsive adenylate cyclase in granulose cells of preantral and antral ovarian follicles: effects of estradiol and follicle-stimulating hormone. Endocrinology 1982;111:74–79.

33. Erickson GF, Case E. Epidermal growth factor antagonizes ovarian theca-interstitial cytodifferention. Mol Cell Endocrinol 1983;31:71–76.

34. Mason HD, Margara R, Winston RML, Beard RW, Reed MJ, Franks S. Inhibition of oestradiol production by epidermal growth factor in human granulosa cells of normal and polycystic ovaries. Clin Endocrinol 1990;33:11–17.

35. Hsu SY, Kubo M, Chun S-Y, Haluska FG, Housman DE, Hsueh AJW. Wilms'tumor protein WTI as an ovarian transcription factor: decreases in expression during follicle development and repression of inhibin-α gene promoter. Mol Endocrinol 1995;9:1356–66.

36. Gougeon A, Lefèvre B. Evolution of the diameters of the largest healthy and atretic follicles during the human menstrual cycle. J Reprod Fertil 1983;69:497–502.

37. Gougeon A. Influence of cyclic variations in gonadotrophin and steroid hormones on follicular growth on the human ovary. In: de Brux J, Gautray JP, eds. Clinical pathology of the endocrine ovary. Lancaster; MTP Press, 1984; 63–72.

38. Gougeon A, Testart J. Influence of human menopausal gonadotropin on the recruitment of human ovarian follicles. Fertil Steril 1990;54:848–52.
39. Sungurtekin U, Fraser IS, Shearman RP. Pregnancy in women with Kallman's syndrome. Fertil Steril 1995;63:494–99.
40. Kousta E, White DM, Piazzi A, Loumaye E, Franks S. Successful induction of ovulation and compleyed pregnancy using recombinant human luteintizing hormone and follicle-stimulating hormone in a woman with Kallmann's syndrome. Hum Reprod 1996;11:70–71.

3

The Graafian Follicle:
A Functional Definition

GREGORY F. ERICKSON

The broad question to be considered in this discussion concerns the functional definition of a Graafian follicle (GF). There are two important reasons why this is a very challenging question. The first is the extreme heterogeneity that exists with respect to the biochemical properties and regulatory pathways of one GF to another. The second is that the very essence of GF development is continuous change in which some functions vary markedly from stage to stage and from follicle to follicle. As a result, it is difficult to come to grips with a simple functional definition. In order to appreciate this complexity, I will consider here the nature and relationship of the structure of a GF to its normal function. Because of the enormity of the topic, my discussion will provide only a selected analysis of some of the structure–function correlates of the GF. I will focus my attention on some important principles and on some advances in follicle biology as they relate to GF function, concentrating on the human and bringing in a few other animals to illustrate particular points.

A GF can be defined structurally as a heterogeneous family of relatively large follicles (400 μm to 2 cm at ovulation) characterized by a cavity or antrum containing a fluid termed *follicular fluid* or *liquor folliculi*. The characteristic structural unit of all GF is the antrum. For this reason, the term *antral follicle* is used correctly as a synonym for GF. The follicular fluid is the medium in which the granulosa cells and oocyte are found and through which regulatory molecules must pass on their way to and from this microenvironment. We surprisingly know almost nothing about the physiological significance of the antrum and follicular fluid in folliculogenesis. It is clear that follicle development and ovulation occur in birds and amphibians despite the absence of an antrum and follicular fluid. One important question that therefore needs to be addressed in GF development concerns the physiological relevance of the antrum. Nonetheless, its presence in all mammalian species testifies to its importance in ovarian physiology.

All GFs can be divided into two groups, healthy and atretic (Fig. 3.1). The main difference between these two groups is whether or not apoptosis is oc-

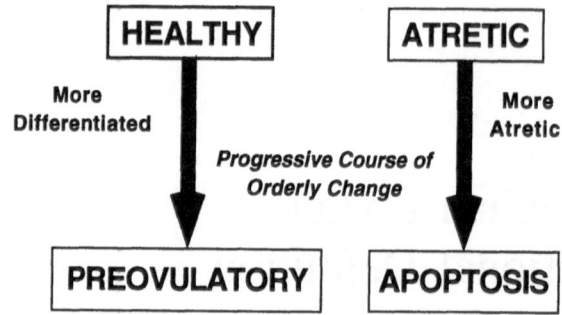

Figure 3.1. The two major classes of Graafian follicles, healthy and atretic. Each undergoes a regulated course of progressive change that results in either ovulation or the fate of apoptosis.

curring in the granulosa cells. An important concept is that the development of the GF (healthy or atretic) follows a progressive course over time. This concept is of paramount importance in formulating the functional definition of a GF because it implies that variability or heterogeneity is a normal consequence of folliculogenesis. In a healthy follicle, the GF becomes progressively more differentiated with increasing time until it attains the preovulatory stage. The time for this process has been calculated to be about 2 months in women (1). When this occurs, there is a temporal and spatial pattern of expression of large numbers of genes that direct the follicle to undergo cytodifferentiation and proliferation as well as follicular fluid formation. In a similar manner, the atretic follicles undergo time-dependent changes in gene expression that cause the GF to stop mitosis and proceed along a pathway of atresia. Under atresia conditions, the oocyte and granulosa cells become committed to undergo a temporal pattern of expression of those genes that lead to apoptosis or programmed cell death (2). In both healthy and atretic GFs, the control mechanisms involve ligand-dependent signaling pathways that act to inhibit or stimulate the expression of differentiation and apoptosis. Understanding the molecular mechanisms and cellular consequences of these ligand–receptor signaling pathways is a major goal of reproductive research.

Following its formation, the process of GF growth and development can arbitrarily be divided into several stages based on follicle size. This is both convenient and important for clinicians and researchers to identify the physiological function of various types of classes of follicles over the cycle. The healthy GF (i.e., the human) has a destiny to complete the transition from the small (1–6 mm), medium (7–11 mm), and large (12–17 mm), to the fully differentiated preovulatory state (18–23 mm). The atretic GF has a destiny to complete the transition from the small to the medium stage (1–10 mm), but is never capable of growing to the large size under normal physiological conditions. Because these processes of GF development are asynchronous, they

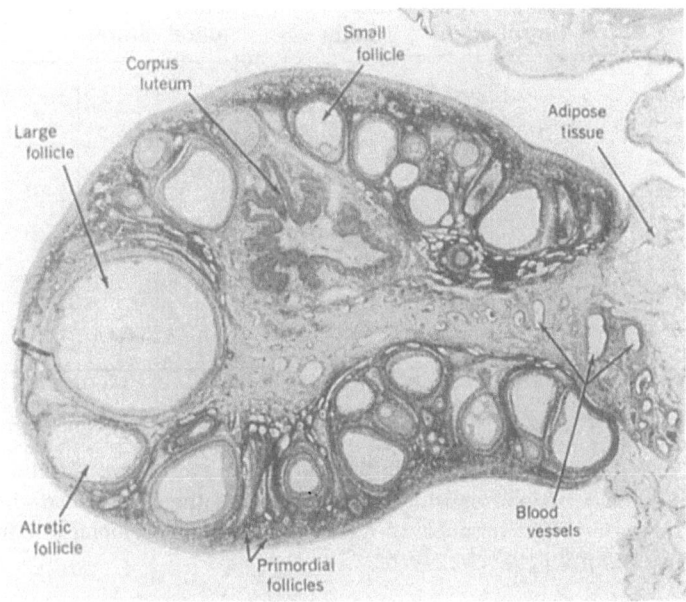

FIGURE 3.2. Photomicrograph of an adult primate ovary showing large numbers of different sized healthy and atretic follicles. Reprinted with permission from Bloom W, Fawcett DW, eds. A Textbook of Histology. Arnold Publishing, 1975.

lead to the presence of a large heterogeneous population of GFs in the ovaries at any moment in time (Fig. 3.2). In a very real sense, each of these morphologically distinct GFs is a dynamic structure undergoing a flow or progression of developmental change on its way to becoming more differentiated or more atretic. It should be kept in mind that this results in the presence of an extremely heterogeneous pool of GF, and it is the heterogeneity that makes it difficult to come to grips with a simple functional definition for the GF.

What determines the size of a GF? The size of a GF is determined largely by the size of the antrum (Fig. 3.3), which is in turn determined by the volume of follicular fluid, which is in turn determined by the availability of follicle stimulating hormone (FSH) in the fluid (3). It should be emphasized that FSH is obligatory for GF development and no other ligand by itself has the ability to induce follicular fluid formation. In the absence of FSH, follicular fluid is not produced and no GFs are formed in the ovaries. The proliferation of the follicle cells also changes dramatically: In healthy follicles, the granulosa and theca cells proliferate extensively (as much as 100-fold) concomitant with the antrum becoming filled with follicular fluid (Fig. 3.3). These events—

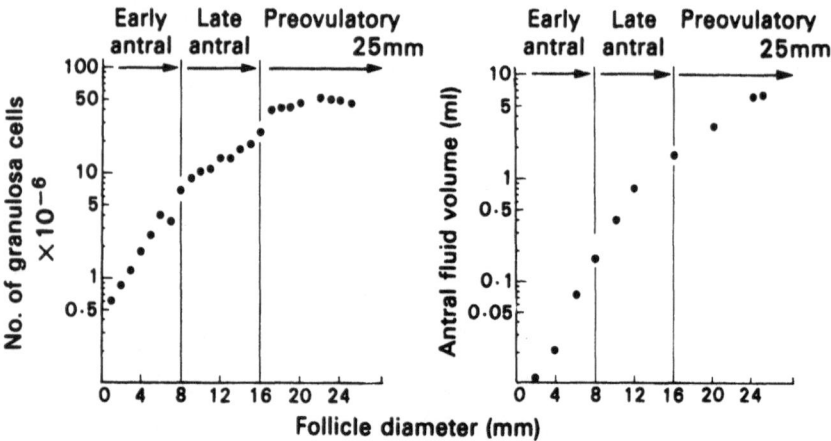

FIGURE 3.3. Changes in the number of granulosa cels and volume of follicular fluid during the growth (size) of a healthy human Graafian follicle. Reprinted with permission from McNatty KP. Hormonal correlates of follicular development in the human ovary. Aust J Biol Sci 1981;34:249–68.

increased follicular fluid accumulation and cell proliferation—are responsible for the tremendous growth of healthy GFs (1,4). In contrast, it is the cessation of mitosis and follicular fluid formation that directly determine the size of the atretic GF.

The first question to be analyzed is when during folliculogenesis does GF development begin? When a preantral follicle reaches the secondary stage in development, it contains five distinct structural units: a fully grown oocyte surrounded by a zona pellucida, six to nine layers of granulosa cells, a basal lamina, a theca interna, and a theca externa (3). The first indication of the onset of GF development is the appearance of a cavity or antrum in the secondary follicle at the end of the preantral stage (3). In response to stimulation, a cavity begins to form at one pole of the oocyte. This process, termed *cavitation* or *beginning antrum formation*, is characterized by the uptake of fluid between the granulosa cells and therefore the formation of an internal cavity (Fig. 3.4). In essence cavitation results in the remodeling of the granulosa cells to form a miniature but complete spatial pattern of a GF. At completion of cavitation, the basic plan of the Graafian follicle is established, and all the various cell types are in their proper position awaiting the stimulation that will shift them along paths of differentiation and proliferation. Based on evidence from polyoocyte follicles it would seem that the specification mechanism is tightly regulated (Fig. 3.5).

What determines antrum formation? It is well known that cavitation occurs in hypophysectomized animals, demonstrating that pituitary hormones like FSH are not required for this morphogenetic event (5). Consistent with this concept is the recent observation that cavitation can occur in secondary follicles in FSHβ-deficient mice (6,7); therefore, this fundamental morphologi-

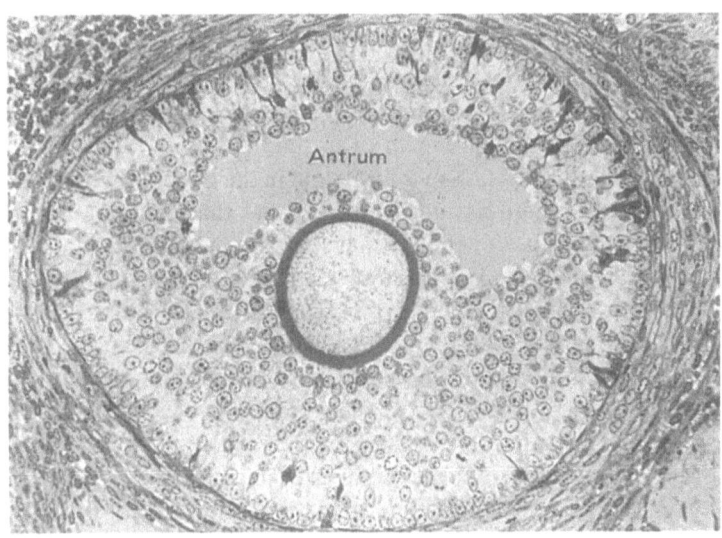

FIGURE 3.4. Photomicrograph of an early tertiary follicle 400 μm in diameter undergoing cavitation or antrum formation. Reprinted with permission from Bloom W, Fawcett DW, eds. A Textbook of Histology. Arnold Publishing, 1975.

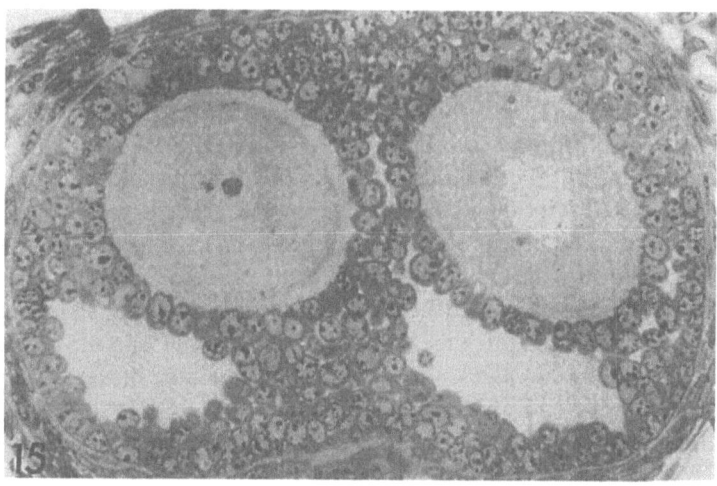

FIGURE 3.5. Photomicrograph of a polyoocyte follicle at cavitation showing two early antra developing simultaneously and at that same pole above each egg. Reprinted with permission from Zamboni L. Comparative studies on the ultrastructure of mammalian oocytes. In: Biggers JD, Schuetz AW, eds. Oogenesis. Baltimore: University Park Press; 1972:5–45.

cal change in the secondary follicle is believed to be mediated by autocrine–paracrine mechanisms. Two growth factors expressed in the follicle itself have been implicated in cavitation: activin and c-kit ligand. Treating cultured granulosa cells with activin causes morphogenetic changes that result in the formation of a histological unit with an antrumlike cavity (8). It has also been found that blocking the action of c-kit ligand in the ovary prevents GF formation; consequently, there are no ovulations and the female is infertile (9). Finally, evidence has been obtained that supports the concept that the oocyte gap junctions are involved in cavitation. Gap junctions are intercellular channels composed of proteins called *connexins* (10,11). There are at least 13 members of the connexin family that directly couple adjacent cells, allowing diffusion of ions, metabolities, and other low molecular weight signaling molecules like cyclic AMP (10,11). Connexin 37 (Cx37) appears to be an oocyte-derived Cx which forms gap junctions between the oocyte and surrounding granulosa cells. Evidence from Cx37-deficient mice assigns to Cx37 an obligatory role in GF formation, ovulation, and fertility (12). This evidence collectively implicates follicular-derived activin, c-kit, and Cx37 as potential players in the autocrine–paracrine mechanisms underlying the initiation (first step) in GF development, namely cavitation.

Once the GF is formed at cavitation, it begins to grow and carry out its differentiated function. A very important concept is that the follicle cells change gradually during the course of GF development, in which new qualities or features appear and disappear in a time-dependent manner (Fig. 3.6). That is, as a GF grows and develops, it proceeds from level to level in an organizational scheme, during which time something new emerges; these changes can be either intrinsically beneficial or destructive. The trigger for the induction of GF development is FSH. At cavitation, plasma FSH is brought to the early tertiary follicle by surrounding blood vessels in the theca interna, where it can diffuse into the follicular fluid (Fig. 3.6).

The entry of FSH into the follicular fluid at cavitation provides the induction stimulus that will initiate the process of GF growth and development. At the cellular level, it is the FSH receptor on the granulosa cell that is the fundamental player in this process. In humans, the period leading up to selection is marked by a progressive time-dependent increase in the size of the GF from 0.4 to ~5mm in diameter (Fig. 3.6), and the process takes about 1 month (1). As the GF moves through the small stage in development, the cells in the follicle wall proliferate and follicular fluid accumulates in the antrum (1). Beginning with the end of luteolysis in the menstrual cycle (1,13), it is believed that FSH increases in concentration in the follicular fluid of one of the small GF in a cohort. When an appropriately high FSH threshold is reached in one GF, it is selected to become dominant. By contrast, the small GFs in the cohort with subthreshold levels of FSH become nondominant (Fig. 3.6). An important point is that the mechanism whereby one small GF is able to concentrate high levels of FSH in its microenvironment remains one of the big mysteries in ovary physiology. The FSH action on the granulosa cells causes

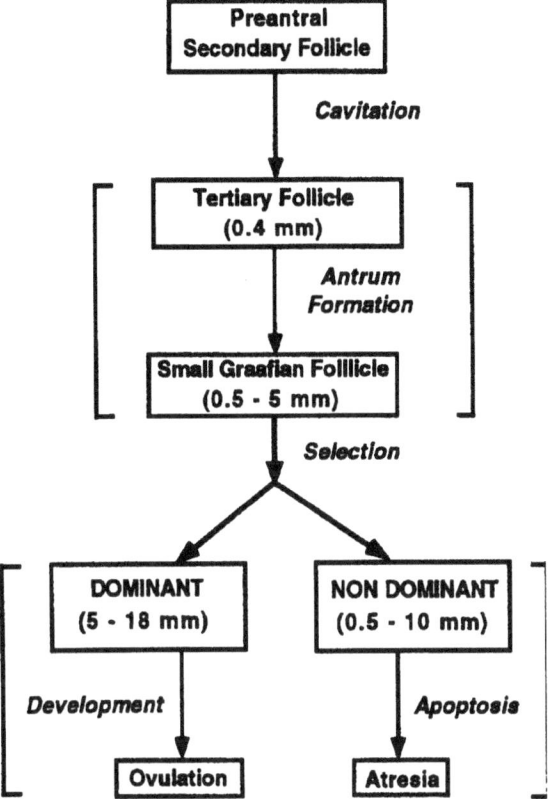

FIGURE 3.6. The principal stage-specific shifts in the life and death of a Graafian follicle.

the dominant follicle to leave the pool of small follicles. Under normal conditions the cells in the dominant GF undergo a predictable temporal pattern of differentiation and proliferation that ultimately results in the expression of a preovulatory follicle (Fig. 3.6). The situation is just the opposite in the nondominant follicle. That is, in the absence of adequate FSH stimulation, the follicle cells stop dividing, apoptosis is triggered, and the nondominant follicles enter an atretic state during which time the granulosa cells and oocyte eventually disappear. During the life of the female, the vast majority (99.9%) of the GF do not survive to complete the process; rather, they die by atresia. This is important because it demonstrates the principle that dominant follicle formation is a highly selective process, and further that atresia is the most common event in the physiology of the mammalian ovary.

The progressive growth and development of a GF is closely tied to the differentiation of the cells in the follicle wall. What is the relationship between the structure of a GF and its function? Before discussing function it is important to consider briefly some structural aspects of the GF. A GF is a

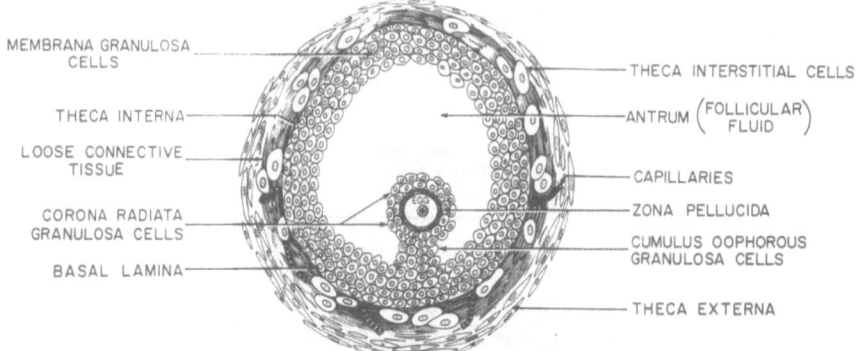

FIGURE 3.7. Diagram portraying a typical Graafian follicle as it might appear frozen in time. Reprinted from Erickson GF. Primary cultures of ovarian cells in serum-free medium as models of hormone-dependent differentiation. Mol Cell Endocrinol 1983;29:21–49, with permission from Elsevier Science.

three-dimensional structure with a central antrum surrounded by a variety of different cell types (Fig. 3.7). There are six distinct histological components in the GF, including the theca externa, theca interna, basal lamina, granulosa cells, oocyte, and follicular fluid. The GFs do not change their morphologic complexity as development proceeds; thus, all healthy GF have this same basic histologic structure. In other words, even though there are dramatic changes in GF size, their appearance remains more or less the same.

The major changes that occur during the stages of GF development involve cytodifferentiation. As the levels of cytodifferentiation become progressively expressed, specific functional activities of the GF emerge, with each cell type in the follicle exhibiting a strikingly different function. A key feature of this process, however, is that all the cellular components seem to be functionally related to one another. A good example is that the production of estrogen by the granulosa cells requires androgen substrate provided by the theca interna. Thus, a GF must be viewed as a whole unit, with no part having a truly separate identity in the functional state. A general principle to emerge from all our knowledge is that the function of a GF is greater than the sum of the functional activities of each cellular component (e.g., the function of a GF is greater than the sum of its parts). To understand this concept more fully we must understand the major differentiated functions of the various cell populations in the GF.

The theca externa is characterized by the presence of smooth muscle cells (14,15), which in turn are innervated by autonomic nerves (reviewed in Ref. 16). Although the physiological significance of the theca externa remains unclear, there is evidence (17,18) that it contracts during ovulation and atresia (Fig. 3.8). These observations suggest that changes in the contractile activity of the theca externa may be involved in these important physiological

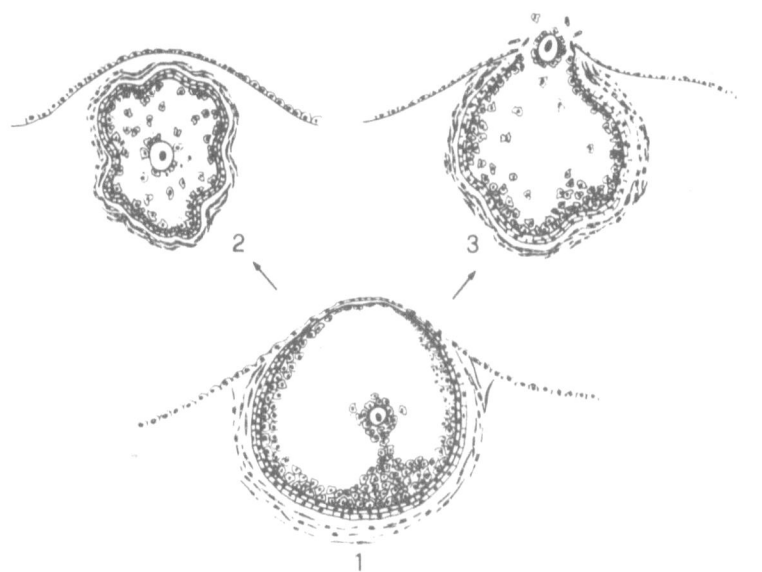

FIGURE 3.8. Diagram illustrating the contraction of the theca externa of a Graafian follicle (1), during atresia (2) and ovulation (3). Note the shortening and contracted smooth muscle cells in the theca externa. Reprinted from Motta PM, Familiari G. Occurrence of a contractile tissue in the theca externa of atretic follicles in the mouse ovary. Acta Anat 1981;109:103–14, with permission from Kreiger Basel.

processes, but this has not been rigorously proven. Some fundamental questions that need to be addressed include: What is the origin of the theca externa and what is the precise nature of its cell types? What are the mechanisms underlying the control of their differentiation? What is their physiological role in GF development and atresia? It is noteworthy that the corpus luteum retains a theca externa throughout its life (19); however, the significance of the theca externa during luteinization and luteolysis is not known.

The theca interna is composed of differentiated theca interstitial cells (TIC) located within a matrix of loose connective tissue and blood vessels. In all GF, LH is a key regulatory hormone for TIC function and its importance in regulating TIC androgen production in vivo and in vitro has been clearly established (16). Beginning at the very early stages of GF development, for example, at or about the time of cavitation, the TIC express their differentiated state as androgen producing cells (16). In situ hybridization and immunocytochemistry studies have demonstrated that this cytodifferentiation (Fig. 3.9) is accompanied by the expression of the LH receptors (20), and specific genes in the androgen biosynthetic pathway including StAR or the steroid acute regulatory protein (21,22), P450 side-chain cleavage, 3β-hydroxysteroid dehydrogenase, and P450$_{c17}$ (23–25). By virtue of the differential expression of this battery of genes, the TIC express their terminal differentiated state as an androstenedione-producing tissue in the GF (Fig. 3.9). Very little is known about the inducers for the differentiation of TIC, most notably the induction of the expression of the gene encoding the LH receptor. In this regard, there is a report that large GFs with well-developed theca interna (hyperplastic and hypertrophied TIC) are present in the ovaries of a patient with an LH-receptor-inactivating mutation (26). This suggests an interesting and important role for yet to be identified regulatory ligands in TIC development (e.g., novel ligands that can stimulate the expression of TIC proliferation and differentiation in the absence of the biological actions of LH). Further studies are necessary to identify the nature of these putative regulatory factor(s) of TIC mitosis and differentiation, and to establish their physiological and pathological significance.

It should be mentioned that we know precious little about the regulatory elements that control the theca vasculature. A functional link between the vasculature and GF development is suggested by the study of Zeleznik (27)

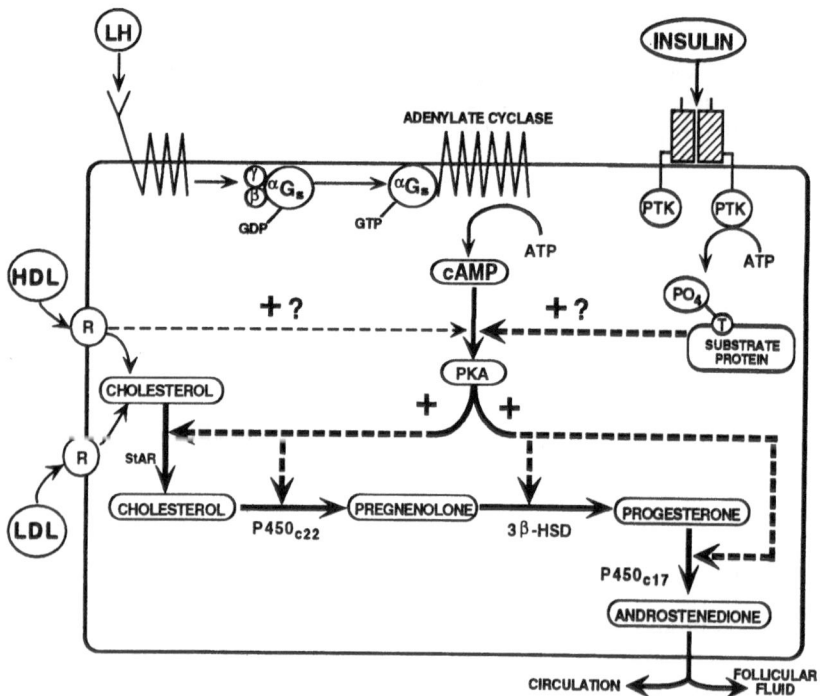

FIGURE 3.9. Diagram of a differentiated theca interstitial cell showing the expression of the key components in the LH receptor signaling pathway that leads to androstenedione production. Redrawn with permission from Erickson GF. Normal regulation of ovarian androgen production. Sem Reprod Endocrinol 1993;11:307–12.

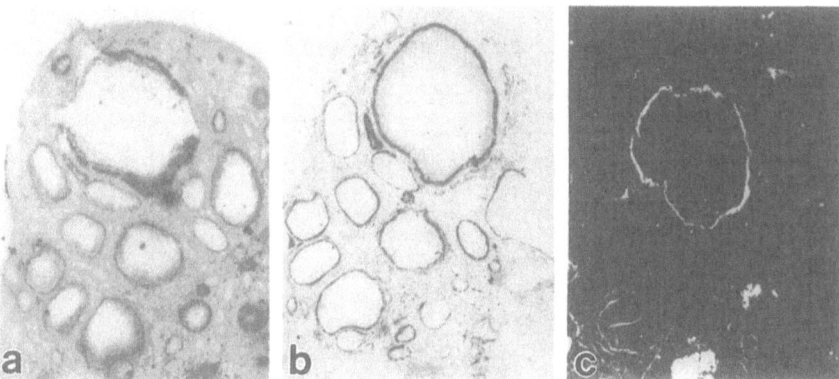

FIGURE 3.10. Photomicrograph showing that all Graafian follicles in the monkey ovary are characterized by the presence of FSH (a) and LH (b) receptors in the granulosa and theca cells, respectively, whereas injected ^{125}I-hCG is detectable only in the theca of the dominant follicle (c). Reprinted from Zeleznik AJ, Schuler HM, Reichert LE. Gonadotropin-binding sites in the Rhesus monkey ovary: role of the vasculature in the selective distribution of human chorionic gonadotropin to the preovulatory follicle. Endocrinology 1981;109:356–62 © The Endocrine Society.

in the monkey. He showed that all monkey GFs express high levels of FSH and LH receptor regardless of size, but when ^{125}I-hCG is injected systemically, only the dominant GF appears to be capable of accumulating ^{125}I-hCG in the theca interna (Fig. 3.10). These results are consistent with the concept that the dominant GF expresses increased vascularization that might in turn play an important role in its selected maturation. In this regard, follicle-derived VEGF (28,29) and other angiogenic factors [e.g., endothelin (30)] are being intensively investigated.

One of the major points of GF development is that the theca compartments (theca externa and interna) express their differentiated functions at the very beginning of GF development (at cavitation), and appear constitutively to express a mature phenotype throughout the life and death of the GF. In a broad sense, there is little or no evidence that major changes occur in the theca layers during the various stages of GF development, beyond those related to vascular and proliferative activities. In other words, the cellular activities of theca externa and theca interna would appear to be more or less the same in all GF, regardless of size or developmental state. This is important because it implies that it is the granulosa cells (and perhaps the oocyte) that are variable and thus responsible for GF diversity.

What do we know about granulosa cell diversity? A detailed examination of the GF reveals that the granulosa cells and oocyte are a mass of precisely shaped and precisely positioned cells (Fig. 3.11). The spatial variation creates at least

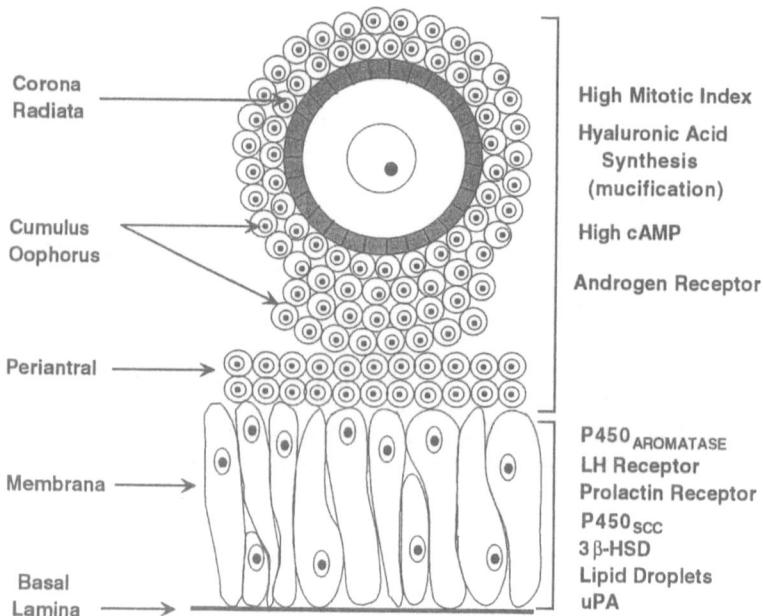

FIGURE 3.11. Diagram of the structural and functional heterogeneity of the granulosa cells in a Graafian follicle. The granulosa cells express different patterns of proliferation and differentiation as a result of their position or location in the unit.

four different granulosa cell layers or domains: The outermost domain is the membrana granulosa, the inner most domain is the periantral, the intermediate domain is the cumulus oophorus, and the domain juxtaposed to the oocyte is the corona radiata. A characteristic histological property of the peripheral domain is that it is composed of a pseudostratified epithelium of tall columnar granulosa cells, all of which are anchored to the basal lamina. It is apparent, therefore, that the granulosa cells are heterogeneous as a result of their position within the GF.

The heterogeneity in the granulosa cells has important implications for GH development. The primary importance of the heterogeneity is that the granulosa cells have the opportunity for specialization (e.g., different granulosa cells within the spatial organization are capable of accomplishing different tasks). Indeed, one of the remarkable features of the granulosa cells in the GF is that one gets different patterns of mitosis and differentiation expressed within the various domains (Fig. 3.11). For example, cells in the membrana domain stop proliferating before those in central domain (31,32) as seen by an absence of cells in S phase or mitosis (Fig. 3.12). The ability of the granulosa cells in the inner domains to continue dividing throughout GF suggests they might be precursor cells. The cessation of mitosis in the membrana domain is characterized by the progressive expression of overt differentiation in which the membrana granulosa cells assume the functional phenotype of

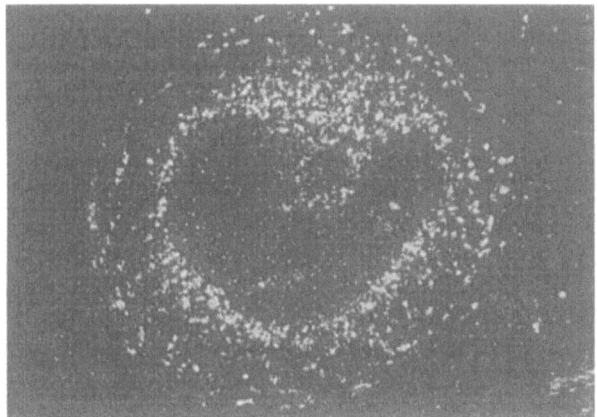

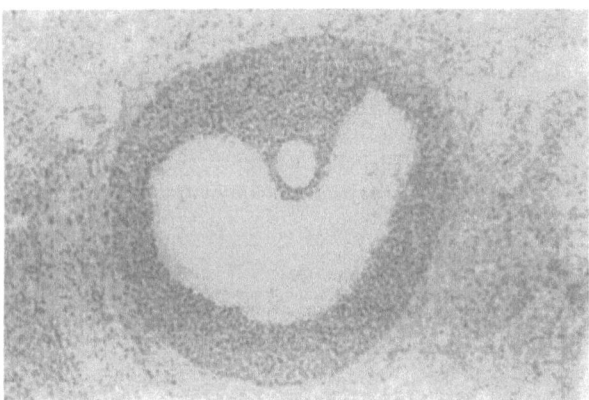

FIGURE 3.12. Proliferative pattern of granulosa cells in a healthy rat Graafian follicle. Top, darkfield of an autoradiogram showing ^{3}H thymidine incorporation; Bottom, brightfield. Reprinted with permission from Hirshfield AN. Patterns of [^{3}H] thymidine incorporation differ in immature rats and mature, cycling rats. Biol Reprod 1986;34: 229–35.

fully differentiated cells. This process requires the temporal and coordinate expression of genes that form the basis of granulosa cytodifferentiation. The mechanisms by which this occurs involves ligand-dependent signaling pathways that are coupled to the activation and inhibition of specific genes. For example, normal differentiation of the membrana granulosa cells requires the activation of specific genes including P450$_{aromatase}$ (33), LH receptor (34), and prolactin receptor (35), as well as the inhibition of structural genes in the apoptotic pathway. By contrast, a very different pattern of synthetic activities occurs in the periantral, cumulus, and corona radiata domains (Fig. 3.11). Here, the granulosa cells in these domains proliferate (Fig. 3.12), but fail to express the genes that are involved in a terminal differentiation (Fig. 3.13).

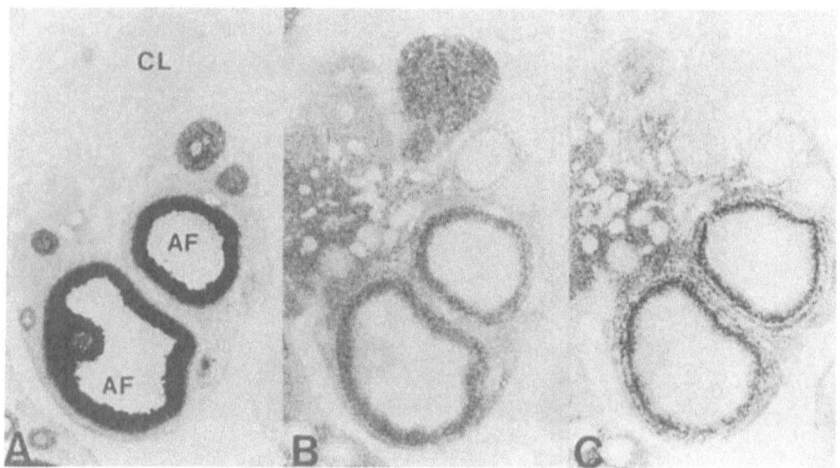

FIGURE 3.13. Photomicrographs showing granulosa heterogeneity. (A) ^{125}I-FSH binding; (B) ^{125}I-hCG binding; (C) ^{125}I-prolactin binding. AF, antral follicle; CL, corpus luteum. Reprinted with permission from Oxberry BA, Greenwald GS. An autoradiographic study of the binding of ^{125}I-labeled follicle-stimulating hormone, human chorionic gonadotropin and prolactin to the hamster ovary throughout the estrous cycle. Biol Reprod 1982;27:505–16.

It is clear that granulosa cytodifferentiation is regulated at the level of position within the GF and with remarkable precision indeed. What are the means in cellular terms by which these various morphogenetic differentiations are affected? What controls it? What is accomplished by the heterogeneity? We know that all the granulosa cells in the healthy GF express FSH receptor mRNA and protein (20,36,37), and it has been shown that the granulosa cells in the membrana and cumulus domains produce cyclic AMP in response to FSH stimulation (38). Considering this fact, together with the evidence that cyclic AMP mediates FSH-dependent granulosa cytodifferentiation, argues that postcyclic AMP regulatory events are involved in the aspects of granulosa heterogeneity (Fig. 3.14).

The idea that the oocyte plays a key role in causing the different patterns of granulosa cytodifferentiation during GF development is supported by studies in rodents (39). It is now apparent that a dialogue takes place between the oocyte and granulosa cells that has great impact on folliculogenesis. In developing murine GFs, the differential pattern of proliferation and differentiation between the granulosa in the membrana and cumulus domains are under the control of a secreted oocyte morphogen (39). What do we know about the nature of the putative oocyte morphogen(s), and how does it control granulosa cell mitotic and differentiation pathways?

Progress in the area of oocyte morphogens has been technically difficult because of the lack of oocyte-specific ligands (Fig. 3.15). A novel TGF-β family

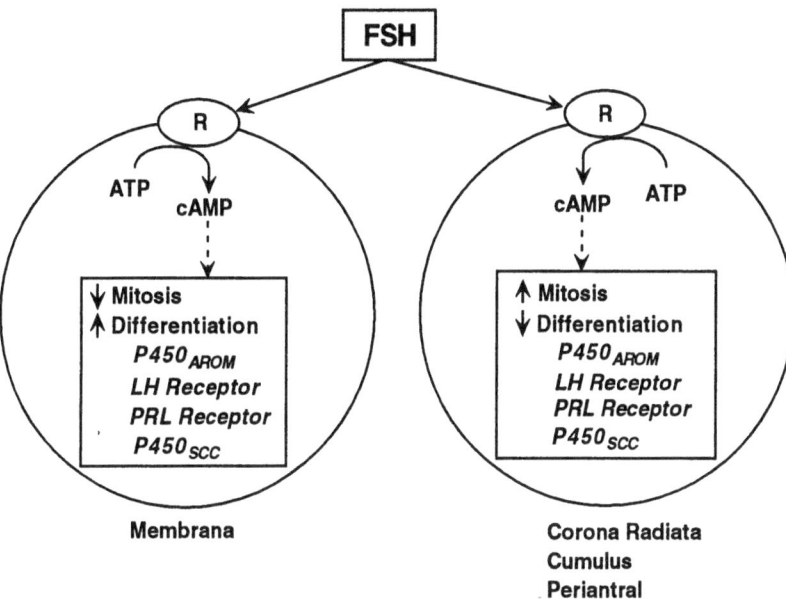

FIGURE 3.14. Diagram showing that FSH receptor signaling information can be translated in a specific manner to give different patterns of gene expression in the various granulosa cell layers. R, receptor.

member, GDF-9 (Growth and Differentiation Factor-9) was discovered in the mouse (40,41). Definitive evidence that GDF-9 is obligatory for folliculogenesis came from studies of GDF-9–deficient mice (42). In these animals, the absence of GDF-9 resulted in the arrest of follicle growth and development at primary stage and the females are infertile. These data support the idea for GDF-9 secreted by the egg is obligatory for GF development, granulosa cytodifferentiation and proliferation, and for female fertility. The clinical relevance of this new concept is demonstrated by the presence of GDF-9 mRNA in the human ovary (41). At present, almost nothing is known about the mechanisms controlling GDF-9 expression and nothing is known about the target cells for GDF-9 and the biological processes that GDF-9 regulates.

In this discussion, we have dissected the GF into its components and have described some selected salient functions of each. In a real sense, we must conclude that the GF is greater than the sum of its parts, and a functional analysis can be misleading if it fails to consider the interrelated nature of the structure and function of the cells. In other words, each cell type in the GF depends on the continuing function of the other follicular components. As such, they do not function in isolation. Thus, in every sense, the function of a GF reflects the specialized actions and interactions of the five different cell types. The major conclusion of this discussion is that continuous change is a general property of all GF; therefore, a functional definition must reflect the progressive changes that occur, most notably in the oocyte and

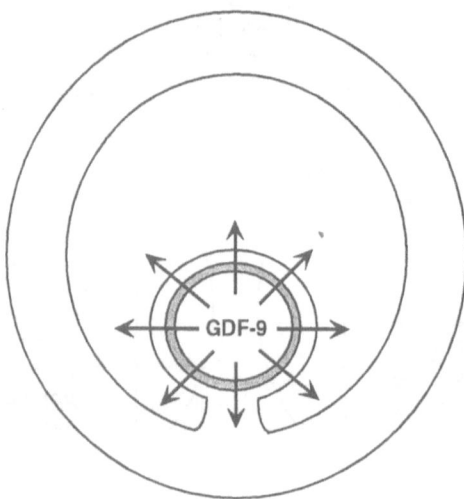

FIGURE 3.15. A hypothetical model showing a linear gradient of a putative oocyte-derived diffusible substance (GDF-9) that may play a role in determining specific patterns of granulosa cytodifferentiation in the Graafian follicle system.

granulosa cells, as the GF becomes either increasingly more differentiated or more atretic. With this in mind, I propose the following definition to be pondered. A Graafian follicle can be functionally defined as a progressively changing diverse tissue capable of transmitting and receiving a wide variety of regulatory ligands that act in a time- and dose-dependent manner to determine the rates of proliferation, cytodifferentiation, and apoptosis, which in turn determines whether it lives to ovulate a mature oocyte or it dies by atresia.

References

1. Gougeon A. Regulation of ovarian follicular development in primates: facts and hypotheses. Endocrinol Rev 1996;17:121–55.
2. Hsueh AJ, Billig H, Tsafriri A. Ovarian follicle atresia: a hormonally controlled apoptotic process. Endocrinol Rev 1994;15:707–24.
3. Erickson GF. The Ovary: basic principles and concepts. In: Felig P, Baxter JD, Broadus AE, Frohman LA, eds. Endocrinology and metabolism, Third ed. New York: McGraw-Hill; 1995:973–1015.
4. McNatty KP. Hormonal correlates of follicular development in the human ovary. Australian J Biol Sci 1981;34:249–68.
5. Erickson GF. Primary cultures of ovarian cells in serum-free medium as models of hormone-dependent differentiation. Mol Cell Endocrinol 1983;29:21–49.
6. Kumar TR, Wang Y, Lu N, Matzuk MM. Follicle stimulating hormone is required for ovarian follicle maturation but not male fertility. Nat Genet 1997;15:201–4.

7. Kumar TR, Low MJ, Matzuk MM. Genetic rescue of follicle-stimulating hormone beta-deficient mice. Endocrinology 1998;139:3289–95.
8. Li R, Phillips DM, Mather JP. Activin promotes ovarian follicle development in vitro. Endocrinology 1995;136:849–56.
9. Yoshida H, Takakura N, Kataoka H, Kunisada T, Okamura H, Nishikawa SI. Stepwise requirement of c-kit tyrosine kinase in mouse ovarian follicle development. Dev Biol 1997;184:122–37.
10. Beyer EC. Gap junctions. Int Rev Cytol 1993;137C:1–37.
11. Kumar NM, Gilula NB. The gap junction communication channel. Cell 1996;84: 381–88.
12. Simon AM, Goodenough DA, Li E, Paul DL. Female infertility in mice lacking connexin 37. Nature 1997;385:525–29.
13. McNatty KP, Moore-Smith D, Osathanondh R, Ryan KJ. The human antral follicle: Functional correlates of growth and atresia. Ann Biol Anim Biochim Biophys 1979;19:1547–58.
14. Amsterdam A, Lindner HR, Groschel-Stewart U. Localization of actin and myosin in the rat oocyte and follicular wall by immunofluorescence. Anat Rec 1977;187: 311–28.
15. Self DA, Schroeder PC, Gown AM. Hamster thecal cells express muscle characteristics. Biol Reprod 1988;39:119–30.
16. Erickson GF, Magoffin DA, Dyer C, Hofeditz C. The ovarian androgen producing cells: A review of structure/function relationships. Endocrinol Rev 1985;6:371–99.
17. Motta PM, Familiari G. Occurrence of a contractile tissue in the theca externa of atretic follicles in the mouse ovary. Acta Anat 1981;109:103–14.
18. Martin GG, Talbot P. The role of follicular smooth muscle cells in hamster ovulation. J Exp Zool 1981;216:469–82.
19. Crisp TM, Dessouky DA, Denys FR. The fine structure of the human corpus luteum of early pregnancy and during the progestational phase of the mestrual cycle. Am J Anat 1970;127:37–69.
20. Yamoto M, Shima K, Nakano R. Gonadotropin receptors in human ovarian follicles and corpora lutea throughout the menstrual cycle. Horm Res 1992;37(suppl. 1):5–11.
21. Kiriakidou M, McAllister JM, Sugawara T, Strauss JF III. Expression of steroidogenic acute regulatory protein StAR in the human ovary. J Clin Endocrinol Metab 1996;81:4122–28.
22. Pollack SE, Furth EE, Kallen CB, Arakane F, Kiriakidou M, Kozarsky KF, et al. Localization of the steroidogenic acute regulatory protein in human tissues. J Clin Endocrinol Metab 1997;82:4243–51.
23. Suzuki T, Sasano H, Tamura M, Aoki H, Fukaya T, Yajima A, et al. Temporal and spatial localization of steroidogenic enzymes in premenopausal human ovaries: in situ hybridization and immunohistochemical study. Mol Cell Endocrinol 1993;97:135–43.
24. Tamura T, Kitawaki J, Yamamoto T, Osawa Y, Kominami S, Takemori S, et al. Immunohistochemical localization of 17α-hydroxylase/C17-20 lyase and aromatase cytochrome P-450 in polycystic human ovaries. J Endocrinol 1993;139:503–9.
25. Takayama K, Fukaya T, Sasano H, Funayama Y, Suzuki T, Takaya R, et al. Immunohistochemical study of steroidogenesis and cell proliferation in polycystic ovarian syndrome. Hum Reprod 1996;11:1387–92.
26. Toledo SP, Brunner HG, Kraaij R, Post M, Dahia PL, Hayashida CY, et al. An inactivating mutation of the luteinizing hormone receptor causes amenorrhea in a 46,XX fcmalc. J Clin Endocrinol Metab 1996;81:3850 54.

27. Zeleznik AJ, Schuler HM, Reichert LE. Gonadotropin-binding sites in the Rhesus monkey ovary: role of the vasculature in the selective distribution of human chorionic gonadotropin to the preovulatory follicle. Endocrinology 1981;109:356–62.
28. Gordon JD, Mesiano S, Zaloudek CJ, Jaffe RB. Vascular endothelial growth factor localization in human ovary and fallopian tubes: possible role in reproductive function and ovarian cyst formation. J Clin Endocrinol Metab 1996;81:353–59.
29. Laitinen M, Ristimäki A, Honkasalo M, Narko K, Paavonen K, Ritvos O. Differential hormonal regulation of vascular endothelial growth factors VEGF, VEGF-B, and VEGF-C messenger ribonucleic acid levels in cultured human granulosa-luteal cells. Endocrinology 1997;138:4748–56.
30. Mancina R, Barni T, Calogero AE, Filippi S, Amerini S, Peri A, et al. Identification, characterization, and biological activity of endothelin receptors in human ovary. J Clin Endocrinol Metab 1997;82:4122–29.
31. Hirshfield AN. Patterns of [^{3}H] thymidine incorporation differ in immature rats and mature, cycling rats. Biol Reprod 1986;34:229–35.
32. Hirshfield AN. Granulosa cell proliferation in very small follicles of cycling rats studied by long-term continuous tritiated-thymidine infusion. Biol Reprod 1989;41:309–16.
33. Whitelaw PF, Smyth CD, Howles CM, Hillier SG. Cell-specific expression of aromatase and LH receptor mRNAs in rat ovary. J Mol Endocrinol 1992;9:309–12.
34. Bortolussi M, Marini G, Reolon ML. A histochemical study of the binding of 125I-HCG to the rat ovary throughout the estrous cycle. Cell Tissue Res 1979;197:213–26.
35. Oxberry BA, Greenwald GS. An autoradiographic study of the binding of I-labeled follicle-stimulating hormone, human chorionic gonadotropin and prolactin to the hamster ovary throughout the estrous cycle. Biol Reprod 1982;27:505–16.
36. Camp TA, Rahal JO, Mayo KE. Cellular localization and hormonal regulation of follicle-stimulating hormone and luteininzing hormone receptor messenger RNAs in the rat ovary. Mol Endocrinol 1991;5:1405–17.
37. Minegishi T, Tano M, Igarashi M, Rokukawa S, Abe Y, Ibuki Y, et al. Expression of follicle-stimulating hormone receptor in human ovary. Eur J Clin Invest 1997;27:469–74.
38. Buccione R, Vanderhyden BC, Caron PJ, Eppig JJ. FSH-induced expansion of the mouse cumulus oophorus in vitro is dependent upon a specific factor(s) secreted by the oocyte. Dev Biol 1990;138:16–25.
39. Eppig JJ, Chesnel F, Hirao Y, O'Brien MJ, Pendola FL, Watanabe S, et al. Oocyte control of granulosa cell development: How and why. Hum Reprod 1997;12:127–32.
40. McPherron AC, Lee S-J. GDF-3 and GDF-9: two new members of the transforming growth factor-β superfamily containing a novel pattern of cysteines. J Biol Chem 1993;268:3444–49.
41. McGrath SA, Esquela AF, Lee S-J. Oocyte-specific expression of growth/differentiation factor-9. Mol Endocrinol 1995;9:131–36.
42. Dong J, Albertini DF, Nishimori K, Kumar TR, Lu N, Matzuk M. Growth differeniation factor-9 is required during early ovarian folliculogenesis. Nature 1996;383:531–35.

4

The Critical Granulosa Cell Complement: Lessons from the Cyclin D2 Knockout

JoAnne S. Richards and Rebecca L. Robker

Interactions of A-Kinase and Cell Cycle Regulated Kinase Cascades

Growth, ovulation, and luteinization of ovarian follicles is regulated by a number of distinct but interacting kinase cascades. Two of these kinase cascades are of paramount importance in regulating ovarian cell proliferation and differentiation. Cyclic AMP(cAMP)-dependent protein kinase (A-kinase) regulates growth and differentiation of ovarian cells by stimulating transcriptional activation of different genes, including those involved in the synthesis of mitogenic steroids (1–3). The myriad cell cycle-associated, cyclin-dependent protein kinases (cdks) control progression through the cell cycle (4–10). This chapter will summarize studies showing how these two cascades interact to regulate ovarian granulosa cell proliferation and ovulation (11,12; Fig. 4.1).

The ovarian A-kinase cascade is stimulated by the pituitary gonadotropins follicle stimulating hormone (FSH) and luteinizing hormone (LH), which bind cognate receptors in granulosa cells and theca cells, respectively, and stimulate the production of cAMP (1–3). Increased responsiveness of small follicles to these hormones is associated with the exponential growth of follicles prior to ovulation (13,14). This exponential growth is largely the result of the increased proliferative activity of the FSH-responsive granulosa cells as reported by studies using tritiated thymidine ûptake (13,14), BrdU labeling (12) and proliferating cell nuclear antigen (PCNA) immunostaining (11,12,15) of dividing cells. This rapid growth is terminated by the LH surge that both stimulates ovulation and initiates terminal differentiation of granulosa cells (1,16,17). These cells rapidly exit the cell cycle and cease dividing (11,12).

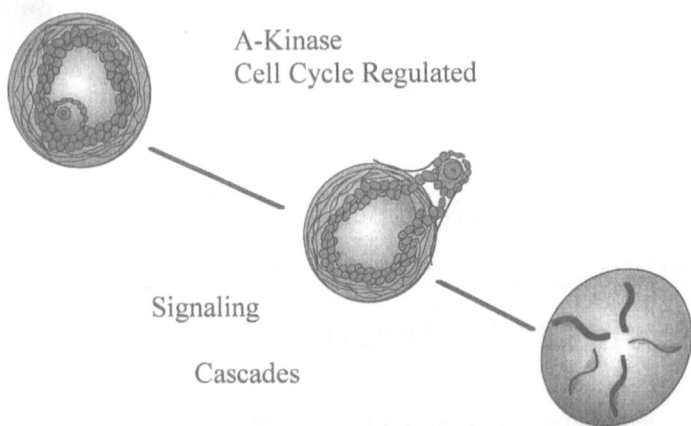

A-Kinase
Cell Cycle Regulated

Signaling

Cascades

FIGURE 4.1. Schematic of signaling cascades that regulate ovulation and luteinization of preovulatory follicles. The A-kinase cascade that regulates gene expression leading to granulosa cell proliferation and terminal differentiation is of paramount importance. See text for discussion.

Within 4 hours of the LH surge, BrdU staining is markedly reduced in granulosa cells contained within the preovulatory follicles that are destined to ovulate (12); by 48 hours PCNA staining is completely absent in corpora lutea (11). Within 7 hours of the LH surge, the granulosa cells have been completely reprogrammed to become luteal cells (16,17). Thus, the A-kinase pathway is involved not only in stimulating proliferation of granulosa cells of antral follicles and for terminating their proliferation leading to luteinization. These two distinct aspects of A-kinase pathway activation impact on regulatory molecules controlling progression through, and exit from, the cell cycle.

The progression through the cell cycle is dependent on the precise, sequential activation of specific protein kinase cascades (Fig. 4.2A). The sequence is initiated by the regulated synthesis of specific regulatory molecules, the cyclins, that bind and control the activation of the cdks and cdk-activating kinase (CAK)(4–10). Progression through the cell cycle can be arrested by specific inhibitory molecules, such as $p27^{KIP1}$ (18,19), $p21^{CIP1}$ (20,21), and others (22,23), that bind and inactivate cdks. The balance of these activators and inhibitors dictates whether cells will progress through G1, enter S, and synthesize DNA, or exit the cell cycle (4–10 and references therein). The schematic shown in Figure 4.2B depicts how this process is presumed to work. Mitogens known to impact ovarian cell proliferation, such as FSH and estradiol (14; and possibly other growth regulators, 24–26) stimulate the synthesis of cyclins that bind to their respective partner cdks. In G1, members of the cyclin D family (cyclins D1, 2, or 3) bind cdk4/6. Once this complex is assembled it can be activated by CAK, which itself is a cyclin-cdk complex.

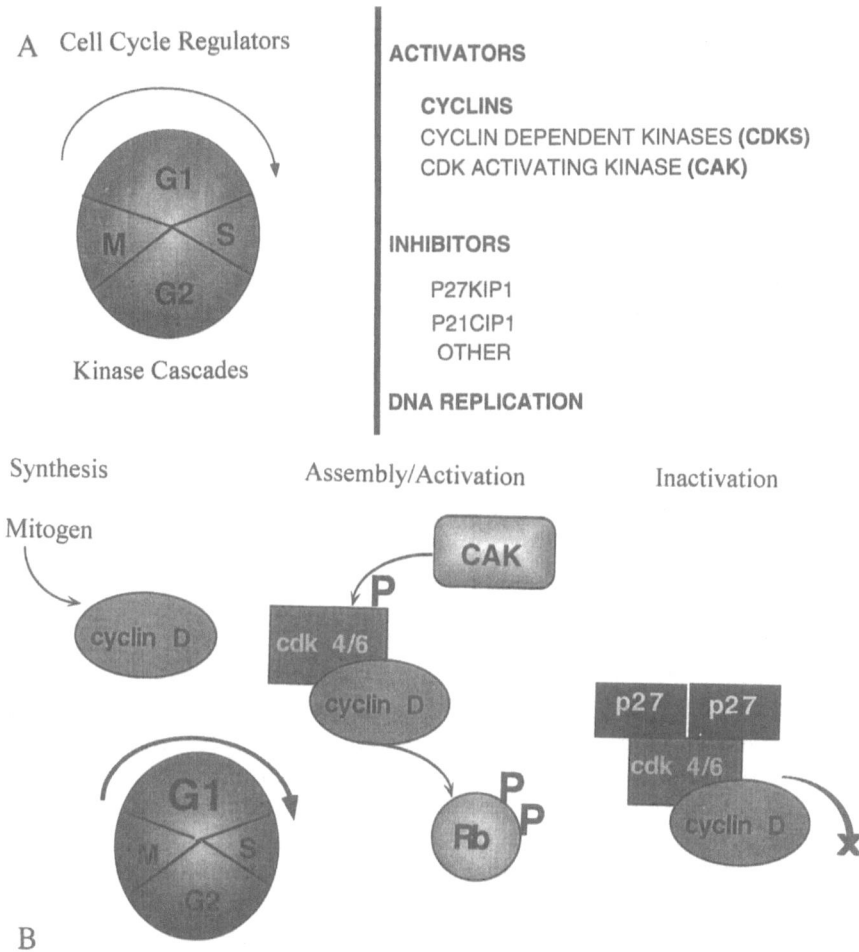

FIGURE 4.2. (A) Schematic of cell cycle regulators that control the progression of cells through G1 of the cell cycle. (B) A model of how the cell cycle regulators are presumed to control the kinase cascades that regulate cell cycle progression and DNA synthesis. See text for discussion.

Once the cyclin D–cdk complex is phosphorylated by CAK, it is active and can phosphorylate specific proteins involved in DNA synthesis (e.g., the retinoblastoma protein, Rb), thereby releasing transcription factors necessary for DNA synthesis. In a similar manner, increased synthesis of cyclin E permits its assembly with cdk2, allowing cells to progress beyond the restriction point in G1 and enter S. Inhibitors (e.g., p27^{KIP1}) bind to the cyclin D-cdk4/6 and cyclin E-cdk2 complexes in such a manner as to block CAK-mediated phosphorylation, thereby preventing completion of these kinase cascades. Cell-cycle progression through G1 is blocked and cells exit the cell cycle.

Cell Cycle Regulators: Hormonal Regulation in Ovarian Cells

Targeted deletion of cell-cycle regulatory molecules in mice has led to specific ovarian phenotypes. Mice null for cyclin D2 are infertile and fail to ovulate (27). Mice null for p27[KIP1] are also infertile and exhibit impaired luteinization (28–30). We have therefore sought to determine how hormones regulate the expression of these molecules in the ovary and to determine what accounts for the anovulatory phenotype of the cyclin D2 null mice.

In situ hybridization analyses show that cyclin D2 is exclusively expressed in granulosa cells of growing follicles, whereas cyclins D1 and D3 are localized to the theca cells of the same follicles (11,12). Northern blot analysis and Western blot analyses have determined that cyclin D2 mRNA and protein are expressed at low levels in granulosa cells of immature, preantral follicles present in ovaries of hypophysectomized (H) rats (4), as well as in mice lacking functional FSHβ (11,31). These observations indicate that cyclin D2 is expressed in these small, slowly growing follicles by mechanisms independent of gonadotropin and steroid stimulation (11,12). Increased levels of cyclin D2 (11) and cyclin E (12) occur in granulosa cells of H rats treated with estradiol (E) and/or FSH, corresponding to increased proliferative activity of the granulosa cells in response to these hormones (11,12,14). Thus, both cyclin D2 and cyclin E are hormonally regulated in granulosa cells of follicles growing exponentially to the preovulatory stage. Expression of cyclin D2 and cyclin E mRNA and protein are also regulated by these hormones in primary cultures of rat granulosa cells (11, data not shown), indicating that FSH/cAMP as well as estradiol act directly via their respective cognate receptors present in granulosa cells (1,32; Fig. 4.3).

When this rapid growth is terminated by administration of an ovulatory dose of hCG (given to mimic the LH surge), cyclin D2 mRNA and protein drop dramatically by 4 hours, when cell proliferation has ceased (11,12). Expression of cyclin D2 remains low in luteal cells that are terminally differentiated and nonproliferative (11,12). Expression of cyclin E is also reduced by the ovulatory LH signal but the rate of decline is more gradual than that of cyclin D2; cyclin E protein remains present for 24 hours but is low at 48 hours when corpora lutea are fully formed (12). Thus, the rapid decline in cyclin D2 appears to be tightly associated with the first evidence (loss of DNA synthesis) that granulosa cells have ceased dividing and have been reprogrammed to express the luteal cell functions.

Cellular localization and hormonal regulation of the inhibitors, p27[KIP1]

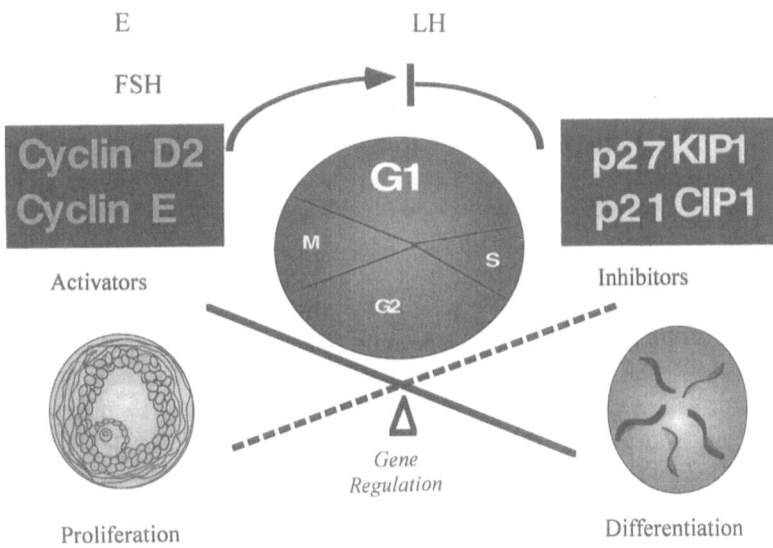

FIGURE 4.3. Schematic of the balance between cell cycle activators and inhibitors that regulate progression through G1. See text for discussion.

and $p21^{CIP1}$, were analyzed by similar approaches (11,12). Whereas $p27^{KIP1}$ was expressed in most ovarian cell types, the highest level of expression was observed in corpora lutea, 48 hours after the LH surge (11,12,29,30). The induction of $p27^{KIP1}$ by elevated levels of cAMP has also been reported for other cell types (33,34), indicating that this may be a fundamental response of cells that terminally differentiate or cease dividing in response to elevated cAMP. The specific role played by $p27^{KIP1}$ in the luteinization process remains to be determined. Unlike $p27^{KIP1}$, the cdk inhibitor $p21^{CIP1}$, was expressed at low (undetectable) levels in follicles but was increased rapidly (within 2 hours) by hCG and remained elevated corpora lutea. These results indicate that rapid increase in $p21^{CIP1}$coupled with the rapid and dramatic loss of cyclin D2 are the initial events that block granulosa cell proliferation (progression through G1) and cause exit from the cell cycle. The terminal differentiated state of luteal cells is associated with markedly low levels of cyclin D2 and cyclin E and elevated levels of $p27^{KIP1}$ and $p21^{CIP1}$ (11,12).

Cyclin D2 and the Anovulaory Phenotype

Based on these observations, how does one explain the anovulatory phenotype of the cyclin D2 null mice? Ovaries of cyclin D2 null mice respond to gonadotropins and exhibit many normal functions (11,27). Although the ovaries of cyclin D2 null mice contain a markedly reduced number of granulosa cells, some of these cells are proliferating and stain immunopositive for PCNA (11), providing evidence to explain the slow growth of follicles of cyclin D2-/- mice in vivo as well as in organ culture (27). This raises the intriguing possibility that low levels of either cyclin D1 or D3 are actually present in granulosa cells, but have not been detected using in situ hybridization, Northern blots, or Western blot techniques (11,12,27). On the other hand, another cyclin may substitute (albeit poorly) for cyclin D2, or the cyclin D2(-/-) granulosa cells may bypass the cyclin D/cdk4/6 step and enter G1 with cyclin E. That the absence of cyclin D2 per se is not associated with rampant apoptosis or luteinization indicates that the loss of cyclin D2 is not synonymous with either cell death or terminal differentiation. Thus, although cyclin D2 expression is rapidly turned off in association with luteinization, loss of cyclin D2 itself does not trigger luteinization. Rather, the granulosa cells of the cyclin D2 null mice appear to luteinize normally in response to PMSG–hCG regimen: The cells cease to divide, hypertrophy, and express P450scc, which are all markers of luteal cell function (11,27). These results indicate that the A-kinase pathway, not the cell-cycle kinase cascades, cause the morphological and functional changes associated with the terminal differentiation to luteal cells (1). In fact, the granulosa cells of the cyclin D2 null mice exhibit other normal biochemical and molecular responses to PMSG and hCG. Aromatase mRNA and estradiol production are induced by PMSG/FSH in a manner similar to wild-type litter mates and is high in "preovulatory" follicles (11,27). Upon stimulation with hCG, normal preovulatory granulosa cells, as well as those deficient in cyclin D2, express several genes in a rapid but transient manner, including progesterone receptor (PR; 1, 27), prostaglandin synthase-2 (PGS-2 or COX-2; 1, 27) as well as C/EBPβ (1). These results are intriguing because mice null for PR (35), PGS-2 (36,37), and C/EBPβ (38,39) are also infertile and fail to ovulate. Based on these observations, cyclin D2, PR, PGS-2, and C/EBPβ appear to exert distinct, non-overlapping effects during the process of ovulation (11, 40; Fig. 4.4).

The apparent normality of granulosa cells in the cyclin D2 null mice and their ability to express genes presumed to control the ovulation process raise many questions about the functional role of cyclin D2 in ovulation (Fig. 4.5). Why is granulosa cell number important for ovulation? How does cell number relate, if at all, to the functions of other factors which mediate the ovulatory process; namely PR (35), PGS-2 (36,37) as well as C/EBPβ, the loss of which also impairs ovulation (38,39)? How does cyclin D2 relate to the proteolytic cascade(s) controlling ovulation? Does cyclin D2 interact with intracellular signaling pathways in addition to the cell-cycle kinase cascades? For, example does it have functions analagous to those of cyclin D1, which has been shown to bind steroid receptors (41) and possibly other transcription factors in a similar paradigm?

At this time, one can only speculate; however, several scenarios might explain the importance of granulosa cell number for successful completion

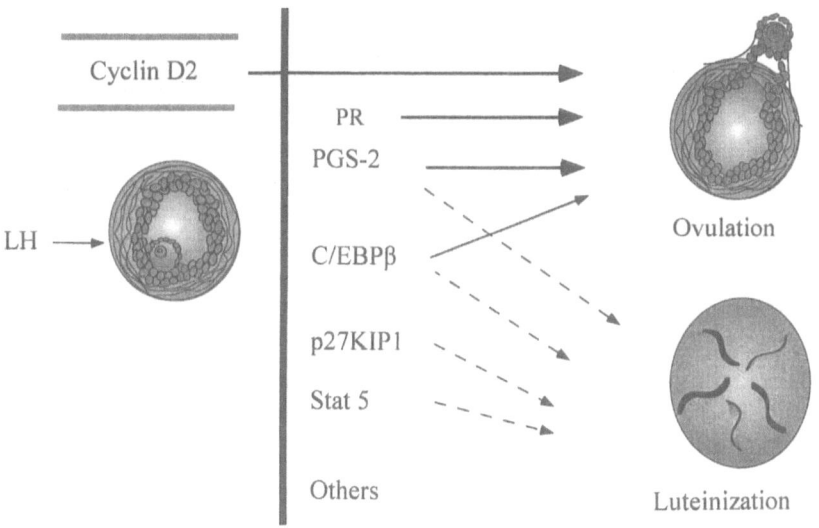

FIGURE 4.4. Schematic showing the relationships among several key factors controling ovulation and luteinization. Cyclin D2 is the only factor expressed in granulosa cells prior to the LH surge that regulates ovulation. PR, PGS-2, and C/EBPβ are all induced by the LH surge. p27^{KIP1} is a regulator of luteinization. See text for discussion.

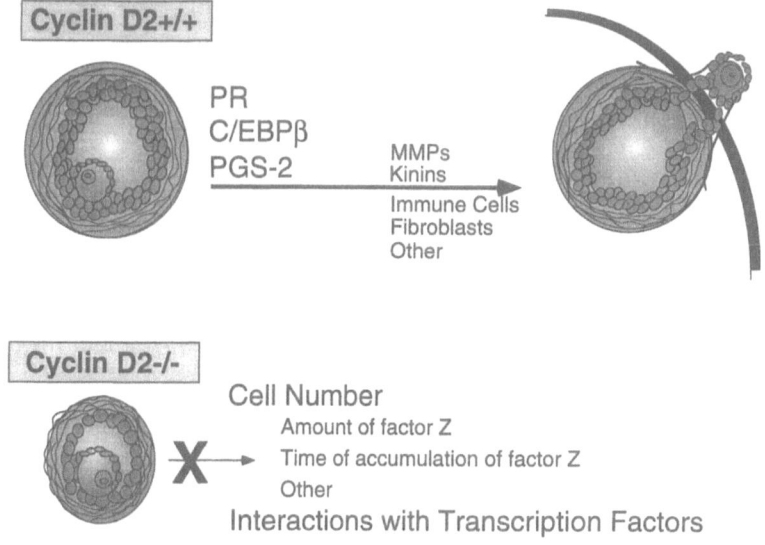

FIGURE 4.5. Schematic of protease cascades and mechanisms controlling ovulation that might be regulated by the number of granulosa cells. See text for discussion.

of ovulation. If granulosa cell number is important, then one must predict that some factor (called factor Z; Fig. 4.5) being secreted by granulosa cells is critical to the ovulatory proteolytic cascade (40,42), or the total amount of the factor produced is insufficient or it is not produced in sufficient amounts within the critical time period required to activate the obligatory proteolytic cascade. It remains to be determined what this activating factor(s) is (are). On the other hand cell number may control the balance of inhibitors relative to activators of the proteolytic cascades. In addition to being infertile, the cyclin D2 null mice may have defects in the immune cells that express cyclin D2 (42). Immune cells, in turn, have been implicated in facilitating ovulation (43,44). These results raise the possibility that a subpopulation of immune cells are critical for ovulation, and that their number or function in the cyclin D2 null ovary is insufficient or inadequate to stimulate a critical step in the ovulation process. On the other hand, if cyclin D2 exerts functions in addition to regulating cell-cycle progression through activation of cdk 4/6, then one would predict functional interactions of cyclin D2 with other intracellular proteins. These interactions either have not yet been tested or have not been observed. What might the candidate proteins be? Their ultimate role would presumably also be linked in some fashion to the protease cascades controlling the ovulatory process. These and many more interesting questions will haunt us until the answer(s) are in. In the meantime, the cyclin D2 null mouse provides a unique model in which to test the expression and effects of factors and proteases presumed to be involved in ovulation. That ovulation involves many steps and cell types necessitates that each of many pieces of information will need to be put in place to solve how each factor impacts the ovulation puzzle.

Acknowledgment. Supported in part by NIH-HD-16272 (JSR)

References

1. Richards JS. Hormonal control of gene expression in the ovary. Endocrinol Rev 1994;15:725–51.
2. Richards JS. Maturation of ovarian follicles: actions and interactions of pituitary and ovarian hormones on follicular cell differentiation. Physiol Rev 1980;60: 51–89.
3. Richards JS, Midgley AR Jr. Protein hormone action: a key to understanding ovarian follicular and luteal cell development. Biol Reprod 1976;14:82–94.
4. Sherr CJ. Cancer cell cycles. Science 1996;274:1672–77.
5. Sherr CJ. G1 progression: cycling on cue. Cell 1994;79:551–55.
6. Sherr CJ. Mammalian G1 cyclins. Cell 1993;73:1059–65.
7. Sherr CJ, Roberts JM. Inhibitors of mammalian G1 cyclin-dependent kinases. Genes Dev 1995;9:1149–63.
8. Hunter T, Pines J. Cyclins and cancer II: cyclin D and cdk inhibitors come of age. Cell 1994;79:573–82.

9. Elledge S. Cell cycle checkpoints: preventing an identity crisis. Science 1996;274: 1664–71.
10. Weinberg RA. E2F and cell proliferation: a world turned upside down. Cell 1996;85:457–59.
11. Robker RL, Richards JS. Hormone-induced proliferation and differentiation of granulosa cells: a coordinated balance of the cell cycle regulators cyclin D2 and p27^{KIP1}. Mol Endocrinol 1998;12:924–40.
12. Robker RL, Richards JS. Hormonal control of the cell cycle in ovarian cells: proliferation versus differentiation. Biol Reprod 1998;59:476–82.
13. Hirshfield AN. Development of follicles in the mammalian ovary. Int Rev Cytol 1991;124:43–101.
14. Rao MC, Midgley AR Jr, Richards JS. Hormonal regulation of ovarian cellular proliferation. Cell 1978;14:71–78.
15. Oktay K, Schenken RS, Nelson JF. Proliferating cell nuclear antigen marks the initiation of follicular growth in the rat. Biol Reprod 1995;53:295–301.
16. Richards JS, Hedin L, Caston L. Differentiation of rat ovarian cells: evidence for functional luteinization. Endocrinology 1986;118:1660–68.
17. Oonk RB, Beattie WG, Richards JS. Cyclic AMP-dependent and -independent regulation of cholesterol side-chain cleavage P450 (P450scc) in rat ovarian granulosa cells and corpora lutea: cDNA and deduced amino acid sequence of rat P450scc. J Biol Chem 1989;264:21934–42.
18. Polyak K, Lee M, Erdjument-Bromage H, Koff A, Roberts JM, Tempst P, et al. Cloning of p27^{Kip1}, a cyclin-dependent kinase inhibitor and a potential mediator of extracellular antimitotic signals. Cell 1994;78:59–66.
19. Coats S, Flanagan WM, Nourse J, Roberts JM. Requirement of p27^{Kip1} for restriction point control of fibroblast cell cycle. Science 1996;272:877–80.
20. Harper JW, Elledge SJ, Keyomarsi K, Dynlacht B, Tsai L-H, Zhang P, et al. Inhibition of cyclin-dependent kinases by p21. Mol Biol Cell 1995;6:387–400.
21. Deng C, Zhang P, Harper JW, Elledge SJ, Leder P. Mice lacking p21$^{CIP1/WAF1}$ undergo normal development, but are defective in G1 checkpoint control. Cell 1995;82: 675–84.
22. Matsuoka S, Edwards MC, Bai C, Parker S, Zhang P, Baldini A, et al. p57^{KIP2}, a structurally distinct member of the p21^{CIP1} cdk inhibitor family, is a candidate tumor suppressor gene. Genes Dev 1995;9:650–62.
23. Zhang P, Liegeois NJ, Wong C, Finegold M, Hou H, Thompson JC, et al. Altered cell differentiation and proliferation in mice lacking p57^{Kip2} indicates a role in Beckwith-Wiedemann syndrome. Nature 1997;387:151–58.
24. Miro F, Hillier SG. Modulation of granulosa cell deoxyribonucleic acid synthesis and differentiation by activin. Endocrinology 1996;137:464–68.
25. Zhou J, Refuerzo J, Bondy C. Granulosa cell DNA synthesis is strictly correlated with the presence of insulin-like growth factor I and absence of c-fos/ c-jun expression. Mol Endocrinol 1995;9:924–31.
26. Risma KA, Hirshfield AN, Nilson JH. Elevated luteinizing hormone in prepubertal transgenic mice causes hyperandrogenemia, precocious puberty, and substantial ovarian pathology. Endocrinology 1997;138:3540–47.
27. Sicinski P, Donaher JL, Geng Y, Parker SB, Gardner H, Park MY, et al. Cyclin D2 is an FSH-responsive gene involved in gonadal cell proliferation and oncogenesis. Nature 1996;384:470–74.
28. Nakayama K, Ishida N, Shirane M, Inomata A, Inoue T, Shishido N, et al. Mice lacking

p27^{Kip1} display increased body size, multiple organ hyperplasia, retinal dysplasia, and pituitary tumors. Cell 1996;85:707–20.

29. Kiyokawa H, Kineman RD, Manova-Todorova KO, Soares VC, Hoffman ES, Ono M, et al. Enhanced growth of mice lacking the cyclin-dependent kinase inhibitor function of p27^{Kip1}. Cell 1996;85:721–32.

30. Fero ML, Rivkin M, Tasch M, Porter P, Carow CE, Firpo E, et al. A syndrome of multiorgan hyperplasia with features of gigantism, tumorigenesis, and female sterility in p27^{Kip1}-deficient mice. Cell 1996;85:733–44.

31. Kumar TR, Wang Y, Lu N, Matzuk MM. Follicle stimulating hormone is required for ovarian follicle maturation but not male fertility. Nat Gen 1997;15:201–4.

32. Byers M, Kuiper GGJM, Gustafsson J-A, Park-Sarge O-K. Estrogen receptor-b mRNA in rat ovary: down regulation by gonadotropins. Mol Endocrinol 1997;11:172–82.

33. Kato J, Matsuoka M, Polyak K, Massague J, Sherr CJ. Cyclic AMP-induced G1 phase arrest mediated by an inhibitor (p27^{Kip1}) of cyclin-dependent kinase 4 activation. Cell 1994;79:487–96.

34. Tikoo R, Casaccia-Bonnefil P, Chao MV, Koff A. Changes in cyclin-dependent kinase 2 and p27^{Kip1} accompany glial cell differentiation of central glial-4 cells. J Biol Chem 1997;272:442–47.

35. Lydon JP, DeMayo FJ, Funk CR, Mani SK, Hughes AR, Montgomery CA Jr, et al. Mice lacking progesterone receptor exhibit pleiotropic reproductive abnormalities. Genes Dev 1995;9:2266–78.

36. Dinchuk JE, Car BD, Focht RJ, Johnston JJ, Jaffee BD, Covington MB, et al. Renal abnormalities and an altered inflammatory response in mice lacking cyclooxygenase II. Nature 1995;378:406–9.

37. Russell DL, Richards JS. Causes of infertility in mice with targeted deletion of the PGS-2 gene. Program of the 30th Annual Meeting of the Society for the Study of Reproduction, Portland, OR: 1997:178 (abstr.).

38. Pall M, Hellberg P, Brannstrom M, Mikuni M, Peterson CM, Sundfeldt K, et al. The transcription factor C/EBPb and its role in ovarian function; evidence for direct involvement in the ovulatory process. EMBO 1997; J. 16:5273–79.

39. Sterneck E, Tessarollo L, Johnson PF. An essential role of C/EBPβ in female reproduction. Genes Dev 1997;11:2153–62.

40. Richards JS, Russell DL, Robker RL, Dajee M, Alliston TN. Molecular Mechanisms of ovulation and luteinization. Mol Cell Endocrinol 1998;145:47–54.

41. Neuman E, Ladha MH, Lin N, Upton TM, Miller SJ, DiRenzo J, et al. Cyclin D1 stimulation of estrogen receptor transcriptional activity independent of cdk4. Mol Cell Biol 1997;17:5338–47.

42. Sherr CJ, Matsushime H, Roussel MF. Regulation of CYL/cyclin D genes by colony-stimulaitng factor 1. Regulation of the Eukaryotic Cell Cycle. Ciba Foundation Sympoiusm 1992;170:209–26.

43. Espey LL. Ovulation as an inflammatory reaction—a hypothesis. Biol Reprod 1980;22:73–106.

44. Norman RJ, Brannstrom M. White cells and the ovary—incidental invaders or essential effectors? J Endocrinol 1994;140:333–36.

5

Ovarian Teratocarcinogenesis: A Consequence of Abnormal Regulation of Meiosis

JOHN J. EPPIG, ALES HAMPL, AND YUJI HIRAO

Introduction

Abnormalities in the regulation of meiosis can lead to several disastrous outcomes, including infertility, birth defects, and teratocarcinogensis. This chapter will discuss abnormalities in oocyte meiosis that lead to the formation of spontaneous ovarian teratomas. Emphasis is placed on ovarian teratocarcinogenesis in strain LT mice, and related strains. The word *teratoma* is derived from the Greek *teras*, meaning monster, because the tumors are composed of a variety of differentiated cell and tissue types including skin, glandular tissue, bone, muscle, neural tissue, and even hair and teeth, which is assembled into a highly disorganized, sometimes bizarre, mass. Ovarian teratomas in both mice and humans often arise from oocytes that undergo parthenogenetic embryo development without ovulation.

Teratomas occur commonly in women and are often referred to as *dermoid cysts*. Although usually benign, malignant transformation occurs in about 2% of the cases (1). In contrast, immature teratomas, which occur more often in girls or young women, frequently contain undifferentiated cells and are usually malignant. Approximately 14% of all ovarian tumors of women 20–50 years old are teratomas, and most are benign (2). In striking contrast, about 58% of ovarian tumors in females younger than 20 years are derived from oocytes, and about 65% of these are malignant (3).

Ovarian teratomas are generally rare in mice but occur commonly in four inherited conditions: (1) strain LT and genetically related mice (4); (2) an insertional mutation referred to as TG.KD (5); (3) transgenic mice overexpressing the human BCL2 gene (TG.BCL2) (6); and (4) *Mos*-null mice (7,8). It is known that teratomas in LT and *Mos*-null mice are derived from oocytes that undergo maturation and spontaneous parthenogenetic activation followed by embryonic development within ovarian follicles (4,9). In both cases abnormalities in the meiotic cell cycle promote parthenogenetic activation; LT oocytes become activated only after atypical arrest at metaphase I (10,11), whereas *Mos*-null oocytes appear to begin mitotic cycles after uninterrupted transit through either metaphase I or II (9,12). The mechanisms of teratoma development in TG.KD and TG.BCL2 mice are unknown.

Knowledge of the mechanisms of teratoma development in mice is greatest for LT and related strains. Dr. Leroy Stevens, who originally described the high incidence of teratoma development in LT mice (4), made recombinant inbred (RI) strains using LT/Sv and C57BL/6J mice. Of the several lines originally produced, only two remain: LTXBO and LTXBJ. Females of these RI strains have significantly higher incidences of parthenogenetic development of oocytes and teratoma formation than LT/Sv females; see (10). In this chapter, LT/Sv, LTXBO, and LTXBJ are all referred to as LT mice. Ovaries of LT females contain normal-appearing preimplantationlike parthenogenetic embryos from the two-cell stage up to early postimplantationlike stages. These embryos become disorganized and can give rise to teratomas containing embryonal carcinoma cells and a variety of differentiated cell types (4,13). Genetic analysis carried out more than 20 years ago showed that LT teratomas are derived from oocytes that complete the first meiotic division (14). Now it is known that the first meiotic division is completed only after parthenogenetic activation of metaphase I-arrested oocytes (10). Metaphase I is transient in fully grown normal oocytes and is followed by anaphase I, telophase, and progression of meiosis to metaphase II without an intervening interphase. Meiosis is arrested again at metaphase II until penetration of a spermatozoan activates the oocyte and triggers entry into anaphase II and the completion of meiosis II. The progression of meiosis in many LT oocytes, however, is abnormal and arrested precociously at metaphase I (10,15–17), It is only these metaphase I-arrested oocytes that undergo spontaneous parthenogenetic activation (10,11).

Regulation of the Meiotic Cell Cycle in Normal Oocytes

Ovarian teratomas are derived from oocytes that undergo aberrant development. In most cases this probably involves defects in the progression of meiosis. Meiosis is a cell-division process occurring only in germ cells. It reduces the number of chromosomes from the diploid to the haploid number. Mammalian oocytes usually become arrested in prophase I of meiosis during the fetal period. Completion of the first meiotic division usually occurs only after oocytes, and the ovarian follicles that encompass them have undergone extensive growth. The nucleus of the oocyte is called the germinal vesicle (GV), and germinal vesicle breakdown (GVB) is an early indication of the reinitiation of meiosis. A fully grown oocyte undergoes an asymmetric cytokinesis in the first meiotic division, producing a secondary oocyte with a polar body. Both secondary oocytes and their polar bodies contain a haploid chromosome complement. The second meiotic division is initiated immediately after completion of the first meiotic division, but oocytes become arrested at metaphase II until penetration by sperm. Oocyte "maturation" is defined as the resumption and completion of the first meiotic division. It encompasses the subsequent progression to metaphase II (nuclear maturation), and the accompanying cytoplasmic processes essential for fertilization and early embryo development (cytoplasmic maturation). Before the reinitiation of meiosis, the oocyte is a primary oocyte. After completion of the first meiotic division, the metaphase II oocyte is a secondary oocyte and is referred to as an *ovum* or *egg*.

Oocyte maturation normally occurs in vivo shortly before gonadotropin-induced ovulation. It can occur spontaneously, however, independent of gonadotropic stimulation, if the fully grown oocyte is removed from the Graafian follicle and cultured. This spontaneous maturation occurs because the oocytes are removed from the maturation-inhibiting influence of the follicular somatic cells; see (18,19) for reviews.

The eukaryotic cell cycle is regulated, in part, by the activity of M-phase Promoting Factor (MPF), which consists of a catalytic subunit, $p34^{cdc2}$, and a regulatory subunit, cyclin B. Entry into metaphase is driven by the activity of MPF, and re-entry into interphase requires cyclin B destruction and decreased MPF activity; see (20–22). for reviews. MPF activity also drives meiosis in mammalian oocytes (23–26). MPF activity is necessary to maintain metaphase II arrest in oocytes, and the function of a multicomponent complex, known as cytostatic factor (CSF), is required to sustain MPF activity. CSF activity is the coordinated function of at least two proteins, MOS and mitogen-activated protein kinase (MAPK). MOS protein is the product of the *Mos* proto-oncogene, and *Mos* mRNA is produced throughout mouse oocyte growth and stored in a dormant form (27–30). Translation of *Mos* mRNA occurs in mouse oocytes mainly after the resumption of meiosis; thus, MOS accumulates during oocyte maturation (31). MOS is not necessary for meiotic resumption in mouse oocytes, as it is in frog oocytes (32,33), because GVB occurs in oocytes of *Mos*-null (knockout) mice (7,8,12). In contrast, MOS is required for metaphase II arrest in mouse oocytes because this arrest does not occur in most oocytes from *Mos*-null mice (7,8,12,34). MOS is also essential for MAPK activity because there is little or no MAPK activity detectable in oocytes of *Mos*-null mice (12,34,35).

Origin of LT Mice and Metaphase I-Arrest Parthenogenesis Phenotypes

Strain LT is actually an inbred strain derived from C58 and BALB/c progenitors. In 1950, MacDowell described a color coat mutation, called "light" (Blt) that arose spontaneously in his colony of C58 mice (36). Blt, a dominant mutation caused by a single base substitution in the tyrosinase-related protein-1, causes premature death of melanocytes due to the production of a toxic product during melanin synthesis (37). This mutation is totally unrelated to teratoma development. Mice carrying Blt were later outcrossed to BALB, and the inbred LT strain was produced by successive brother–sister matings making LT an RI strain derived from strains C58 and BALB/c. The traits of metaphase I-arrest, spontaneous parthenogenesis, and ovarian teratoma formation, which character- ize LT mice, may have resulted from the fortuitous combination of alleles present in BALB/c and C58 mice, or from mutation(s) that arose during inbreeding of the LT strain. To reconstruct the derivation of LT mice, BALB/c × C58/J (CX8) recombinant inbred strains were constructed by Dr. Eva Eicher and Dr. Joe Nadeau at the Jackson Laboratory. We assessed oocytes of these strains for incidence of metaphase I-arrest and parthenogenetic activation (10).

The oocytes of both parental strains, BALB/cJ and C58/J, and oocytes of the hybrid mice, (BALB/cJ × C58/J)F1 surprisingly also arrested at metaphase I at a high frequency. Unlike LT oocytes, however, the frequency of parthenogenetic activation was low. Although both BALB/cJ and C58/J showed a high frequency of metaphase I-arrest, the genetic control mechanism is probably not identical in both strains. If the genetic mechanism for metaphase I-arrest was identical, all CX8 strains should have a high frequency of metaphase I-arrest, but they do not. Oocytes of 2 of the CX8 strains, CX8-1 and –2, became parthenogenetically activated at a high frequency and exhibit a frequency of metaphase I-arrest higher than normal. Likewise, frequencies of metaphase I-arrest and parthenogenetic activation higher than normal were found in (C57BL/6J × LT)F1 oocytes and oocytes from recombinant inbred strains LTXBJ and LTXBO, which are derived from C57BL/6J and LT/Sv parental strains, and RI lines CX8-3 -4, -5A, -5B, -6, -7, -9, and -15. Oocytes with a high incidence of parthenogenetic activation occurred only in strains with oocytes having a high incidence of metaphase I- arrested oocytes. In fact, only metaphase I-arrested oocytes became spontane- ously activated. Strains with oocytes arrested at metaphase I, however, do not necessarily show a high frequency of spontaneous parthenogenetic activation. Thus, metaphase I-arrest is a necessary but not sufficient prerequisite for sponta- neous parthenogenetic activation. A cell cycle abnormality in the regulation of the first meiotic division, which results in arrest at metaphase I rather than metaphase II, is therefore necessary for spontaneous parthenogenetic activation of oocytes and teratoma formation. Moreover, the traits of metaphase I-arrest, spontaneous parthenogenesis, and ovarian teratoma formation expressed by LT mice probably resulted from the fortuitous combination of alleles present in BALB/c and C58 mice (10).

Regulation of Meiosis in Strain LT Oocytes

Metaphase I-arrest in LT oocytes is correlated with a sustained elevation of $p34^{cdc2}$ kinase activity (26). In fact, $p34^{cdc2}$ kinase activity continued to in- crease when it normally decreased. In addition, cyclin B, which is degraded in normal oocytes with meiotic progression beyond metaphase I, is stable in metaphase I-arrested LT oocytes (26). These results suggest that the progression of meiosis in LT oocytes is arrested at metaphase I by continued p34^{cdc2} kinase activity sustained, at least in part, by restricted degradation of cyclin B. Although there is a restriction of cyclin B degradation in metaphase I-arrested LT oocytes, it is possible that other factors underlie the failure to enter anaphase. Thus, it is possible that the failure to enter anaphase does not reflect a deficiency of the p34^{cdc2} kinase inactivating system per se; rather, it shows a deficiency in an upstream process that results in failure to trigger the p34^{cdc2} kinase inactivating system.

Given the established role of MOS in maintaining metaphase II-arrest, the hypothesis that MOS participates in initiating or sustaining metaphase I-arrest in LT oocytes was tested (38). The amount of MOS accumulated during maturation of LT oocytes is similar to that of normal oocytes. Moreover, MOS in LT oocytes is probably functional because MAPK appeared normally activated (38). It is well established that there is no MAPK activity in the absence of functional MOS (12,34,35). These results suggest that there are no abnormalities in the temporal production of functional MOS per se that contribute to metaphase I-arrest in LT oocytes.

Two experimental paradigms were used to reduce or delete MOS in LT oocytes and assess the effects on metaphase I-arrest (38). First, sense (control) and antisense *Mos* oligonucleotides were microinjected into metaphase I-arrested oocytes. Antisense, but not sense, *Mos* oligonucleotides promoted the activation of metaphase I-arrested oocytes. Second, a *Mos*-null mutation (8) was introduced by backcrossing into the LT strain; *Mos+/-* N$_3$ mice were intercrossed to produce *Mos-/-*, *Mos+/-*, and *Mos+/+* N$_3$F$_2$ mice. An identical backcross experiment was performed using the CX8-4 RI strain in which many fully grown oocytes become arrested at metaphase I, but the frequency of spontaneous parthenogenetic activation is very low (10). (CX8-4 is a useful model to study the possible participation of MOS in the maintenance of metaphase I-arrest, because progression of oocytes beyond metaphase I in the absence of MOS cannot be due to LT-related spontaneous parthenogenetic activation.) Oocytes from all mice surprisingly exhibited a very high occurrence of metaphase I-arrest, inferring that the instigation of metaphase I-arrest is not initially MOS dependent. Metaphase I-arrest of *Mos*-null oocytes from N$_3$F$_2$ females, however, was temporary and gradually reversed (38). This observation, in combination with the reversal of metaphase I-arrest by antisense *Mos* oligonucleotides, suggests that MOS participates in sustaining metaphase I-arrest in LT oocytes. Although MOS does not instigate metaphase I-arrest, MOS does therefore function to sustain it.

From these findings, we hypothesize that there is a two-step mechanism for metaphase I-arrest in LT oocytes. The first step reflects the fundamental lesion in LT oocytes; this step initiates metaphase I-arrest. The second step is the maintenance of metaphase I-arrest by CSF-like activity, which presumably functions subsequent to the metaphase I-arrest instigating lesion. We hypothesize that Step 1 involves a delay in the acquisition of competence by maturing metaphase I oocytes to enter anaphase I. By the time metaphase I LT oocytes are competent to initiate anaphase I, CSF-like activity may reach a level sufficient to prevent cyclin degradation, MPF activity remains high, and progression beyond metaphase I is arrested. In support of this hypothesis, preliminary experiments indicate that LT oocytes acquire competence to enter anaphase I approximately 1 hour after normal oocytes. This delay may participate in Step 1 instigating metaphase I-arrest by allowing the increasing CSF-like activity to reach levels sufficient to prevent cyclin B degradation and other processes required for initiation of anaphase I.

Conclusion

Arresting the progression of oocyte meiosis at metaphase I provides a necessary, though insufficient, condition for activation of LT oocytes without fertilization and subsequent parthenogenetic embryonic development. Moreover, sustaining metaphase I-arrest involves high MPF activity, failure to degrade cyclin B, and the participation of MOS, which suggests a CSF-like activity. When this occurs in oocytes that are not ovulated, and therefore remaining within the ovary, a likely consequence is teratocarcinogenesis. Resolution of the processes underlying aberrant metaphase I-arrest will reveal both a fundamental lesion to leading to ovarian teratocarcinogenesis as well as the mechanisms that drive normal meiosis in oocytes.

Acknowledgment. This research was supported by grant CA62392 from the National Cancer Institute.

References

1. Peterson WF. Malignant degeneration of benign cystic teratomas of the ovary. A Collective review of the literature. Obstet Gynecol Surg 1957;12:793–830.
2. Abell MR. The nature and classification of ovarian neoplasaams. Can Med Assoc J 1966;94:1102–24.
3. Norris HJ, Jensen RD. Relative frequency of ovarian neoplasms in children and adolescents. Cancer 1972;30:713–19.
4. Stevens LC, Varnum DS. The development of teratomas from parthenogenetically activated ovarian mouse eggs. Dev Biol 1974;37:369–80.
5. Fafalios MK, Olander EA, Melhem MF, Chaillet JR. Ovarian teratomas associated with the insertion of an imprinted transgene. Mamm Genome 1996;7:188–93.
6. Hsu SY, Lai RJM, Finegold M, Hsueh AJW. Targeted overexpression of bcl-2 in ovaries of tranagenic mice leads to decreased follicle apoptosis, enhanced folliculogenesis, and increased germ cell tumorigenesis. Endocrinology 1996;137:4837–43.
7. Hashimoto N, Watanabe N, Furuta Y, Tamemoto H, Sagata N, Yokoyama M, et al. Parthenogenetic activation of oocytes in c-mos deficient mice. Nature 1994;370:68–71.

8. Colledge WH, Carlton MBL, Udy GB, Evans MJ. Disruption of c-mos cause parthenogenetic development of unfertilized mouse eggs. Nature 1994;370:65–68.

9. Hirao Y, Eppig JJ. Parthenogenetic development of *Mos*-deficient mouse oocytes. Mol Reprod Dev 1997;48:391–96.

10. Eippig JJ, Wigglesworth K, Varnum DS, Nadeau JH. Genetic regulation of traits essential for spontaneous ovarian teratocarcinogenesis in strain LT/Sv mice: aberrant meiotic cell cycle, oocyte activation, and partheogenetic development. Cancer Res 1996;56:5047–54.

11. Malezewski M, Yanagimachi R. Spontaneous and sperm-induced activation of oocytes in LT/Sv strin mice. Dev Growth Differ 1995;37:679–85.

12. Verlhac MH, Kubiak JZ, Weber M, Geraud G, Colledge WH, Evans MJ, et al. Mos is required for MAP kinase activation and is involved in microtubule organization during meiotic maturation in the mouse. Development 1996;122:815–22.

13. Stevens LC. Teratocarcinogenesis and spontaneous parthenogenesis in mice. In: Market CL, Papaconstantinou J, eds. The developmental biology of reproduction. New York: Academic Press; 1975:93–106.

14. Eppig JJ, Kozak LP, Eicher EM, Stevens LC. Ovarian tertomas in mice are derived from oocytes that have completed the first meiotic division. Nature 1977; 269:517–18.

15. Kaufman MH, Howlett SK. The ovulation and activation of primary and secondary ooctes in LT/Sv strain mice. Gamete Res 1986;14:255–64.

16. West JD, Webb S, Kaufman MH. Inheritance of a meiotic abnormality that causes the ovulation of primary oocytes and the production of digynic triploid mice. Gen Res 1993;62:183–93.

17. Eppig JJ, Wigglesworth K. Atypical maturation of oocytes of strain I/LnJ mice. Hum Reprod 1994;9:1136–42.

18. Eppig JJ. Intercommunication between mammalian oocytes and companion somatic cells. BioEssays 1991;13:569–74.

19. Eppig JJ. Regulation of mammalian oocyte maturation. In: Adashi EY, Leung PCK, eds. The ovary. New York: Raven Press; 1993:185–208.

20. Norbury C, Nurse P. Animal cell cycles and their control. Ann Rev Biochem 1992;61:441–70

21. Jacobs T. Control of the cell cycle. Dev Biol 1992;153:1–15.

22. Murray A. Cyclin ubiquitination: the destructive end of mitosis. Cell 1995;81:149–52.

23. Hashimoto H, Kishimoto T. Regulation of meiotic metaphase by a cytoplasmic maturation-promoting factor during mouse oocyte maturation. Dev Biol 1988;126:242–52.

24. Choi T, Aoki F, Mori M, Yamashita M, Nagahama Y, Kohomoto K. Activation of p34cdc2 protein kinase activity in meiotic and mitotic cell cycles in mouse oocytes and embryos. Development 1991;113:789–95.

25. Hampl A, Eppig JJ. Translational regulation of the gradual increase in histone H1 kinase activity in maturing mouse oocytes. Mol Reprod Dev 1994;40:9–15.

26. Hampl A, Eppig JJ. Analysis of the mechanism(s) of metaphase I arrest in maturing mouse oocytes. Development 1995;121:925–33.

27. Goldman DS, Kiessling AA, Millette CF, Cooper GM. Expression of c-mos RNA in germ cells of male and female mice. Proc Nat Acad Sci USA 1987;84:4509–13.

28. Keshet E, Rosenberg MP, Mercer JA, Propst F, Vande Woude GF, Jenkins NA, et al. Developmental regulation of ovarian-specific Mos expression. Oncogene 1988;2: 235–40.

29. Mutter GL, Wolgemuth DJ. Distinct developmental patterns of c-mos protooncogene

expression in female and male mouse germ cells. Proc Nat Acad Sci USA 1987;84: 5301–5.

30. Gebauder F, Xu WH, Cooper GM, Richter JD. Translational control by cytoplasmic polyadenylation of c-*mos* mRNA is necessary for oocyte maturation in the mouse. EMBO J 1994;13:5712–20.

31. Paules RS, Buccione R, Moschel RC, Vande Woude GF, Eppig JJ. Mouse Mos protooncogene product is present and functions during oogenesis. Proc Natl Acad Sci USA 1989;86:5395–99.

32. Sagata N, Daar I, Oskarsson M, Showalter SD, Vande Woude GF. The product of the mos proto-oncogene as a candidate "initiator" for oocyte maturation. Science 1989;245:643–46.

33. Yew N, Mellini ML, Vande Woude GF. Meiotic initiation by the *mos* protein in *Xenopus*. Nature 1992;355:649–52.

34. Araki K, Naito K, Haraguchi S, Suzuki R, Yokoyama M, Inoue M, et al. Meiotic abnormalities of c-mos knockout mouse oocytes: activation after first meiosis or entrance into third meiotic metaphase. Biol Reprod 1996;55:1315–24.

35. Choi TS, Fukasawa K, Zhou RP, Tessarollo L, Borror K, Resau J, et al. The Mos/ mitogen-activated protein kinase (MAPK) pathway regulates the size and degradation of the first polar body in maturing mouse oocytes. Proc Natl Acad Sci USA 1996;93:7032–35.

36. MacDowell EC. "Light"—A new mouse color. J Hered 1950;41:35–36.

37. Johnson R, Jackson IJ. *Light* is dominant mouse mutation resulting in premature cell death. Nat Gen 1992;1:226–29.

38. Hirao Y, Eppig JJ. Analysis of the mechanism(s) of metaphase I arrest in strain LT mouse oocytes: participation of MOS. Development 1997;124:5107–13.

6

The Role of the Oocyte in Ovulation

ANTONIETTA SALUSTRI, CSABA FULOP, VINCENT C. HASCALL,
ANTONELLA CAMAIONI, AND MONICA DI GIACOMO

Introduction

Ovulation requires tight control of extracellular matrix modifications, within both the follicle wall and the inner mass of granulosa cells surrounding the oocyte, namely the cumulus cells. In most mammals, prior to ovulation, mural granulosa cells promote selective degradation of perifollicular matrix, resulting in the formation of a thinner area at the follicular apex. At the same time, the cumulus cells synthesize and deposit a large and viscoelastic extracellular matrix around the oocyte, a process known as cumulus expansion or mucification. As ovulation approaches, the apical follicle wall breaks, and a hole is formed that is sufficiently large to allow a portion of the cumulus mass to pass through it. Deformation of the cumulus matrix allows the passage of the first cumulus cells through the rupture site, after which the oocyte, surrounded by the remaining cumulus cells, is rapidly extruded from the follicle. Cumulus cells and the oocyte remain firmly bound within the matrix so that they are not dispersed during the extrusion.

The mucoid and elastic matrix of the expanded cumulus appears to provide an essential vehicle for oocyte protrusion. When the synthesis of this matrix by the cumulus cells was inhibited in mice stimulated to ovulate, only 5–10% of oocytes were released from the mature follicles even though rupture sites in their walls occurred normally (1). In addition, the few ovulated cumuli remained within the ovarian bursa and were not transferred to the oviduct. This result supports the hypothesis that specific components of the expanded cumulus matrix are also required for pickup and transfer of ova by the ciliated epithelium of the fimbria (2). Further, oocytes developing in ZP3-/- mutant mice lack a zona pellucida and are often separated from the expanding cumuli in the preovulatory follicles (3,4). After ovulation, expanded cumulus cell masses were always recovered in the oviducts, but the large majority contained no ovum. It is likely that most of the cumulus cell-denuded oocytes remained trapped in the ruptured follicles. Some other zona-free oocytes may dissociate from the cumulus during ovulation and stick to the epithelium of the reproductive tract where they degenerate.

Restriction of the formation of the mucoid extracellular matrix to the cumulus cells in the preovulatory follicle appears to be the result of paracrine influence by the oocyte. Our research indicates that the oocyte modulates the response of the cumulus cells to an ovulatory gonadotropin stimulus and has a crucial role both in promoting synthesis and in preventing degradation of the cumulus matrix. Although gonadotropins are essential for triggering the complex events involved in ovulation, the oocyte therefore appears to orchestrate this process through paracrine interaction with the surrounding cumulus cells, thereby ensuring its transfer from the ovary to the oviduct.

Components of the Expanded Cumulus Matrix

The dominant component of the expanded cumulus matrix is hyaluronan, a glycosaminoglycan that consists of a long polymer of repeating glucuronic acid-N-acetylglucosamine disaccharides. These large, polyanionic macromolecules (typically, 1–5 million D) have extended hydrodynamic domains that occupy large solvent volumes and yield solutions with high viscosities (5). Their ability to attract solvent is most likely responsible for the increase of the intercellular spaces between cumulus cells and, consequently, for the expansion of the preovulatory cumulus. By ultrastructural analysis, hyaluronan strands appear to be organized through interactions with proteins to form a fibrillar network anchored to cumulus cell surface (6) and extended into the oocyte zona pellucida (7). Molecules that interact with hyaluronan are required for such matrix assembly (8).

We have identified two proteins with such characteristics that are expressed by cumulus cells during expansion: CD44 (preliminary results) and tumor necrosis factor stimulated gene-6 TSG-6 (9). CD44 may serve to anchor the hyaluronan matrix to the surfaces of the cumulus cells because this molecule is a known hyaluronan-binding cell surface receptor involved in cell-matrix adhesion in several cell types (10). TSG-6 is a matrix protein that can form a stable complex with inter-α-trypsin inhibitor (ITI) (11), a serum protease inhibitor present in the follicular fluid that is known to be required for forming the expanded matrix (12). The ITI/TSG-6 complexes may form cross-bridges between hyaluronan strands because both molecules have the ability to bind to hyaluronan, although ITI does so weakly (13). On the other hand, TSG-6 may potentiate the antiproteolytic activity of ITI (14) by localizing it on the hyaluronan strands, thereby preventing degradation of important structural proteins. Indeed, increased synthesis and secretion of proteases (e.g., plasminogen activator by mural granulosa cells in response to gonadotropins) increases the proteolytic activity in the follicular fluid during the preovulatory period. On the other hand, the cumulus cells express lower levels of plasminogen activator and higher levels of protease nexin-1, a protease inhibitor (15,16). These findings suggest that cumulus cells, in addition to synthesizing and organizing the matrix, activate several mechanisms for protecting the expanding matrix from degradation.

Gonadotropin Influence on Cumulus Expansion

When large ovarian follicles are punctured under a dissecting microscope, the cumulus cell layers remain closely associated with the oocyte, and intact cumulus cell-oocyte complexes (COCs) can be isolated. Culture of the COCs in defined medium conditions has allowed molecular mechanisms involved in cumulus expansion to be studied in more detail. In all examined species, gonadotropins are potent inducers of COC expansion in vitro, although the cumulus cells are more sensitive to follicle stimulating hormone (FSH) than to luteinizing hormone (LH) or human chorionic gonadotropin (hCG) (17–20). In reality, highly purified LH and hCG fail to induce expansion of isolated mouse COCs (21). These findings are consistent with the low or undetectable levels of LH receptors in the cumulus cells in the preovulatory follicle (22–25).

We have shown that hyaluronan synthesis correlates closely with the expansion of mouse COCs in vitro. Hyaluronan synthesis is first detected 2–3 hours after stimulation, increases to a maximum rate sustained between 4–10 hours, and then declines and ceases by 12–18 hours when maximum expansion has been reached (26). Several lines of evidence suggest that FSH exerts its influence on hyaluronan synthesis via cAMP. Dibutyryl cAMP, a cyclic AMP analogue, shows a potency and temporal course of hyaluronan induction similar to that observed with FSH (26). In addition, FSH stimulates cAMP production by the cumulus cells (27). Maximum hyaluronan synthesis occurs when a concentration of 14 fmol of cAMP/COC is reached. Similar cAMP levels (8–12 fmol/COC) are reached in vivo 2–4 hours after hCG injection into PMSG-primed mice (28,29), a time at which hyaluronan synthesis is initiated (30). As discussed earlier, because mouse cumulus cells do not appear to have LH/hCG receptors, the hCG-dependent cAMP elevation observed in cumulus cells in vivo is likely mediated by mural granulosa either by direct transfer of cAMP via gap junctions or by the synthesis or activation of a molecule that can activate adenylate cyclase in the cumulus cells (28,31–34). Based on in vitro results, it is reasonable to hypothesize a primary role for cAMP in regulating hyaluronan synthesis and in promoting cumulus expansion in vivo.

Regulation of hyaluronan synthesis in cumulus cells is primarily controlled at the level of hyaluronan synthase-2 (Has2) mRNA transcription (35). The Has2 mRNA is at very low levels in the compact COCs isolated from

PMSG-primed mice, but reaches high levels 2–3 hours after hCG injection into the animals. By the time hyaluronan synthesis ceases, the Has2 mRNA returns to the basal levels observed initially. If transcription of mRNA is inhibited in FSH-stimulated COCs by adding actinomycin D at 6 hours of culture, when the rate of hyaluronan production is maximum, hyaluronan synthesis rapidly declines, only producing an amount equivalent to that which would be achieved if the maximal rate was sustained for an additional ~2 hours (27). Thus, the half-lives of Has2 mRNA and of Has2 enzyme activity appear to be short during the COC expansion process.

Influence of Oocyte on Synthesis and Stability of the Cumulus Matrix

Although the oocyte does not synthesize hyaluronan, it has an essential role in mouse cumulus expansion. When the oocyte is mechanically removed from the COC, isolated cumulus cells synthesize low levels of hyaluronan in the presence of FSH, and they do not form an expanded matrix (36,37). Further, in the absence of oocytes, FSH-stimulated cumulus cells secrete much higher levels of the protease urokinase plasminogen activator (uPA) than intact COCs (15). Both a high level of hyaluronan synthesis and a low level of uPA activity are restored in FSH-stimulated cumulus cells by adding back either oocytes or oocyte-conditioned medium to the cultures. Soluble factors released by the oocyte, therefore, appear to be important paracrine regulators of endocrine action on cumulus cells surrounding the oocyte, facilitating hyaluronan-matrix production, and stabilizing the matrix by inhibiting the synthesis of degradative enzymes.

Preliminary characterization of the oocyte factors that regulate hyaluronan and uPA synthesis suggests that they are heat-labile proteins with an apparent molecular weight above 100 kDa (15,38). They also show a similar pattern of secretion during oogenesis (15,39,40). Thus, it is possible that both hyaluronan and uPA synthesis activities are regulated by a single factor produced by the oocyte. Identification of the oocyte factor(s) remains elusive, however, because it is unstable in solution and difficult to obtain in adequate amounts. Transforming growth factor (TGF) β1, among several growth factor tested, is the only one able to substitute for the oocyte factor(s) that promotes hyaluronan synthesis by FSH-stimulated cumulus cells (41); however, this growth factor is less effective than the oocyte factor(s), and neutralizing antibodies against TGFβ1 do not inhibit the response to the oocyte factor(s), which indicates that they are different. Their effects, however, are not additive at optimal doses, and they show identical patterns of induction of hyaluronan synthesis (27). Thus, it is possible that the oocyte factor(s) that promotes hyaluronan synthesis is a member of the TGFβ family that differs from TFGβ1, but which triggers similar intracellular signals.

Similar to mouse, rat cumulus expansion depends upon the presence of the oocyte factor, but porcine and bovine cumulus expansion apparently does not, because their isolated cumulus cells can synthesize an expanded matrix with only FSH treatment (42–45). It has been reported that pig cumulus cells synthesize a factor similar to the oocyte factor that would act as an autocrine factor to promote hyaluronan synthesis (46). Quantitative analyses, however, show that pig cumulus cells synthesize significantly less hyaluronan when stimulated with FSH in the absence of the oocyte (47). In addition, pig and cattle oocytes can substitute for mouse oocytes in inducing mouse cumulus expansion indicating that they also synthesize the factor that promotes hyaluronan synthesis (43–46). It is possible, then, that in the larger cumulus cell masses (20,000 cells in pig versus 3000 cells in mouse) the oocyte factor and the cumulus cell factor cooperate to achieve an optimal concentration of hyaluronan for full cumulus expansion. At present, no information is available on uPA activity in species other than mouse.

We have investigated the intracellular mechanisms in cumulus cells through which the oocyte factor(s) operates to modulate hyaluronan and uPA synthesis in the presence of gonadotropins. Cyclic AMP elevation induced by FSH through its receptor is not influenced by the presence or the absence of oocytes (37). Mouse cumulus cells produce maximal hyaluronan synthesis if they are exposed to FSH for only 2 hours, indicating that its action is completed within this time and before hyaluronan synthesis is actually apparent (27). On the other hand, the presence of the oocyte is not required during this initial phase, but its continuous presence is required thereafter to promote and sustain maximal hyaluronan synthesis. It is, therefore, likely that the oocyte factor(s) does not interact directly with the FSH signal transduction pathway.

The level of uPA mRNA achieved under FSH stimulation is significantly lower in the presence of oocytes suggesting that the oocyte factor(s) decreases the steady-state level of uPA mRNA (15). We have found that Has2 mRNA levels increase when cumulus cells are stimulated in vitro with FSH in the presence of oocytes; however, cumulus cells cultured with FSH in the absence of oocytes show only a minor, transient increase in the amount of the Has2 transcript, which implies that the paracrine factor secreted by the oocyte is essential to obtain and/or maintain high levels of Has2 mRNA (preliminary results). These data suggest the following model for regulation of Has2 and uPA synthesis by FSH and the oocyte factor(s): FSH activates a cyclic AMP responsive element binding protein that acts as a transcription factor for Has2 and uPA genes. The oocyte factor operates through a separate receptor and signalling pathway to activate other proteins which regulate the cyclic AMP-dependent transcription factor activity positively on Has2 and negatively on uPA gene. On the other hand, or in addition, the oocyte factor(s) can modulate the degradation of Has2 and uPA mRNAs (Fig. 6.1).

Acknowledgments. This work was supported by a joint grant CRG 950829 from the NATO, by a grant from MURST 40% (to A.S.); and by NIH grant HD34831 and the Cleveland Clinic Foundation (to V.C.H.).

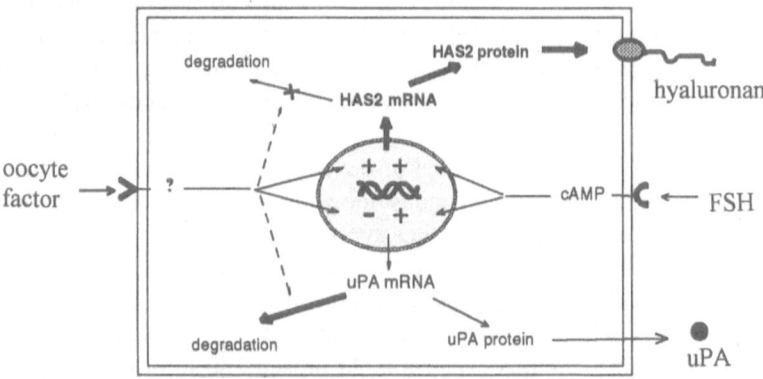

FIGURE 6.1. A model for regulation of hyaluronan and uPA synthesis by FSH and the oocyte factor in mouse cumulus cells. See text for details.

References

1. Chen L, Russell PT, Larsen WJ. Functional significance of cumulus expansion in the mouse: roles for the preovulatory synthesis of hyaluronic acid within the cumulus mass. Mol Reprod Dev 1993;34:87–93.
2. Mahi-Brown CA, Yanagimachi R. Parameters influencing ovum pickup by oviductal fimbria in the golden hamster. Gamete Res 1983;8:1–10.
3. Rankin T, Familiari M, Lee E, Ginsberg A, Dwyer N, Blanchette-Mackie J, et al. Mouse homozygous for an insertional mutation in the Zp3 gene lack a zona pellucida and are fertile. Development 1996;122:2903–10.
4. Liu C, Litscher ES, Mortillo S, Sakai Y, Kinloch RA, Stewart CL, et al. Targeted disruption of the mZP3 gene results in production of eggs lacking a zona pellucida and infertility in female mice. Proc Natl Acad Sci 1996;93:5431–36.
5. Fraser JR, Laurent TC, Laurent UB. Hyaluronan: its nature, distribution, functions and turnover. J Intern Med 1997;242:27–33.
6. Cherr GN, Yudin AI, Katz DF. Organization of the hamster cumulus extracellular matrix: a hyaluronate-glycoprotein gel which modulates sperm access to the oocyte. Dev Growth Differ 1990;32:353–65.
7. Talbot P. Sperm penetration through oocyte investments in mammals. Am J Anat 1985;174:331–46.
8. Camaioni A, Hascall VC, Yanagishita M, Salustri A. Effect of exogenous hyaluronic acid and serum on matrix organization and stability in the mouse cumulus cell-oocyte complex. J Biol Chem 1993;268:20473–81.
9. Fulop C, Kamath RV, Li Y, Otto JM, Salustri A, Olsen BR, et al. Coding sequence, exon-intron structure and chromosomal localization of murine TNF-stimulated gene 6 that is specifically expressed by expanding cumulus cell-oocyte complexes. Gene 1997;202:95–102.
10. Lesley J, Hyman R, Kincade PW. CD44 and its interaction with extracellular matrix. Adv Immunol 1993;54:271–335.
11. Wisniewski HG, Burgess WH, Oppenheim JD, Vilcek J. TSG-6, an arthritis-associ-

ated hyaluronan binding protein, form a stable complex with the serum protein inter-alpha-trypsin inhibitor. Biochemistry 1994; 33:7423–29.

12. Chen LC, Mao SJT, Larsen WL. Identification of a factor in fetal bovine serum that stabilizes the cumulus extracellular matrix. J Biol Chem 1992;267:12380–86.

13. Chen L, Mao SJ, McLean LR, Powers RW, Larsen WJ. Proteins of the inter-alpha-trypsin inhibitor family stabilize the cumulus extracellular matrix through thier direct binding with hyaluronic acid. J Biol Chem 1994;269:28282–87.

14. Wisniewski HG, Hua JC, Poppers DM, Naime D, Vilcek J, Cronstein BN. TNF/IL-1 inducible protein TSG-6 potentiates plasmin inhibition by inter-alpha-inhibitor and exerts a strong anti-inflammatory effect in vivo. J Immunol 1996;156:1609–15.

15. Canipari R, Epifano O, Siracusa G, Salustri A. Mouse oocytes inhibit plasminogen activator production by ovarian cumulus and granulosa cells. Dev Biol 1995;167: 371–78.

16. Hagglund AC, Ny A, Liu K, Ny T. Coordinated and cell-specific induction of both physiological plasminogen activators creates functionally redundant mechanisms for plasmin formation during ovulation. Endocrinology 1996;137:5671–77.

17. Thibault CG. Final stages of mammalian oocyte maturation. In: Biggers JD, Schuetz AW, eds. Ooogenesis. Baltimore: University Park Press; 1972:397–411.

18. Ball GD, Bellin ME, Ax RL, First NL. Glycosaminoglycans in bovine cumulus-oocyte complexes: morphology and chemistry. Mol Cell Endocrinol 1982;28:113–22.

19. Singh B, Barbe GJ, Armstrong DT. Factors influencing resumption of meiotic maturation and cumulus expansion of porcine oocyte-cumulus cell complexes in vitro. Mol Reprod Dev 1993;36:113–19.

20. Armstrong DT, Xia P, de Gannes G, Tekpetey FR, Khamsi F. Differential effects of insulin-like growth factor-1 and follicle-stimulating hormone on proliferation and differentiation of bovine cumulus cells and granulosa cells. Biol Reprod 1996;54: 331–38.

21. Eppig JJ. FSH stimulates hyaluronic acid synthesis by oocyte-cumulus cell complexes from mouse preovulatory follicles. Nature 1979;281:483–84.

22. Amsterdam A, Koch Y, Lieberman ME, Lindner HR. Distributions of binding sites for human chorionic gonadotropin in the preovulatory follicle of the rat. J Cell Biol 1975;67:894–900.

23. Lawrence TS, Dekel N, Beers WH. Binding of human chorionic gonadotropin by rat cumuli oophori and granulosa cells: a comparative study. Endocrinology 1980;106:1114–18.

24. Channing CP, Bae IH, Stone SL, Anderson LD, Edelson S, Fowler SC. Porcine granulosa and cumulus cell properties. LH/hCG receptors, ability to secrete progesterone and ability to respond to LH. Mol Cell Endocrinol 1981;22:359–70.

25. Oxberry BA, Greenwald GS. An autoradiographic study of the binding of ^{125}I-labeled follicle stimulating hormone, human chorionic gonadotropin, and prolactin to the hamster ovary throughout the estrous cycle. Biol Reprod 1982;27:505–16.

26. Salustri A, Yanagishita M, Hascall VC. Synthesis and accumulation of hyaluronic acid and proteoglycans in the mouse cumulus cell-oocyte complex during follicle stimulating hormone-induced mucification. J Biol Chem 1989;264:13840–47.

27. Tirone E, D'Alessandris C, Hascall VC, Siracusa G, Salustri A. Hyaluronan synthesis by mouse cumulus cells is regulated by interactions between follicle-stimulating hormone (or epidermal growth factor) and a soluble oocyte factor (or transforming growth factor beta 1). J Biol Chem 1997;272:4787–94.

28. Schultz RM, Montgomery RR, Belanoff JR. Regulation of mouse oocyte meiotic maturation: implication of a decrease in oocyte cAMP and protein dephosphorilation in commitment to resume meiosis. Dev Biol 1983;97:264–73.

29. Eppig JJ, Downs SM. Gonadotropin-induced murine oocyte maturation in vivo is not associated with decreased cyclic adenosine monophosphate in the oocyte-cumulus cell complex. Gamete Res 1988;20:125–31.

30. Salustri A, Yanagishita M, Underhill C, Laurent TC, Hascall VC. Localization and synthesis of hyaluronic acid in the cumulus cells and mural granulosa cells of the preovulatory follicles. Dev Biol 1992;151:541–51.

31. Eppig JJ. Regulation of cumulus oophorus expansion by gonadotropins in vivo and in vitro. Biol Reprod 1980;23:545–52.

32. Eppig JJ. Prostaglandin E2 stimulates cumulus expansion and hyaluronic acid synthesis by cumuli oophori isolated from mice. Biol Reprod 1981;25:191–95.

33. Downs SM, Longo FJ. Effects of indomethacin on preovulatory follicles in immature, superovulated mice. Am J Anat 1982;164:265–74.

34. Salustri A, Petrungaro S, Siracusa G. Granulosa cells stimulate in vitro the expansion of isolated mouse cumuli oophori: involvement of prostaglandin E2. Biol Reprod 1985;33:229–34.

35. Fulop C, Salustri A, Hascall VC. Coding sequence of a hyaluronan synthase homologue expressed during expansion of the mouse cumulus-oocyte complex. Arch Biochem Biophys 1997;337:261–66.

36. Salustri A, Yanagishita M, Hascall VC. Mouse oocytes regulate hyaluronic acid synthesis and mucification by FSH-stimulated cumulus cells. Dev Biol 1990;138:26–32.

37. Buccione R, Vanderhyden BC, Caron PJ, Eppig JJ. FSH-induced expansion of the mouse cumulus oophorus in vitro is dependent upon a specific factor(s) secreted by the oocyte. Dev Biol 1990;138:16–25.

38. Eppig JJ, Peters AHFM, Telfer E, Wigglesworth K. Production of cumulus expansion enabling factor by mouse oocytes grown in vitro: preliminary characterization of the factor. Mol Reprod Dev 1993;34:450–56.

39. Vanderhyden BC, Caron PJ, Buccione R, Eppig JJ. Developmental pattern of the secretion of cumulus-expansion enabling factor by mouse oocytes and the role of oocytes in promoting granulosa cell differentiation. Dev Biol 1990;140:307–17.

40. Eppig JJ, Wigglesworth K, Chesnel F. Secretion of cumulus expansion enabling factor by mouse oocytes: relationship to oocyte growth and competence to resume meiosis. Dev Biol 1993;158:400–9.

41. Salustri A, Ulisse S, Yanagishita M, Hascall VC. Hyaluronic acid synthesis by mural granulosa cells and cumulus cells in vitro is selectively stimulated by a factor produced by oocytes and by transforming growth factor-beta. J Biol Chem 1990;265:19517–23.

42. Prochazka E, Nagyova E, Rimkeviova T, Nagai T, Kikuchi K, Motlik J. Lack of effect of oocytectomy on expansion of the porcine cumulus. J Reprod Fertil 1991;93:569–76.

43. Vanderhyden BC. Species differences in the regulation of cumulus expansion by an oocyte-secreted factor(s). J Reprod Fertil 1993;98:219–27.

44. Singh B, Zhang X, Armstrong DT. Porcine oocytes release cumulus expansion-enabling activity even though porcine cumulus expansion in vitro is independent of the oocyte. Endocrinology 1993;132:1860–62.

45. Ralph JH, Telfer EE, Wilmut I. Bovine cumulus cell expansion does not depend on the presence of an oocyte secreted factor. Mol Reprod Dev 1995;42:248–53.

46. Prochazka R, Nagyova E, Brem G, Schellander K, Motlik J. Secretion of cumulus expansion-enabling factor (CEEF) in porcine follicles. Mol Reprod Dev 1998;49:141–49.
47. Nakayama T, Inoue M, Sato E. Effect of oocytectomy on glycosaminoglycan composition during cumulus expansion of porcine cumulus-oocyte complexes cultured in vitro. Biol Reprod 1996;55:1299–304.

Part II

The Gonadotropin Surge

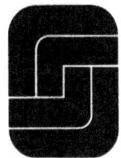

7

The Physiology of the Human Midcycle Gonadotropin Surge

ANN E. TAYLOR, JANET E. HALL, JUDITH M. ADAMS,
KATHRYN A. MARTIN, CORRINE K. WELT, AND
WILLIAM F. CROWLEY, JR.

Introduction

The human menstrual cycle requires a tightly integrated series of neuroendocrine and peripheral hormonal signals involving the hypothalamus, pituitary, and ovaries for normal folliculogenesis, ovulation, and maintenance of the corpus luteum. From many human, animal, and cellular models, we now understand that pulsatile secretion of hypothalamic gonadotropin releasing hormone (GnRH) is absolutely required for and sufficient to induce pulsatile pituitary luteinizing hormone (LH) secretion. The pattern of pulsatile LH secretion changes significantly in both frequency and amplitude across the normal menstrual cycle, at least partly reflecting negative feedback of ovarian estradiol, progesterone, and inhibins; however, the mechanism of the dramatic increase in LH secretion that occurs in response to estrogen positive feedback at the time of the midcycle surge (MCS) is still poorly understood. This midcycle surge is absolutely required for final follicular maturation and initiation of follicular rupture and is therefore a crucial component of the human menstrual cycle.

In this chapter, we will first review the neuroendocrine changes that occur across the menstrual cycle, then describe the features of the LH surge in detail. We will then review the relative roles of increased GnRH secretion versus increased pituitary sensitivity, ending with an evaluation of the role of ovarian sex steroids and other factors in initiation and termination of the surge. Overall, the preponderance of evidence indicates that the human midcycle surge of gonadotropins occurs independent of any increase in GnRH secretion, which suggests that the surge represents a dramatic change in pituitary sensitivity, induced by changes in both ovarian sex steroids and perhaps other ovarian factors.

The Normal Menstrual Cycle

The human menstrual cycle is dependent on a specific pattern of episodic gonadotropin secretion controlled by the hypothalamic pituitary axis. Because direct assessment of GnRH secretion is not possible in women, the assessment of peripheral gonadotropin secretion remains the best tool to investigate the hypothalamic–pituitary axis. Validation of frequent peripheral LH measurements as a marker of pulsatile GnRH secretion comes from many animal models. In the rhesus monkey (1,2), as well as the sheep (3) and the rat (4), each episode of LH secretion is preceded by a burst of GnRH release as measured directly in the hypothalamus or the hypophyseal–portal blood. In addition, ablation of specific hypothalamic areas in animal models eliminates gonadotropin secretion, whereas replacement of GnRH alone restores pulsatile gonadotropin secretion (5,6). In women, absence and derangement of pulsatile LH secretion are both associated with amenorrhea (7). Thus, a normal pattern of GnRH secretion is absolutely required for normal menstrual cycles.

To characterize normal gonadotropin secretion across the human menstrual cycle and at the time of the midcycle surge, strict criteria were applied to the selection of normal women volunteers for study. All were healthy, aged 18–40, with regular menstrual cycles of 26–34 day duration. Each had a normal physical examination with body weight within 15% of normal by the Sargent scale, and no significant acne, hirsutism, or galactorrhea. No women exercised more than 1 hour/day or ran more than 20 miles/week. None had taken any hormonal or other medications (except stable thyroid hormone replacement) for at least 3 months prior to study. In addition, all subjects had normal prolactin and TSH levels, as well as a luteal phase length greater than 10 days and a peak luteal phase serum progesterone level greater than 6 ng/mL. Blood was sampled daily from the onset of menses until the next menses. A subset of subjects underwent frequent pelvic ultrasonography during the follicular phase with daily scans around the time of ovulation until follicular rupture was documented. Another subset underwent 12–48 hours of q5 to q10 minute blood sampling for measurement of pulsatile LH secretion. LH, follicle stimulating hormone (FSH), estradiol, progesterone, inhibin A and inhibin B were measured in each sample by radioimmunoassay. From these results, the day of ovulation was determined as the day on which at least 3 of the following four criteria were met: LH peaked, FSH peaked, progesterone doubled or exceeded 0.6 ng/mL, and/or the day of or the day after the estradiol peaked, as previously described (8).

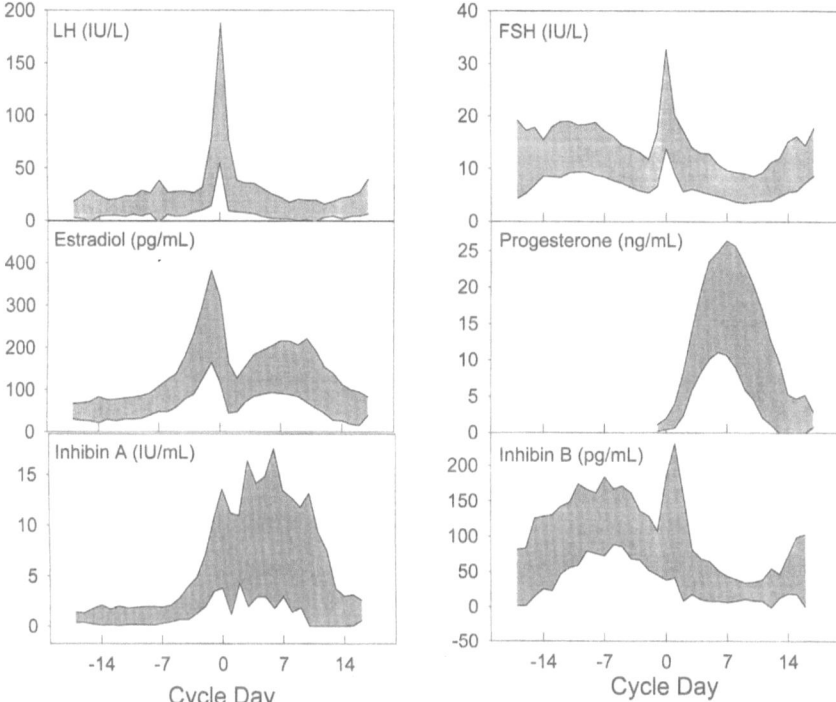

FIGURE 7.1. The normal menstrual cycle: Estradiol, progesterone, LH, and FSH were obtained from 118 normal cycles in 109 women. Thirty-seven women are included for Inhibin A values, and 28 women are included for Inhibin B values. All data are presented as +/– SEM and centered to the day of ovulation as defined in the text.

From these studies, we have described the hormonal changes across the normal menstrual cycle in 118 women as shown in Figure 7.1. The menstrual cycle begins with low levels of estradiol, progesterone, and LH, whereas FSH levels are about 30% higher than they are during the previous luteal phase. Due to this increased FSH stimulation, estradiol levels slowly begin to rise as the dominant follicle is selected approximately 7 days before ovulation (9). Concomitant with rising estradiol levels, the dominant follicle begins to grow as documented by frequent pelvic ultrasonographic examinations (Fig. 7.2). Estradiol peaks the day before the midcycle surge when the first small increase in progesterone is detectable. Inhibin A begins to rise a day or two after estradiol and reaches its first peak on the day of the LH surge.

The gonadotropin surge is quite dramatic. Within a period of 2–3 days as detected by daily samples, LH levels acutely increase more than 10 fold, whereas

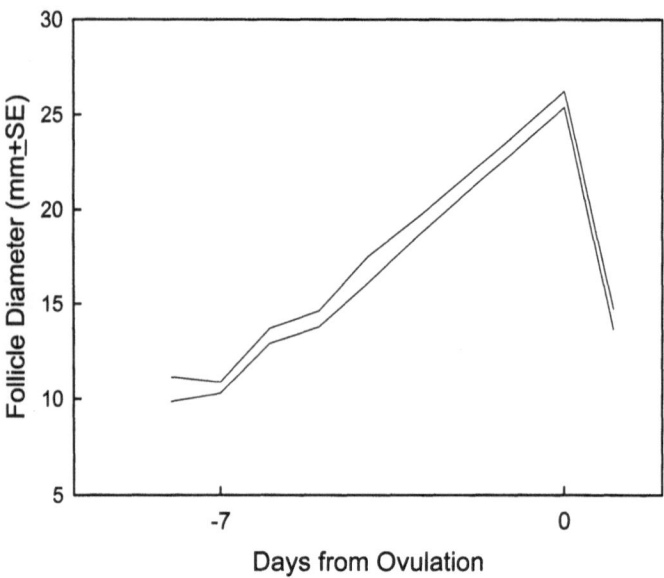

FIGURE 7.2. Follicular growth as defined by ultrasonography in 42 normal menstrual cycles, centered to the day of ovulation as defined in the text.

FSH levels rise about four fold. Progesterone continues to rise after the surge, whereas estradiol transiently dips before rising again in the luteal phase. The dominant follicle collapses within 1 day of the surge, as the oocyte is released. It is interesting that if the surge is delayed by up to 3 days by the use of RU486 to block progesterone receptors (10), the follicle continues to grow and estradiol levels continue to rise until the surge occurs, demonstrating both that the surge is dependent on progesterone production from the growing follicle, and that the process of follicular ovulation requires the gonadotropin surge. Progesterone peaks approximately 7 days after the midcycle surge and falls to baseline over the next 7 days, initiating menses and the next menstrual cycle.

Frequent blood sampling was performed in 49 cycles of 34 women at six different stages of the menstrual cycle (early, mid-, and late follicular, and early, mid-, and late luteal) (8). Cycle phase was assigned from the daily hormone values, centered to the LH peak, and normalized to a 28 day cycle (EFP days −13 to −9, MFP days −8 to −5, LFP days −4 to −1, ELP days +1 to +4, MLP days +5 to +9, and LLP days +10 to +14). Representative examples of the pulsatile LH secretory patterns at each cycle phase are shown in Figure 7.3, and summary data in Figure 7.4. There is clear evidence of slowing of pulsatile LH secretion during sleep in the early follicular phase, which is lost during the rest of the cycle. The LH pulse frequency peaks in the mid- and late follicular phase, then slows dramatically after progesterone exposure in the mid- and late luteal phase. LH pulse amplitude for the most part follows an inverse pattern to that of pulse frequency, consistent with experimental evidence in GnRH-deficient subjects that LH pulse amplitude is significantly increased after long interpulse intervals, even when the dose of GnRH replacement is maintained constant (11).

Description of the Midcycle Surge

To understand the neuroendocrine dynamics of the midcycle surge of LH better, we studied 18 additional normal women (12). Subjects underwent frequent pelvic ultrasonography commencing approximately 5 days before the anticipated day of ovulation as determined by menstrual cycle history and basal body temperature charts from preceding cycles. Ultrasound scans were repeated every 1–2 days during the periovulatory period to assess follicle growth and endometrial thickness to predict the day of the surge and therefore the day of study. Because we anticipated that the surge would last at least 48 hours and that the frequency of LH pulsations would be maximal at this time in the cycle, we increased the sampling duration to 36 hours (the maximal practical before significant anemia occurred) and the sampling interval to q5 minute to optimize the detection of rapid pulses (13,14). Both LH and the gonadotropin free α subunit were measured in all frequent blood samples so that rapid pulsatility could be confirmed in both hormones. Subjects also obtained daily blood samples across the cycle, so the exact day of study could be confirmed endocrinologically. Using these parameters, 14 studies were determined to have occurred on the day of the peak LH, whereas five others occurred between days −3 and +1 after the surge.

There was a highly variable but often quite striking increase in the amplitude of LH pulsations at the time of the surge (Fig. 7.5). Analysis of the pulsatile secretion demonstrated that the LH pulse amplitude increased significantly from the late follicular phase to the midportion of the surge, and then fell. There was no difference in the interpulse interval of LH between the late follicular phase and the early and midportions of the surge (70±8, 67.5±7, and 65±5 minutes, respectively). Pulse frequency then slowed significantly in the late portion of the surge to 87±6 minutes, presumably a response to the inexorably increasing progesterone levels. Similar results were obtained when α subunit pulses were analyzed (Fig. 7.6). We conclude that the midcycle surge of gonadotropins in humans is associated with a dramatic increase in LH pulse amplitude, but no change in LH pulse frequency. The absence of a change in pulse frequency, however, does not allow the determination of whether changes in the amount of hypothalamic GnRH secretion contribute to the surge. The increase in LH pulse amplitude could be explained by either an increase in pituitary sensitivity to GnRH or an increase in the amount of GnRH released per pulse, or by a combination of both.

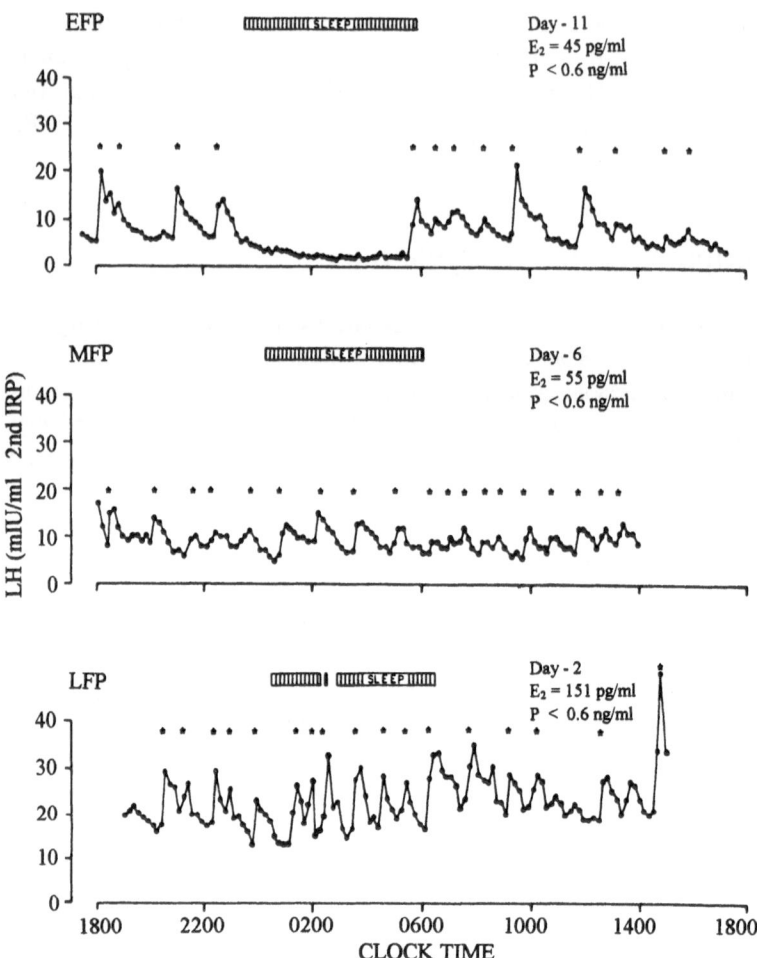

FIGURE 7.3. Patterns of episodic LH secretion from representative subjects throughout the follicular phase of the menstrual cycle, including the early- (EFP), mid- (MFP) and late- (LFP) follicular phases, and from early- (ELP), mid- (MLP), and late- (LLP) luteal phases. Cycle day is represented as days from ovulation as defined in the text. Statistically identified LH pulsations are identified by asterisks. Sleep is indicated by hatched bars. Derived from Figures 2 and 4 in Ref. 8, with permission © The Endocrine Society.

Maintenance of the Surge Requires GNRH

We and others have demonstrated that blockade of GnRH activity with a specific GnRH receptor antagonist results in a dramatic fall in LH levels at all times of the menstrual cycle (15). Administration of the antagonist at the onset of the LH surge results in termination of the menstrual cycle (Fig. 7.7) (15–17). Thus, GnRH is absolutely required for maintenance of the midcycle surge.

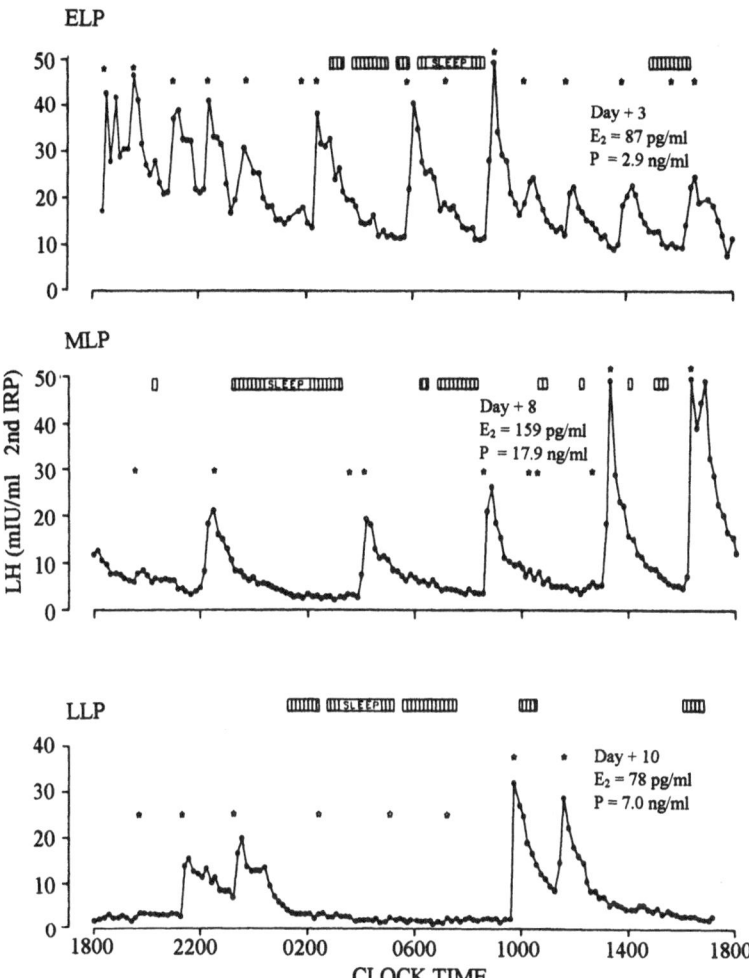

Figure 7.3. *Continued.*

GNRH Is Sufficient to Maintain the Midcycle Surge

Once the physiologic pattern of GnRH secretion in women was determined, this information could be used to provide physiologic replacement of GnRH to women with GnRH deficiency, in whom endogenous pulsatile LH secretion was absent. Exogenous administration of low-dose, pulsatile GnRH in a physiologic pattern effectively restores pituitary and ovarian function, and fertility, to normal (18,19). In particular, pituitary hormone secretion, follicular growth, ovulation, and luteal function are normalized when pulsatile GnRH is administered at 75 ng/kg/pulse (19) at a frequency that changes to match that seen in the normal menstrual cycle (q90 minutes in the early follicular phase (EFP), increasing to q60 minutes in the midfollicular phase (MFP) once

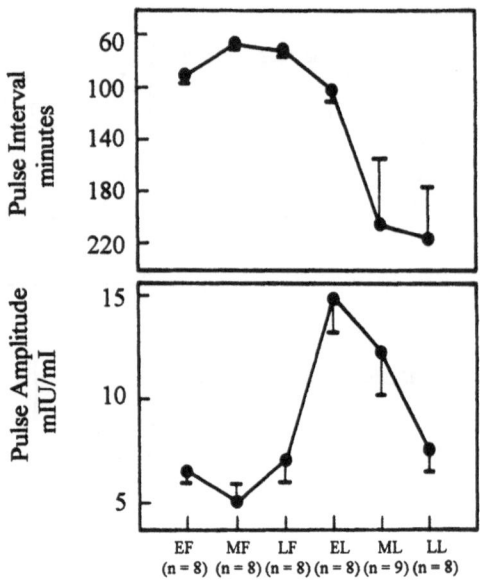

FIGURE 7.4. The LH interpulse interval and amplitude in the different stages of the menstrual cycle. Data are expressed as the mean ± SE. Reprinted, with permission, from Ref. 8 © The Endocrine Society.

a dominant follicle is documented, decreasing to q90 minutes 48 hours after the LH surge is documented and to q240 minutes 7 days after ovulation to mimic the normal luteal phase slowing) (Fig. 7.8). Thus, pulsatile GnRH is the *only* factor required to recreate a normal menstrual cycle in GnRH deficient subjects. It is important to note that there is a dramatic increase in LH and FSH secretion at the time of the surge, identical to normal cycles, without any increase in the amount of GnRH per bolus. This data indicates that a normal surge can be re-created without an increase in GnRH stimulation of the pituitary, which suggests that the surge is entirely explained by increased pituitary sensitivity.

An Increase in GNRH Is *Not* Required to Initiate the Surge

To address further the issue of whether the amount of GnRH is increased during the midcycle surge, we used incomplete GnRH receptor blockade with the Nal–Glu GnRH receptor antagonist to provide a semi-quantitative estimate of endogenous GnRH secretion in normal women (15). Variable doses of the antagonist were administered to normal women in the EFP and late follicular phase (LFP), in the early luteal phase, and at the midcycle surge when baseline LH levels were at least 2 SEMs above mean late follicular phase LH

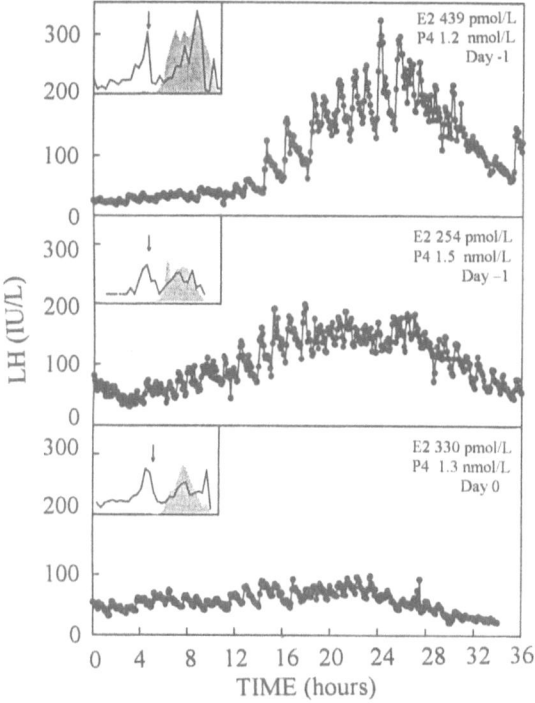

FIGURE 7.5. Pulsatile LH secretion across the midcycle surge in three individual studies. Daily values for estradiol (solid line) and progesterone (shaded area) shown as insets in each panel indicate that each cycle was ovulatory despite considerable interindividual variation in amplitude of the midcycle surge. The day of the frequent sampling study is indicated by the arrow in relation to the sex steroid levels (inset). Reprinted, with permission, from Ref. 12 © The Endocrine Society.

values. Maximal percent inhibition of LH secretion occurred approximately 8 hours after antagonist administration and reached 80% suppression at the highest dose (150 μg/kg). There was a consistently greater degree of LH inhibition by GnRH antagonism at the midcycle surge at submaximal degrees of GnRH receptor blockade than at other phases of the menstrual cycle in normal women (Fig. 7.9). At submaximal doses, a competitive binding situation should occur, allowing a semi-quantitative estimate of the amount of endogenous GnRH available for receptor binding to be derived in comparison to a baseline physiologic state. Thus, the observed leftward shift of the dose–response relationship to GnRH receptor blockade compared with other cycle stages suggests that the overall amount of GnRH secreted at the midcycle surge is *less* than it is at other cycle stages. Thus, the antagonist data again demonstrates the importance of increased pituitary sensitivity to GnRH at the midcycle.

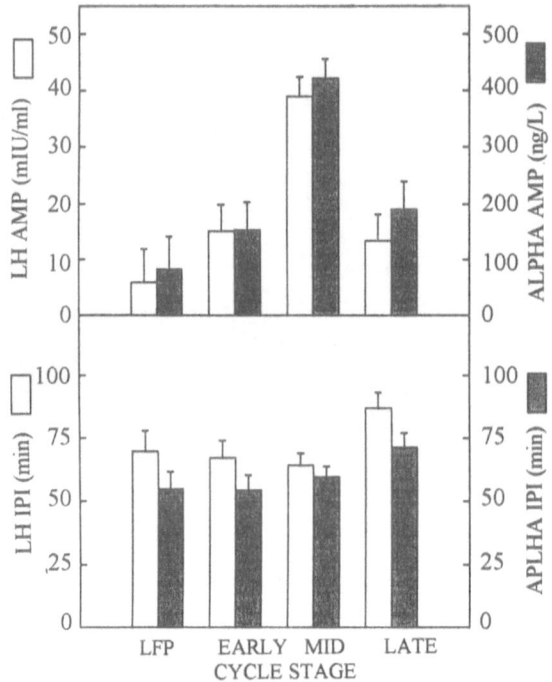

FIGURE 7.6. Amplitude (upper panel) and interpulse interval (lower panel) of LH (open bars) and free α subunit (filled bars) during the LFP and the early, mid-, and late portions of the midcycle surge, expressed as mean±SE. The mean pulse amplitude of both LH and free α subunit increased significantly from the LFP and early portion of the surge to the midportion of the surge, and decreased significantly from the mid- to the late portion of the surge. There was no difference in the interpulse interval of LH or free α subunit between the LFP and the early and midportions of the surge. There was, however, a significant slowing of pulse frequency from the mid- to the late portion of the surge. Reprinted, with permission, from Ref. 12 © The Endocrine Society.

To validate this indirect method of assessing the quantity of GnRH secretion using another experimental model, we then studied seven GnRH-deficient women during two cycles of a physiologic regimen of intravenous pulsatile GnRH therapy to induce ovulation (20). In the control cycle, 75 ng/kg/bolus of GnRH was administered throughout the cycle using the physiologic frequencies described earlier. In a second cycle, the bolus dose of GnRH was decreased by one-half log order to 25 ng/kg/bolus just prior to the LH surge, and returned to 75 ng/kg/bolus after ovulation was documented. Consistent with our hypothesis that the amount of GnRH is decreased at the human midcycle surge, the peak LH level did not differ between the control and decreased GnRH (77.4±9.7 vs. 67.5±17.6 IU/L), and all cycles were ovu-

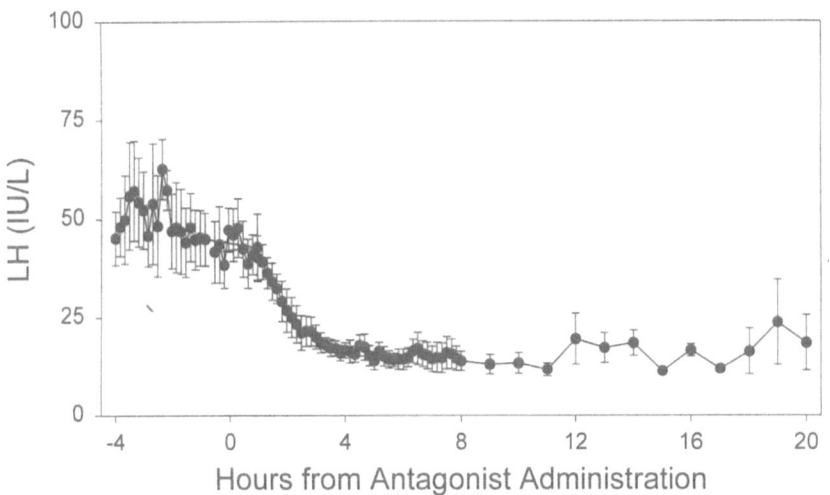

FIGURE 7.7. LH before and after administration of the Nal–Glu GnRH antagonist at a dose of 150 µg/kg in three normal women at the onset of the midcycle surge. Modified from Ref. 15, with permission.

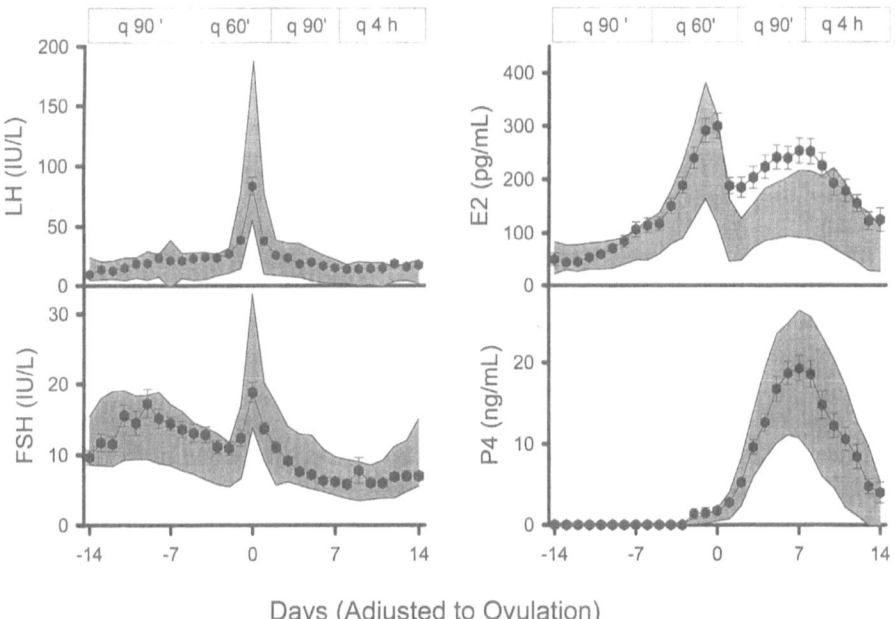

FIGURE 7.8. Estradiol, progesterone, LH, and FSH levels (± SEM) from daily blood samples in 48 GnRH-deficient women (filled circles) receiving physiologic pulsatile GnRH therapy at 75 ng/kg, compared with the mean ± SD of 118 spontaneous normal menstrual cycles (shaded areas).

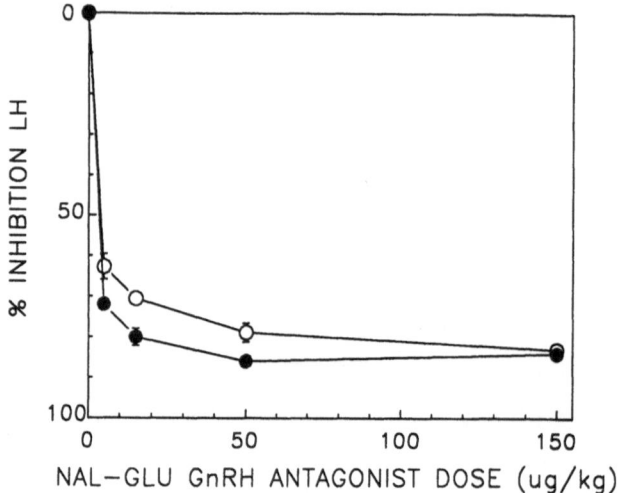

FIGURE 7.9. Maximum percent inhibition of LH in response to the Nal-Glu GnRH antagonist at doses of 5, 15, 50, and 150 μg/kg. Data for the early follicular phase, late follicular phase, and early luteal phase have been combined (open circles) as there was no difference between the dose–response curves for these cycle phases. There was signficantly greater inhibition of LH at submaximal dose at the midcycle surge (filled circles). Where not obvious, the SE is included in the symbol. From Ref. 15, with permission.

latory, (Fig. 7.10). There was no difference in the peak serum estradiol level, follicular phase length, or progesterone level on day 6 of the luteal phase. In addition, three pregnancies were achieved in each of the control and reduced-GnRH cycles. We concluded that a decreased overall amount of exogenous GnRH generates a normal midcycle gonadotropin surge in GnRH-deficient women and has no significant impact on luteal phase adequacy or fertility, providing further evidence that a reduction in endogenous hypothalamic GnRH secretion may occur at the midcycle in normal women.

Midcycle Levels of Sex Steroids Are Insufficient to Replicate the Surge

Once an increase in pituitary sensitivity to GnRH was established as the major determinant of the human midcycle surge, we wished to understand more clearly the role of positive feedback from ovarian steroids. Experimental evidence had previously demonstrated that exogenous estradiol administration to normal women in the early follicular phase could induce an increase in both basal and GnRH-stimulated LH release that was both dose- and time-dependent (21–24). Other evidence suggested that a small amount of proges-

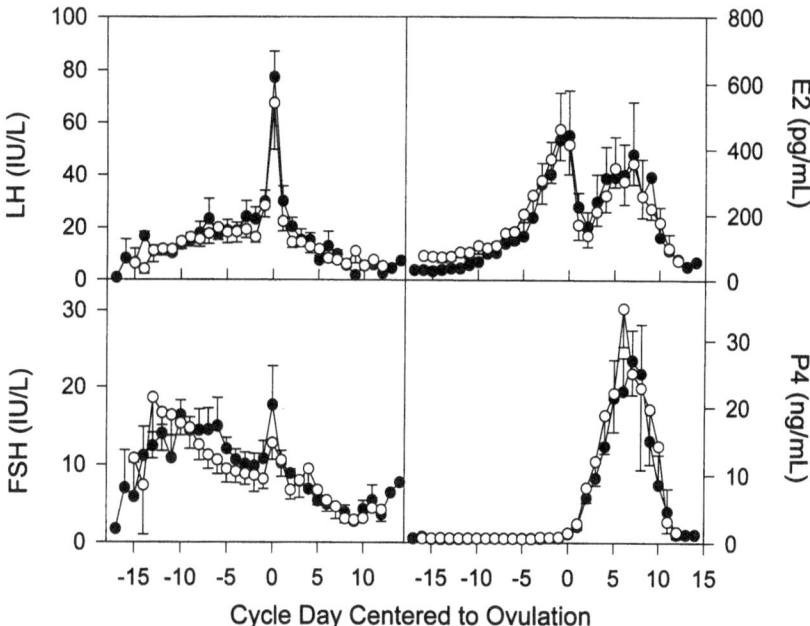

FIGURE 7.10. LH, FSH, estradiol, and progesterone levels (± SEM) in control cycles (filled circles) and cycles in which the dose of GnRH was reduced from 75 to 25 ng/kg at the surge (open circles) in five subjects centered to ovulation. There is no significant difference in the levels of gonadotropins or sex steroids at any time between the two cycles. LH, FSH, estradiol, and progesterone levels during the luteal phase after day +7 reflect only two subjects in each group due to the occurrence of pregnancies. Reprinted from Ref. 20, with permission.

terone could augment this estradiol-induced surge (25). In previous studies, however, the LH responses to exogenous steroids were variable depending on the dose, duration, and form of estrogen administered. In addition, estrogen levels were either not measured or not matched to those of normal women, and LH responses were not compared with normal. We reasoned that if estradiol and progesterone in appropriate doses are the only factors required to induce the normal surge, then administration of physiologic levels of sex steroids to normal women in the absence of a dominant follicle should reproduce all the characteristics of the spontaneous surge.

Stepwise steroid infusions (24) were initiated between 5 and 7 days after the onset of menses in eighteen normal female volunteers (26). A pelvic ultrasound examination was performed at admission and at the completion of the study to verify the absence of a dominant follicle (<12 mm) whose presence would obscure interpretation of the results. In subjects unable to have an ultrasound, lack of a dominant follicle was assumed by a baseline estradiol level below 40 pg/mL. All subjects had blood sampled every 4 hours throughout the study. Results were compared with daily blood samples across the menstrual cycle in 118 normal women. In all subjects, estradiol was infused starting at 1330 hours on the day of admission, increasing incrementally every 12 hours for the first 36 hours, then remaining constant for the next 60 hours, for a total duration of 96 hours. This resulted in serum estradiol levels that precisely matched those obtained on days –3–0 of the spontaneous men-

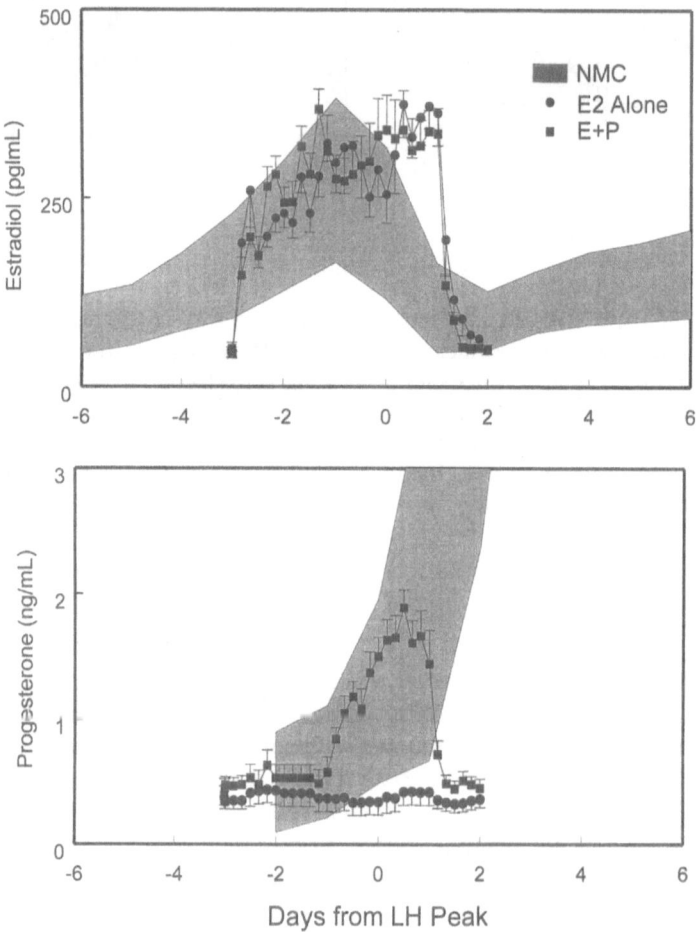

FIGURE 7.11. Mean and 1 SE of estradiol (top) and progesterone (bottom) levels in women who received steroid infusions. The serum sex-steroid levels achieved match those observed at the time of the spontaneous LH surge in 118 normal menstrual cycles. The normal menstrual cycle data is aligned with the induced surge data by centering the day of the spontaneous surge on an average surge time of 72 hours in the infused subjects. Reprinted, with permission, from Ref. 26 © The Endocrine Society.

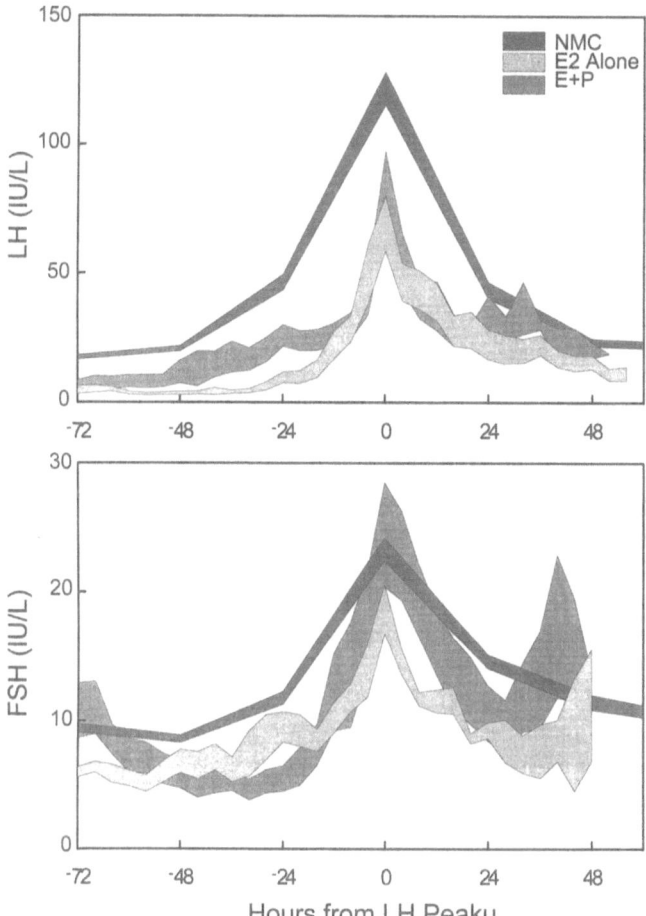

FIGURE 7.12. One SE above and below mean peak LH (top) and FSH (bottom) levels in women who received steroid infusions compared with levels in normal women. Data are centered by time of peak LH. Reprinted, with permission, from Ref. 26 © The Endocrine Society.

strual cycle (Fig. 7.11). In nine subjects, an incremental infusion of progesterone was added from 48 to 96 hours, and serum progesterone matched those from days –2 to +1 of the normal cycle (Fig. 7.11).

All subjects demonstrated both early negative feedback of estradiol on LH levels within 4 hours after initiation of the infusion, and later positive feedback. There was considerable variability in the LH responses, especially in those receiving estradiol alone. The peak LH occurred at 96.0±5.5 hours in those receiving estradiol alone, and at 70.2±1.2 hours in those receiving estradiol plus progesterone ($p < 0.001$). When LH values were centered on the maximum for each individual, there was no significant difference in peak LH levels between the two groups (Fig. 7.12). LH peaks of both groups, however, were significantly lower than were those of the normal menstrual cycle ($p < 0.05$ for estradiol infusions alone and $p < 0.005$ for estradiol plus progesterone infusions). When FSH was centered to the day of the LH peak, the FSH peaks tended to be lower than normal with estradiol alone ($p = 0.07$); however, were indistinguishable from normal during estradiol plus progesterone infusions. In four additional subjects who received both estradiol and progesterone, the estradiol infusion rate was decreased 8 hours before the expected LH peak in an attempt to mimic the fall in estradiol seen immediately before the LH peak in normally menstruating women. This manipulation was unable to restore a normal amplitude to the midcycle LH peak. Thus, the addition of small amounts of progesterone to physiologic levels of estradiol is able to induce a normal FSH surge and improve the synchronization of the induced LH surge; however, gonadal sex steroids alone fail to stimulate a normal midcycle surge of LH.

The inability of physiologic estradiol and progesterone to induce a normal midcycle LH peak in normal women suggests several alternative explanations. The fact that the FSH surge is normal suggests that the sex steroids are able to maintain normal hypothalamic GnRH dynamics, but that the missing factor has a pituitary site of action that is specific for LH. Although it is possible that the duration and pattern of achieved estradiol levels did not exactly match the slower increase observed in the normal menstrual cycle, some normal women certainly achieve normal LH surges despite similarly short spontaneous follicular phases (27). Some evidence suggests an alternate hypothesis that the growing follicle secretes a surge-inhibiting factor (28), which could have been present in our mid-follicular phase subjects but which cannot yet be measured in serum. Our major hypothesis is that the normal dominant follicle secretes another factor at the midcycle that augments the LH surge. An attractive candidate for such a factor is dimeric inhibin A, which begins to rise in serum approximately five days before the midcycle LH peak, reaching a plateau in the midluteal phase (Fig. 7.1) (29). This hypothesis is particularly intriguing given evidence that inhibin increases the LH response to GnRH in sheep pituitary cells as well as increasing GnRH binding and GnRH receptor number and expression (30), with further augmentation by estradiol (31). Inhibin-immunized sheep have a decreased LH response to GnRH (32). In summary, we hypothesize that sex steroids are sufficient to induce a normal midcycle GnRH response and a normal pituitary FSH response, but that another ovarian factor is required for normal LH priming and release at the midcycle.

Conclusions

The combination of a large database of normal menstrual cycles from rigorously defined reproductive-age women in combination with replacement studies in women with GnRH deficiency and interventional studies with a GnRH antagonist and with sex-steroid infusions has permitted us carefully to delineate the features of the normal midcycle surge in the intact human. Our studies have confirmed several important observations about the human midcycle surge. In contrast to evidence for the monkey, sheep, and rat, the midcycle surge in humans appears to occur without either an increase in GnRH pulse frequency or an increase in the total amount of GnRH. Thus, it must reflect entirely an increase in pituitary sensitivity to GnRH. The sex steroid infusion studies demonstrate that the normally rising ovarian sex steroids estradiol and progesterone are insufficient to explain completely the increase in pituitary sensitivity, which could require another ovarian factor (e.g., inhibin). This complex neuroendocrine phenomenon is critical for normal oocyte maturation, follicle rupture, and fertility. The difference between results in human and animal models, unfortunately, suggests that animal models will not always be useful in understanding difficult aspects of this most important moment in the menstrual cycle.

References

1. Levine JE, Norman RL, Gliessman PM, Oyama TT, Bangsberg DR, Spies HG. In vivo gonadotropin-releasing homrone release and serum luteinizing hormone measurements in ovariectomized, estrogen-treated rhesus macaques. Endocrinology 1985;117:711–21.

2. O'Byrne KT, Thalabard J-C, Grosser PM, Wilson RC, Williams CL, Chen M-D, et al. Radiotelemetric monitoring of hypothalamic gonadotropin-releasing hormone pulse generator activity throughout the menstrual cycle of the rhesus monkey. Endocrinology 1991;129:1207–14.

3. Clarke IJ, Thomas GB, Yao B, Cummins JT. GnRH secretion throughout the ovine estrous cycle. Neuroendocrinology 1987;46:82–88.

4. Levine JE, Bauer-Dantoin AC, Besecke LM, Conaghan LA, Legan SSJ, Meredith JM, et al. Neuroendocrine regulation of the luteinizing hormone-releasing hormone pulse generator in the rat. Rec Prog Horm Res 1991;47:97–153.

5. Belchetz PE, Plant TM, Nakai Y, Keogh EJ, Knobil E. Hypophysial responses to continuous and intermittent delivery of hypothalamic gonadotropin-releasing hormone. Science 1978;202:631–33.

6. Knobil E, Plant TM, Wildt L, Belchetz PE, Marshall G. Control of the rhesus monkey menstrual cycle: permissive role of hypothalamic gonadotropin-releasing hormone. Science 1980;207:1371–73.

7. Santoro N, Filicori M, Crowley WF Jr. Hypogonadotropic disorders in men and women: diagnosis and therapy with pulsatile gonadotropin-releasing hormone. Endocrinol Rev 1986;7:11–23.

8. Filicori M, Santoro N, Merriam GR, Crowley WF Jr. Characterization of the physiological pattern of episodic gonadotropin secretion throughout the human menstrual cycle. J Clin Endocrinol Metab 1986;62:1136–44.

9. Gougeon A. Dynamics of follicular growth in the human: A model from preliminary results. Human Reprod 1986;1:81–87.

10. Batista MC, Cartledge TP, Zellmer AW, Nieman LK, Merriam GR, Loriaux DL. Evidence for a critical role of progesterone in the regulation of the midcycle gonadotropin surge and ovulation. J Clin Endocrinol Metab 1992;74:565–70.

11. O'Dea LSL, Finkelstein JS, Schoenfeld DA, Butler JP, Crowley WF Jr. Interpulse

interval of GnRH stimulation independently modulates LH secretion. Am J Physiol 1989;256:E510–15.

12. Adams JM, Taylor AE, Schoenfeld DA, Crowley WF Jr, Hall JE. The midcycle gonadotropin surge in normal women occurs in the face of an unchanging gonadotropin-releasing hormone pulse frequency. J Clin Endocrinol Metab 1994;79:858–64.

13. Crowley WF Jr, Filicori M, Spratt DI, Santoro NF. The physiology of gonadotropin-releasing hormone (GnRH) secretion in men and women. Rec Prog Horm Res 1985;41:473–525.

14. Filicori M, Flamigni C, Crowley WF Jr. The critical role of blood sampling frequency in the estimation of episodic luteinizing hormone secretion in normal women. In: The episodic secretion of hormones. Crowley WF Jr, Hofler JG, eds. New York: John Wiley; 1987:5–13.

15. Hall JE, Taylor AE, Martin KA, Rivier J, Schoenfeld D, Crowley WF Jr. Decreased release of gonadotropin-releasing hormone during the preovulatory midcycle luteinizing hormone surge in normal women. Proc Natl Acad Sci USA 1994;91: 6894–98.

16. Dubourdieu S, Charbonnel B, D'Acremont M-F, Carreau S, Spitz IM, Bouchard P. Effect of administration of a gonadotropin-releasing hormone (GnRH) antagonist (Nal-Glu) during the periovulatory period: the luteinizing hormone surge requires secretion of GnRH. J Clin Endocrinol Metab 1994;78:343–47.

17. Leroy I, d'Acremont M, Brailly-Tabard S, Frydman R, de Mouzon J, Bouchard P. A single injection of a gonadotropin-releasing hormone (GnRH) antagonist (Cetrorelix) postpones the luteinizing hormone (LH) surge: further evidence for the role of GnRH during the LH surge. Fertil Steril 1994;62:461–67.

18. Santoro N, Wierman ME, Filicori M, Waldstreicher J, Crowley WF Jr. Intravenous administration of pulsatile gonadotropin-releasing hormone in hypothalamic amenorrhea: Effects of dosage. J Clin Endocrinol Metab 1986;62:109–16.

19. Martin K, Santoro N, Hall J, Filicori M, Wierman M, Crowley WF Jr. Management of ovulatory disorders with pulsatile gonadotropin-releasing hormone. J Clin Endocrinol Metab 1990;71:1081A–G.

20. Martin KA, Welt CK, Taylor AE, Smith JA, Crowley WF Jr, Hall JE. Is GnRH reduced at the midcycle surge in the human? Evidence from a GnRH-deficient model. Neuroendocrinology 1998;67:363–69.

21. Monroe SE, Jaffe RB, Midgley AR Jr. Regulation of human gonadotropins. XII. Increase in serum gonadotropins in response to estradiol. J Clin Endocrinol Metab 1972;34:342–47.

22. Yen SSC, Tsai CC. Acute gonadotropin release induced by exogenous estradiol during the mid-follicular phase of the menstrual cycle. J Clin Endocrinol Metab 1972;34:298–305.

23. Young JR, Jaffe RB. Strength-duration characteristics of estrogen effects on gonadotropin response to gonadotropin-releasing hormone in women. II. Effects of varying concentrations of estradiol. J Clin Endocrinol Metab 1976;42:432–42.

24. Liu JH, Yen SSC. Induction of midcycle gonadotropin surge by ovarian steroids in women: a critical evaluation. J Clin Endocrinol Metab 1983;57:797–802.

25. Chang RJ, Jaffe RB. Progesterone effects on gonadotropin release in women pretreated with estradiol. J Clin Endocrinol Metab 1978;47:119–25.

26. Taylor AE, Whitney H, Hall JE, Martin K, Crowley WF. Midcycle levels of sex steroids are sufficient to recreate the follicle-stimulating hormone but not the luteinizing

hormone midcycle surge: Evidence for the contribution of other ovarian factors to the surge in normal women. J Clin Endocrinol Metab 1995;80:1541–47.

27. Sherman BM, West JH, Korenman SG. The menopausal transition: analysis of LH, FSH, estradiol and progesterone concentrations during menstrual cycles of older women. J Clin Endocrinol Metab 1976;42:629.

28. Busbridge NJ, Chamberlain GVP, Griffiths A, Whitehead SA. Non-steroidal follicular factors attenuate the self-priming action of gonadotropin-releasing hormone on the pituitary gonadotroph. Neuroendocrinology 1990;51:493–99.

29. Lambert-Messerlian GM, Hall JE, Sluss PE, Taylor AE, Martin KA, Groome NP, et al. Relatively low levels of dimeric inhibin circulate in men and women with polycystic ovary syndrome using a specific two-site enzyme-linked immunosorbent assay. J Clin Endocrinol Metab 1994;79:45–50.

30. Laws SC, Beggs MJ, Webster JC, Miller WL. Inhibin increases and progesterone decreases receptors for gonadotropin-releasing hormone in ovine pituitary culture. Endocrinology 127:373–80.

31. Laws SC, Webster JC, Miller WL. Estradiol alters the effectiveness of gonadotropin-releasing hormone (GnRH) in ovine pituitary cultures: GnRH receptors versus responsiveness to GnRH. Endocrinology 1990;127:381–86.

32. Wrathall JH, McLeod BJ, Glencross RG, Beard AJ, Knight PG. Inhibin immuno-neutralizaiton by antibodies raised against synthetic peptide sequences of inhibin alpha subunit: effects on gonadotrophin concentrations and ovulation rate in sheep. J Endocrinol 1990;124:167–76.

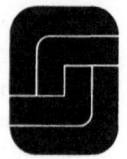

8

Duration, Amplitude, and Specificity of the Midcycle Gonadotropin Surge in Nonhuman Primates

MARY B. ZELINSKI-WOOTEN, YASMIN A. CHANDRASEKHER, AND RICHARD L. STOUFFER

Introduction

The midcycle luteinizing hormone (LH) surge signals key changes within the mature, preovulatory follicle,including resumption of oocyte meiosis, luteinization of the follicle wall, ovulation, and early development of the corpus luteum (1). The duration of the LH surge during normal ovarian cycles is considerably longer (48 hours) in women (2) and rhesus monkeys (3) compared with many nonprimate species (rats and rabbits, 4–6 hours; sheep and cattle, 10–16 hours). The concept that surge requirements vary for periovulatory events has emerged from studies in nonprimate species with resumption of oocyte meiosis requiring less LH exposure than that for optimal luteal development (4–6).

Follicular stimulation protocols in women and nonhuman primates routinely include a pharmacologic bolus of human chorionic gonadotropin (hCG) to mimic the LH surge, thereby initiating periovulatory events in vitro fertilization (IVF)-related cycles. Due in part to its long half-life in the circulation, a large bolus of hCG has a longer duration (7,8) than the typical 48-hours surge in a normal, spontaneous menstrual cycle. The long circulating half-life of hCG presents several clinical disadvantages that include a major concern for increased risk of ovarian hyperstimulation syndrome (8). In nonprimate species oocyte maturation can be attained with doses of LH/hCG that correspond to lower amplitudes of the endogenous gonadotropin surge than those required for follicular rupture (4–6). Supraphysiologic doses of hCG induce ovulatory maturation in IVF-related cycles in women (9), but prospective dose-ranging studies to evaluate the relationship between injected dose of hCG and occurrence of LH/hCG-dependent periovulatory events have only more recently been conducted in primates (9). Understanding the optimal duration and amplitude of the gonadotropin surge required for periovulatory events in primates is necessary to devise methods that produce a more physiogical surge in IVF-related cycles and decrease risk of ovarian hyperstimulation syndrome.

Although the midcycle gonadotropin surge in women (2) and nonhuman primates (3) includes a rise in circulating levels of both follicle stimulating hormone (FSH) as well as LH, the physiological events occurring in the ovulatory follicle are attributed mainly to LH. However, data in rodents treated with recombinant (r) FSH, devoid of LH activity, as a midcycle stimulus confirmed follicle rupture can occur in the absence of a LH surge (10; see Chap. 9). The efficacy of FSH relative to LH/CG for induction of periovulatory events has also been compared in primates (11).

In search of a means to induce a more physiologic gonadotropin surge following follicular stimulation–IVF-related protocols, a series of prospective studies in nonhuman primates evaluated the relationship between the duration, amplitude and specificity of the gonadotropin surge and the induction of periovulatory events (e.g., reinitiation of oocyte meiotic maturation, IVF, granulosa cell luteinization, and subsequent corpus luteum function). Results of these studies will be summarized in this chapter.

Titrating the Duration of the Midcycle Gonadotropin Surge: Does the Interval Vary for Different Periovulatory Events?

Studies in adult rhesus monkeys were conducted to determine the duration of the LH surge elicited endogenously with native gonadotropin releasing hormone (GnRH) or GnRH agonists (12,13), or exogenously with human LH/CG (14) and its relationship to the resumption of oocyte meiosis, oocyte fertilizability, early events in granulosa cell luteinization, and corpus luteum function. Animals received exogenous urinary (u) gonadotropins (hFSH [Metrodin] ± hLH [Pergonal], Serono Laboratories, Inc., Norwell, MA) to promote development of multiple large antral follicles, followed by (1) no ovulatory stimulus; (2) a single injection of 100 µg GnRH (Relisorm, Serono Laboratories, Inc.), three injections of GnRH at 3-hours intervals or two injections of 50 µg of the GnRH agoinist, leuprolide acetate (Lupron, TAP Pharmaceutical, North Chicago, IL) to induce endogenous LH surges; (3) a single or two injections (18 h apart) of r-hLH (2500 IU; Laboratoires Serono SA, Aubonne, Switzerland); or (4) a standard ovulatory dose of u-hCG (1000 IU; Profasi; Serono Laboratories, Inc.). Follicles were aspirated to obtain oocytes and granulosa cells 27 hours after the last gonadotropin injection in animals receiving no ovulatory stimulus, following the initial GnRH/GnRH agonist and r-hLH injection, and post-hCG. Circulating levels of bioactive LH/CG levels were determined at various intervals postinjection, and steroids were measured daily during the treatment cycle. In these studies, a surge was defined as ≥100 ng/ml of circulating bioactive LH, which are concentrations known to saturate LH receptors on macaque ovarian cells.

A single injection of GnRH elicited a gonadotropin surge of 4–6 hours, which could be extended to 8–10 hours or longer than 14 hours by multiple injections of GnRH or GnRH agonist, respectively. Comparable to animals receiving no ovulatory stimulus, oocytes aspirated from these groups typically had not resumed meiosis, granulosa cells produced little progesterone during short-term culture, and a functional luteal phase wherein serum progesterone levels rose above baseline was absent (Table 8.1). In contrast, a single injection of hLH generated an 18- to 24-hour surge that caused resumption of meiosis and granulosa cell luteinization; although serum progesterone levels were elevated within 24 hours, peak levels and the duration of the luteal phase was subnormal (Table 8.1). Gonadotropin surges longer than 36–48 hours generated by two injections of 2500 IU hLH as well as 1000 IU u-hCG resulted in comparable proportions of oocytes resuming meiosis and undergoing IVF, as well as luteal phases displaying normal duration (Table 8.1). Peak progesterone levels, however, tended to be lower and to decline prematurely following two injections of r-hLH relative to u-hCG.

These data suggest that LH exposure reminiscent of gonadotropin surges in rodents (4–8 hours) and domestic animals (10–16 hours) is insufficient to initiate periovulatory events in primates. A surge interval half (18–24 hours) that in the normal, spontaneous menstrual cycle stimulates oocyte meiosis but fails to sustain development and function of the corpus luteum, whereas a surge duration (36 hours) approaching that in spontaneous menstrual cycles elicited normal levels and pattern of progesterone production during the luteal phase. Titration of LH surge requirements in macaques supports the concept derived from nonprimate species (4,5) that surge requirements vary for periovulatory events, with resumption of meiosis requiring less LH exposure than that for optimal luteal development. Studies in the rat (6) propose that the duration, rather than the amplitude, of the LH surge is most critical for ovulatory events. The surge requirements for bona fide ovulation of primate follicles awaits investigation.

Evaluating the Amplitude of the Midcycle Gonadotropin Surge: Are Supraphysiologic Doses of hCG Required for Periovulatory Events?

A prospective study was performed in gonadotropin-treated rhesus monkeys to alter the amplitude of the LH surge using various doses of hCG (9). Animals

TABLE 8.1. Periovulatory events following midcycle gonadotropin surges of various durations during IVF-related cycles in rhesus monkeys.[a]

Ovulatory stimulus	Surge duration (h)	Oocyte maturation (% MI + MII)[b]	Fertilization (%)[c]	In vitro P production (ng/ml)[d]	PR (%)[e]	Luteal phase (days)[f]
None	0	0[g]	0	19	–	0
GnRH, 100 µg × 1	6	0	0	35	–	0
GnRH, 100 µg × 3	10	0[g]	0	61	–	0
GnRH agonist	+14	12	0	105	–	0
r-hLH, 2500 IU × 1	18–24	67	26	300	+/–	1–6
r-hLH, 2500 IU × 2	36–48	75	26	300	+	8–18
u-hCG, 1000 IU	>48	86	50	450	+	11–13

[a]Adapted from Ref. 12–14.
[b]Percentage of total cohort retrieved as metaphase I or II (MI + MII).
[c]Number of oocytes fertilized/number inseminated.
[d]Basal progesterone production by granulosa cells over 24 hours.
[e]Based on percentage of granulosa cells exhibiting nuclear staining for progesterone receptor; – = none, + = detected.
[f]Interval of circulating progesterone > 1 ng/ml from the ovulatory stimulus to menses.
[g]One animal in the no ovulatory stimulus and GnRH × 3 groups exhibited an endogenous LH surge such that some periovulatory events (i.e., oocyte maturation) were observed. Typical responses are indicated in the table.

received the GnRH antagonist Antide (Laboratoires Serono SA) daily beginning at midluteal phase of a spontaneous menstrual cycle through the day of the ovulatory stimulus to prevent an endogenous LH surge. After 7 days of Antide, animals received r-hFSH (Gonal-F, 30 IU, twice daily, IM) until ultrasound revealed ≥6 preovulatory follicles. The following morning, animals received a single, IM injection of 100 IU, 300 IU or 1000 IU, r-hCG (Laboratoires Serono SA), or 1000 IU u-hCG (Profasi, Serono Laboratories). Oocytes and granulosa cells were collected via follicle aspiration 27 hours post-hCG injection. Circulating levels of bioactive hCG were determined at various intervals post-injection, and steroids were measured daily during the treatment cycle.

A dose-dependent increase in the amplitude of the gonadotropin surge following r-hCG was observed (100 < 300 < 1000 IU; Table 8.2). Following 100 IU r-hCG, the surge amplitude achieved at 2 hours (75 ng/ml) was less than the peak values of 300 ng/ml typically observed during the spontaneous midcycle LH surge during the normal menstrual cycle in rhesus monkeys (15). The surge amplitude 2 hours after 300 IU r-hCG (270 ng/ml) was equivalent to that of the spontaneous LH surge; it was exceeded following administration of 1000 IU r- or u-hCG (824 and 1267 ng/ml, respectively). Although the peak level of bioactive hCG at 2 hours following 1000 IU u-hCG was ≈40% less than that after 1000 IU r-hCG, this was consistent with evidence that less in vitro bioactivity was administered (9). The dose of hCG injected was also proportional to the duration of "surge" concentrations (≥ 100 ng/ml) of bioactive hCG (0 hours, 100 IU; 24 hours, 300 IU; >48 hours 1000 IU r- and u-hCG; Table 8.2). The shortened surge of bioactive hCG following 300 IU is reminiscent of those previously observed after three injections of GnRH (12) or a single injection of either u- (7,14) or r-LH (14), whereas 1000 IU r- and u-hCG elicited surge durations equivalent to that of the normal menstrual cycle.

Some periovulatory responses were similar following administration of 3–10-fold lower doses of hCG relative to 1000 IU hCG. Proportions of oocytes resuming meiosis to MI as well continuing meiosis to MII in vivo (Table 8.2), fertilization rates (Table 8.2) and promotion of granulosa cell luteinization (Table 8.3), assessed by acute progesterone production in vitro and progesterone receptor expression, were comparable among doses. Notable dose-related differences in ovarian responses were also observed. Fewer animals yielded fertilizable oocytes following 100 and 300 IU r-hCG compared with 1000 IU r- or u-hCG, despite retrieval of mature oocytes at the lower doses (Table 8.2). Perhaps the lower doses are insufficient to promote final maturation of a cohort of follicles to sizes amenable to oocyte aspiration and cytoplasmic maturation of oocytes necessary for fertilization. The development and function of corpora lutea also differed among doses (Table 8.3). Although peak levels of serum progesterone were similar, they declined 2 days earlier during midluteal phase after 100 and 300 IU relative to 1000 IU

TABLE 8.2. Pharmacokinetic parameters, oocyte maturation and fertilization and periovulatory events after increasing doses of r- and u-hCG administered at midcycle in gonadotropin-stimulated rhesus monkeys.[a]

Dose (IU) of r- or u-hCG	Surge amplitude (ng/ml)[b]	t_{max} (h)[c]	Surge duration (h)	Oocyte recovery (%)[d]	Oocyte maturation (% MI + MII)[e]	IVF/animal[f]	Fertilization (%)[g]
100 r-hCG	106 ± 5[h]	2 (2-8)	0	49 ± 5[h]	94	3/5	34 ± 20
300 r-hCG	266 ± 135[i]	4 (2-8)	24	51 ± 16[h,i]	88	2/4	25 ± 15
1000 r-hCG	1588 ± 633[j]	4 (4-6)	48	90 ± 23[i]	88	4/5	50 ± 17
1000 u-hCG	1113 ± 366[j]	6 (2-8)	48	76 ± 11[i]	89	5/5	50 ± 18

[a]Derived from Ref. 9.

[b]C_{max}; maximum concentration of bioactive hCG; mean ± SD.

[c]Time from administration of r- or u-hCG at which C_{max} was observed; median followed by range in parentheses.

[d]Number of oocytes recovered/total number of follicles observed; mean ± SEM.

[e]Percentage of total cohort collected at metaphase I and II (MI + MII).

[f]Number of animals yielding oocytes that fertilized in vitro/total number of animals per group.

[g]Number of oocytes fertilized/number of oocytes inseminated; mean ± SEM.

[h,i,j]Values with different superscripts differ significantly ($p < 0.05$) within column (event) between rows (dose).

TABLE 8.3. Granulosa cell luteinization and corpus luteum function following increasing doses of hCG administered at midcycle in gonadotropin-treated rhesus monkeys.[a]

Dose (IU) of of r- or u-hCG	In vitro P production (ng/ml)[b]	PR (%)[c]	Peak levels of P in vivo (ng/ml)	Duration of peak P (days)	Luteal phase (days)
100 r-hCG	916 ± 197	73 ± 5	24 ± 7	2	11
300 r-hCG	547 ± 209	81 ± 6	37 ± 10	2	11
1000 r-hCG	530 ± 159	67 ± 4	26 ± 9	4	11
1000 u-hCG	620 ± 186	76 ± 8	22 ± 6	4	12

[a]Derived from Ref. 9.
[b]Basal progesterone production by granulosa cells over 24 hours; mean ± SEM.
[c]Percentage of cells with positive nuclear staining for progesterone receptor; mean ± SEM.

r- or u-hCG, which may be related to the lower amplitude and duration (≤ 24 hours) of circulating bioactive hCG levels at the lower doses relative to 1000 IU hCG.

Our previous studies presumed that the "surge" level (i.e., the amplitude of circulating bioactive LH required for initiation of periovulatory events) was ≥ 100 ng/ml (7,12–14; see earlier); however, results from the dose-ranging study indicate that our previous definition of the minimal amplitude of the LH surge in macaques is incorrect. Circulating bioactive hCG levels of ≤ 75 ng/ml observed after injection of 100 IU r-hCG promoted oocyte maturation, fertilization, and granulosa cell luteinization comparable to hCG levels ≥ 100 ng/ml elicited by 300 and 1000 IU hCG. The inability of a 10-hour exposure to 100 ng/ml LH to elicit optimal oocyte maturation (12) and granulosa cell luteinization (13) following 3 injections of GnRH in macaques may be related to the pulsatile pattern of endogenous LH secretion during the surge, relative to maintenance of constant amounts of bioactive hCG produced after injection or 100 IU r-hCG. Although similar fertilization rates were achieved following 3–10-fold lower doses of r-hCG, it remains to be determined whether attenuated LH surges of low or normal amplitude are optimal for early embryogenesis and production of live offspring.

In summary, the amplitude and duration of the LH/hCG surge in gonadotropin-stimulated macaques following midcycle injection with 100, 300, or 1000 IU r-hCG or 1000 IU u-hCG increased proportionately with the dose of hCG injected. Whereas attenuated surges of ≤ 24 hour elicited by 3–10-fold lower doses of r-hCG reinitiate oocyte meiosis and promote granulosa cell luteinization, surges of higher amplitude and/or longer duration (> 48 hours) may be required for optimal oocyte recovery and fertilization as well as normal luteal function in primates.

Specificity of the Midcycle Gonadotropin Surge: Can FSH Substitute for hCG to Induce Periovulatory Events?

The efficacy of pure FSH to induce periovulatory events when administered as a bolus at midcycle was evaluated in comparison to a standard ovulatory bolus of hCG (11). In this study, Antide was administered as described earlier. Animals received r-hFSH (Gonal-F, 30 IU, twice daily, IM) until ultrasound revealed ≥6 preovulatory follicles. The following day, a single IM injection of either 1000 IU r-hCG (Laboratoires Serono SA) or 2500 IU r-hFSH (Laboratoires Serono SA) was administered, and follicles were aspirated 27 hours later for retrieval of oocytes and granulosa cells. Peak levels of bioactive CG were sustained for 8–12 hours, with "surge levels" evident for > 48 hours postinjection as described above. Levels of immunoreactive FSH increased from baseline within 30 miniutes postinjection, and remained at peak levels (1800 mIU/ml) for 8 hours. High FSH levels (>100 mIU/ml) were evident for 48 hours subsequent to administration.

Oocyte maturation and fertilization, as well as indexes of granulosa cell luteinization and corpus luteum function following administration of r-hCG or r-hFSH are summarized in Table 8.4. A midcycle bolus of r-hFSH was equivalent to r-hCG for the reinitiation of oocyte meiosis, fertilization, progesterone production in vitro, and progesterone receptor expression by granulosa cells. Patterns of serum progesterone levels, however, differed during the luteal

TABLE 8.4. Periovulatory events following a midcycle bolus of r-hCG (1000 IU) versus r-hFSH (2500 IU) during IVF-related cycles.[a]

	r-hCG	r-hFSH
Oocyte maturation and fertilization		
MI (%)[b]	4 4	3 6
MII (%)[b]	4 4	5 3
Overall fertilization rate (mean ± SEM)	50 ± 18	47 ± 19
Granulosa cell luteinization		
Progesterone production (ng/ml)[c]	530 ± 185	958 ± 464
Progesterone receptor (%)[d]	67 ± 9	76 ± 5
Corpus luteum function		
Progesterone on day 6 (ng/ml)	22 ± 6[e]	6 ± 3
Luteal phase length (days)	11 ± 0.2	10 ± 0.2

[a] Derived from Ref. 11.
[b] Percentage of total cohort collected at metaphase I (MI) or II (MII).
[c] Basal production in vitro over 24 hours; mean ± SEM.
[d] Percentage of cells with positive nuclear staining for progesterone receptor; mean ± SEM.
[e] $p < 0.05$ between treatments.

phase following r-hCG relative to r-hFSH. After the r-hCG bolus, peak levels of progesterone were sustained between days 4–8 of the luteal phase. They decreased to baseline thereafter. Although peak levels of progesterone achieved by day 4 were similar, progesterone declined more rapidly during mid-to-late luteal phase following the bolus of r-hFSH relative to r-hCG in a pattern reminiscent of that observed with two injections of 2500 IU r-hLH as described earlier (14). The length of the luteal phase did not differ between animals receiving a midcycle bolus r-hCG or r-hFSH.

Thus, results in nonhuman primates are consistent with those from rodent models wherein administration of FSH at midcycle can substitute for LH/CG to initiate periovulatory events (16–19; see Chap. 9). Oocytes were recovered at follicle aspiration; therefore, it is not known whether a bolus of FSH at midcycle in primates can evoke ovulation as demonstrated in rodents (10). Because FSH receptors reside exclusively on granulosa cells of the preovulatory follicle (20), granulosa cells may play a predominant role during luteinization and ovulation, with a lesser role, if any, for theca cells in promoting these events. On the other hand, a bolus of FSH at midcycle may induce granulosa cell responses that alter thecal function in a paracrine manner as shown in the rat (21). Evidence that neutralization of FSH during the follicular phase in vivo prevented in vitro responsiveness of both granulosa cells to FSH and theca cells to LH supports this mechanism in primates (22).

It is not known whether FSH and LH act in concert or are redundant signals to insure periovulatory events that occur during spontaneous ovarian cycles in primates. Our data in gonadotropin-stimulated macaques support the hypothesis that granulosa cells display different functional responses when exposed to low versus high levels of cAMP; the former stimulated primarily by FSH to evoke follicular growth, maturation, and estradiol production, and the latter to elicit periovulatory events regardless of the gonadotropin stimulus (23).

Conclusions and Clinical Considerations

These data support the concept that gonadotropin surge requirements vary for different processes within the periovulatory follicle in primates. Consistent with evidence from nonprimate species, oocyte nuclear maturation requires a LH surge of lesser duration or amplitude than that for optimal development and function of the corpus luteum. Whereas oocyte maturation occurs with surge durations < 24 hours, surges of ≥36 hours are necessary to sustain luteal development and function. Although 3–10-fold lower doses of r-hCG were sufficient to promote oocyte meiosis, optimal fertilization and luteal function may require surges of higher amplitude. Although the strength–duration of the surge necessary for follicle rupture in primates is not currently known, the temporal expression and regulation during the periovulatory interval of genes responsible for tissue remodeling (i.e., matrix metallo-proteinases and their inhibitors) will provide insight into surge requirements for ovulation as well as luteinization (see Chap. 11). It will be important to verify the surge requirements for periovulatory events derived from artificial polyovular cycles in primates undergoing spontaneous, monovular ovarian cycles. Studies designed to achieve a low amplitude surge of long (>48 hours) duration in primates are needed to test the hypothesis (6) that these characteristics are more efficacious than a high amplitude of short duration for periovulatory events and corpus luteum function.

The current studies also suggest that GnRH agonists (12,13) or r-hLH (14) could be useful alternatives to conventional hCG as a periovulatory stimulus in IVF-related follicular stimulation protocols (see Chap. 25). Stimulation of an endogenous LH surge of a duration and amplitude adequate for oocyte maturation and ovulation with GnRH agonists has been reported in women (8). As in the nonhuman primate, however, some GnRH agonist regimens provide inadequate luteotropic support for the development and maintenance of postovulatory corpora lutea and would require supplementation with LH during the luteal phase (8). GnRH agonist administration at midcycle would not be efficacious for triggering an LH surge in patients downregulated with GnRH agonist to prevent an endogenous LH surge (8). Due to its shorter half-life, a treatment regimen of r-hLH as a periovulatory stimulus must differ from that for hCG. Two injections of r-hLH were superior to a single injection with respect to increasing the number of mature oocytes collected and promoting the development and function of corpora lutea (14). Although the pattern of circulating LH differed from a spontaneous LH surge following two injec-tions of r-hLH, this regimen was more physiological in terms of the duration (48 hours) of the surge relative to that of hCG (14). Supplementation with hLH during the luteal phase should be useful in supporting the function of the corpus luteum and preventing a premature decline in progesterone levels (7) without increasing the chance for errors in detection of pregnancy initia-tion associated with hCG administration. Although induction of periovulatory events with GnRH agonist or r-hLH may provide a more physiologic LH surge, the ability of these regimens to prevent symptoms associated with ovarian hyperstimulation syndrome remains to be demonstrated.

A bolus of FSH as an ovulatory stimulus, following low-dose FSH to pro-mote multiple follicular development will result in oocyte maturation, fertili-zation, and early events in granulosa cell luteinization in primates (11). It is not clear whether the premature decline in progesterone production follow-ing the single midcycle dose of FSH tested is physiologically relevant for establishing pregnancy. Whether normal embryonic development and live offspring can be produced following ovarian stimulation solely with FSH is currently unknown. Regimens composed exclusively of FSH offer potential clinical utility for improving IVF outcome in patients with polycystic ova-rian syndrome, preventing allergic reactions to urinary preparations of FSH

(24), and alleviating infertility in women with ovarian failure due to LH insensitivity (25).

Acknowledgments. The authors thank Dr. Don Wolf and associates in the Assisted Reproductive Core Laboratory, Dr. David Hess and staff in the Endocrine Services Laboratory, and animal technicians and surgical staff of the Division of Animal Resources at the Oregon Regional Primate Research Center. The contributions of Dr. Jim Hutchison and his integral role as liaison with Ares-Serono are gratefully acknowledged. Pharmacokinetic analyses of recombinant hCG were performed by Dr. Isabel Trinchard-Lugan, Ares Serono, Geneva, Switzerland. These studies were supported by Ares Advanced Technology, Inc., Randolph, MA, a member of the Ares-Serono group of companies, and NIH HD20869 (to RLS), HD18185, and RR00163.

References

1. Stouffer RL. Corpus luteum formation and demise. In: Adashi EY, Rock JA, Rosenwaks Z, eds. Reproductive endocrinology, surgery, and technology. Philadelphia: Lippincott-Raven Publishers; 1996:251–69.
2. Hoff JD, Quigley ME, Yen SSC. Hormonal dynamics at midcycle: a reevaluation. J Clin Endocrinol Metab 1983;57:792–96.
3. Weick RF, Dierschke DJ, Karsch FJ, Butler WR, Hotchkiss J, Knobil E. Periovulatory time courses of circulating gonadotropic and ovarian hormones in the rhesus monkey. Endocrinology 1973;93:1140–47.
4. Bomsel-Helmreich O, Huyen LVN, Durand-Gasselin I. Effects of varying doses of HCG on the evolution of preovulatory rabbit follicles and oocytes. Hum Reprod 1989;4:636–42.
5. Peluso JJ. Role of the amplitude of the gonadotropin surge in the rat. Fertil Steril 1990;53:150–54.
6. Ishikawa J. Luteinizing hormone requirements for ovulation in the rat. Biol Reprod 1992;46:1144–50.
7. Zelinski-wooten MB, Hutchison JS, Aladin Chandresekher Y, Wolf DP, Stouffer RL. Administration of human luteinizing hormone (hLH) to macaques after follicular development: further titration of LH surge requirements for ovulatory changes in primate follicles. J Clin Endocrinol Metab 1992;75:502–7.
8. Shoham Z, Schachter M, Loumaye E, Weissman A, MacNamee M, Insler V. The luteinizing hormone surge—the final stage in ovulation induction: modern aspects of ovulation triggering. Fertil Steril 1995;64:237–51.
9. Zelinski-Wooten MB, Hutchison JS, Trinchard-Lugan I, Hess DL, Wolf DP, Stouffer RL. Initiation of periovulatory events in gonadotrophin-stimulated macaques with varying doses of recombinant human chorionic gonadotrophin. Hum Repod 1997;12:1877–85.
10. Galway AB, LaPolt PS, Tsafriri A, Dargan CM, Boime I, Hsueh AJW. Recombinant follicle-stimulating hormone induces ovulation and tissue plasminogen activator expression in hypophysectomized rats. Endocrinology 1990;127:3023–28.
11. Zelinski-Wooten MB, Hutchison JS, Hess DL, Wolf DP, Stouffer RL. A bolus of

recombinant human follicle stimulating hormone at midcycle induces periovulatory events following multiple follicular development in macaques. Hum Reprod 1998;13:554–60.

12. Zelinski-Wooten MB, Lanzendorf SE, Wolf DP, Aladin Chandrasekher Y, Stouffer RL. Titrating luteinizing hormone surge requirements for ovulatory changes in primate follicles. I. Oocyte maturation and corpus luteum function. J Clin Endocrinol Metab 1991;73:577–83.

13. Chandrasekher YA, Brenner RM, Molskness TA, Yu Q, Stouffer RL. Titrating luteinizing hormone surge requirements for ovulatory changes in primate follicles. II. Progesterone receptor expression in luteinizing granulosa cells. J Clin Endocrinol Metab 1991;73:584–89.

14. Chandresekher YA, Hutchison JS, Zelinski-Wooten MB, Hess DL, Wolf DP, Stouffer RL. Initiation of periovulatory events in primate follicles using recombinant and native human luteinizing hormone to mimic the midcycle gonadotropin surge. J Clin Endocrinol Metab 1994;79:298–306.

15. Pau K-Y, Berria M, Hess DL, Spies HG. Preovulatory gonadotropin-releasing hormone surge in ovarian-intact rhesus monkeys. Endocrinology 1993;133:1650–56.

16. Galway AB, Hsueh AJW, Keene JL, Yamoto M, Fauser BCJM, Boime I. In vitro and in vivo biological activity of recombinant human follicle-stimulating hormone and partially deglycosylated variants secreted by transfected eukaryotic cell lines. Endocrinology 1990;127:93–100.

17. Tapanainen JS, LaPolt PS, Perlas E, Hsueh AJW. Induction of ovarian follicle luteinization by recombinant follicle-stimulating hormone. Endocrinology 1993:2875–80.

18. Wang X-N, Greenwald GS. Human chorionic gonadotropin or human recombinant follicle stimulating hormone (FSH)-induced ovulation and subsequent fertilization and early embryo development in hypophysectomized FSH-primed mice. Endocrinology 1993;132:2009–16.

19. Montgomery-Rice VC, Zusmanis K, Malter H. Pure FSH alone induces ovulation and subsequent pregnancy in the mouse resulting in fetal development. Life Sci 1993;53:31–39.

20. Yamamoto M, Shima K, Nakano R. Gonadotropin receptors in human ovarian follicles and corpora lutea throughout the menstrual cycle. Horm Res 1992;37(suppl. 1):5–11.

21. Smyth CD, Miro F, Howles CM, Hillier SG. Effect of luteinizing hormone on follicle stimulating hormone-activated paracrine signalling in rat ovary. Hum Reprod 1995;10:33–39.

22. Selvaraj N, Moudgal NR. In vivo and in vitro studies on the differential role of luteinizing hormone and follicle-stimulating hormone in regulating follicular function in the bonnet monkey (*Macaca radiata*) using specific gonadotropin antibodies. Biol Reprod 1994;51:246–53.

23. Yong EL, Baird DT, Hillier SG. Mediation of gonadotrophin-stimulated growth and differentiation of human granulosa cells by adenosine-3′,5′-monophosphate: one molecule, two messages. Clin Endocrinol 1992;37:51–58.

24. Phipps WR, Holden D, Sheehan RK. Use of recombinant human follicle-stimulating hormone for in vitro fertilization-embryo transfer after severe systemic immunoglobulin E-mediated reaction to urofollitropin. Fertil Steril 1996;66:148–50.

25. Latronico AC, Anasti JA, Arnhold IJP, Rapaport R, Mendonca BB, Bloise W, et al. Testicular and ovarian resistance to luteinizing hormone caused by inactivating mutations of the luteinizing hormone-receptor gene. N Engl J Med 1996;334:507–12.

9

The Many Faces of FSH

AARON J.W. HSUEH

FSH as a Follicle Stimulating Hormone

Follicle stimulating hormone (FSH) was originally discovered based on its ability to synergize with luteinizing hormone (LH) in the stimulation of ovarian follicle development. FSH is a globular glycoprotein with a molecular weight of 28,000–30,000. It consists of a common α and specific β subunits that form a dimer without covalent linkage. In both subunits, there are two asparagine-linked glycosylation sites, which allow the attachment of oligosaccharide side chains. After secretion by the anterior pituitary cells, FSH acts exclusively on granulosa cells in the ovary and Sertoli cells in the testis by binding to specific FSH receptors found in these cells.

In this chapter the multitude of actions of FSH in the ovary and testis will be discussed. Because several reviews have already summarized the role of FSH in gonadal cell growth and differentiation (1–3), the present review will focus only on studies performed in my laboratory.

FSH as a Follicle Survival Hormone

It is clear that FSH is a differentiation factor for ovarian granulosa cells and testicular Sertoli cells, but studies have additionally indicated that FSH is also a survival factor for ovarian follicles and testicular tubules (4–6).

Normal development of both female and male gonads is characterized by massive cell death. More than 99% of ovarian follicles endowed at early life are destined to undergo apoptosis and the exhaustion of these follicles serves as a "clock" for female reproductive senescence. In the testis, up to 75% of male germ cells also undergo apoptosis, perhaps as a mechanism to delete superfluous or defective germ cells. Preovulatory or early antral follicles were dissected and cultured for 24 hours with or without hormonal treatments. After culture, DNA was extracted from follicles, and the degree of apoptotic

DNA fragmentation was determined using 3'-end labeling and gel electrophoresis. In situ analysis of apoptotic DNA fragmentation revealed that granulosa cells in these follicles are the main cell type undergoing apoptosis. Follicles cultured in the absence of hormones showed an increase in the level of apoptotic DNA fragmentation that was prevented by treatment with FSH in a dose-dependent manner (Fig. 9.1). In the preovulatory follicles, FSH acts together with estrogens, growth hormone, growth factors (IGFI, EGF/TGF-a, basic FGF), cytokine (interleukin-1β) and nitric oxide to ensure the survival of preovulatory follicles (7,8). In contrast, FSH is the major determinant for the survival of early antral follicles (4).

Although the somatic granulosa cell is the major cell type that undergoes apoptosis in the ovary, germ cells in the testis also exhibit signs of apoptotic cell demise. In the testis, FSH and androgens act as survival factors (5). The hormonal control of apoptotic cell death was studied in testicular cells collected from immature rats after hypophysectomy. After surgery, animals were treated with daily injections of 20 IU long-acting FSH agonist (FSH-CTP) or 50 IU hCG for 2 days. Hypophysectomy decreased testis weight by 25%, but treatment with FSH-CTP or hCG prevented the effect of hypophysectomy. Testes of intact animals contained a predominantly high molecular weight DNA, whereas hypophysectomy increased DNA cleavage into the low mo-

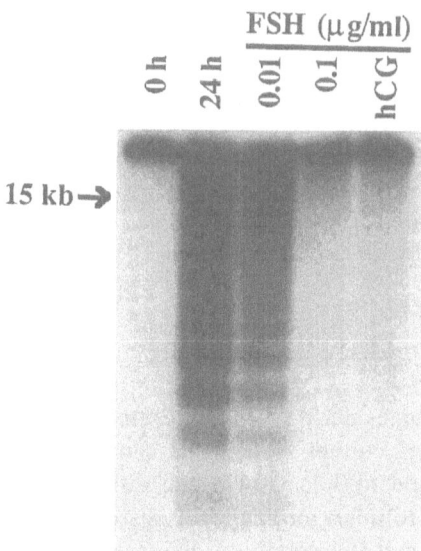

FIGURE 9.1. FSH treatment suppresses apoptosis of preovulatory follicles in culture. Preovulatory follicles were cultured in serum-free media for 24 hours with or without increasing doses of FSH. DNA fragmentation in cultured cells was analyzed following 3'-end labeling and gel fractionation. Reprinted with permission from Endocrinology 1994;135:1845–53 © The Endocrine Society.

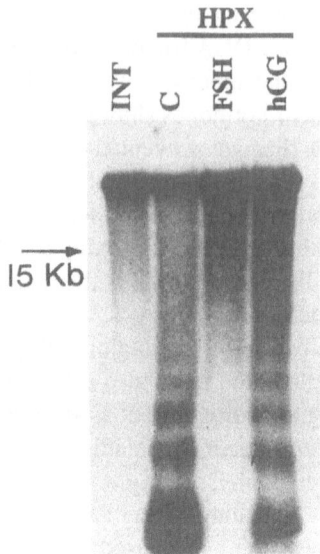

FIGURE 9.2. FSH treatment suppresses testicular germ cell apoptosis in hypophysecto-mized rats. Immature hypophysectomized male rats were treated FSH or hCG for 2 days before analysis of DNA fragmentation in testis cells. Reprinted with permission from Mol Endocrinol 1993;7:643–50 © The Endocrine Society.

lecular weight ladders (< 15 kilobases) characteristic of apoptosis (Fig. 9.2). In contrast, treatment with FSH-CTP or hCG inhibited hypophysectomy-in-duced apoptotic DNA cleavage (5). In the seasonally breeding hamster model, photoperiod-entrained regression and recrudescence of testis tissue serves as a unique natural model of apoptosis. Changes in testis germ-cell apoptosis are highly correlated with circulating levels of FSH in these animals (9).

FSH as a Follicle Growth Hormone

The role of FSH changes during follicle development. We have developed a serum-free rat follicle culture system that can be used to characterize the regulation of preantral follicle growth and differentiation (10). Culture of individual preantral follicles mechanically dissected from ovaries of 12- or 14-day-old rats in serum-free conditions led to major increases in follicle cell apoptosis, similar to that seen in cultures of antral and preovulatory follicles. In contrast to antral and preovulatory follicles, treatment of preantral fol-licles with FSH did not prevent apoptosis; however, treatment with 8-bromo-cGMP suppressed apoptosis by 75%. Taking advantage of the ability of the cGMP analog to suppress apoptosis, we evaluated the potential of FSH as a growth factor. In the absence of serum, FSH treatment for 48 hours did not affect follicle size as compared with the controls; however, treatment with the cGMP analog together with FSH increased follicle diameter and viable cells compared with control values (10). Immunoblot analysis further indicated that the inhibin-α content of the cultured follicles was increased by treatment with the combination of FSH and 8-bromo-cGMP, demonstrating the induction of follicle cell differentiation during culture. Thus, we demonstrated that FSH is a growth and differentiation factor for preantral follicles.

Taking advantage of the relatively uniform development of the first wave of follicles in the postnatal rat ovary, we further evaluated the role of endogenous and exogenous FSH on preantral follicle development in vivo (11). Reduction of the high levels of FSH and LH present in juvenile rats by either hypophysectomy (at day 15 of age) or GnRH antagonist treatment (starting from day 11) resulted in decreased ovarian weight at day 19 that was associated with a reduced number of developing follicles and increased atresia of remaining follicles. In contrast, treatment with FSH-CTP (a long-acting FSH agonist) in intact (days 5–19), hypophysectomized (days 15–19), or GnRH antagonist-treated animals (days 11–19), resulted in increased ovarian weight and follicle development as determined histologically and by inhibin-α expression (Fig. 9.3). These findings demonstrate the important role of endogenous gonadotropins in preantral follicle development and indicate that preantral follicles are highly responsive to exogenous gonadotropins.

FSH as a Follicle Rupture Hormone

Ovulation in mammals is preceded by surges of the two pituitary gonadotropins, LH and FSH. Although previous studies have shown that purified FSH induces ovulation when administered to hypophysectomized rats, proof that FSH has inherent ovulatory potential is lacking because all FSH preparations have varying degrees of residual LH. To determine if FSH alone can induce ovulation, we generated LH-free recombinant FSH (RCFSH). Immature hypophysectomized rats were implanted with estrogen and then primed with PMSG. Fifty-two hours later, either RCFSH or hCG was injected to induce ovulation. A dose-dependent increase in the ovulation rate, comparable to that achieved with hCG (12) (Fig. 9.4) was stimulated by RCFSH. Ovulation induced by either RCFSH or hCG was time-dependent and associated with a periovulatory increase in the ovarian activity and message levels of tissue-type plasminogen activator, a protease important in the preovulatory degradation of the follicle wall. These results demonstrate that FSH is capable of inducing ovulation in hypophysectomized rats, with associated increases in ovarian tissue-type plasminogen activator gene expression. Thus, FSH may be involved in follicular rupture in addition to its role in follicle survival, growth, and maturation. The present finding serves as the basis to formulate new ovulation induction protocols.

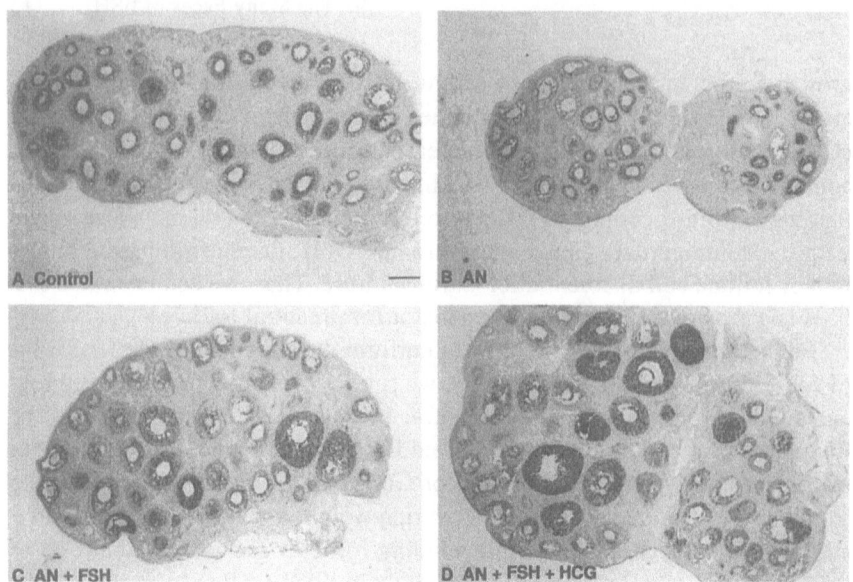

FIGURE 9.3. FSH treatment stimulates follicle growth and inhibin-α expression in immature female rats treated with a GnRH antagonist. Immature female rats were treated with a GnRH antagonist (AN) with or without gonadotropins (FSH or FSH plus hCG) from day 11 to 19. Inhibin-α immunostaining was performed in ovarian sections to determine the ability of gonadotropins to regulate granulosa cell differentiation. (A) Control. (B) GnRH antagonist-treated. (C) FSH and GnRH antagonist-treated. (D) hCG, FSH and GnRH antagonist-treated.

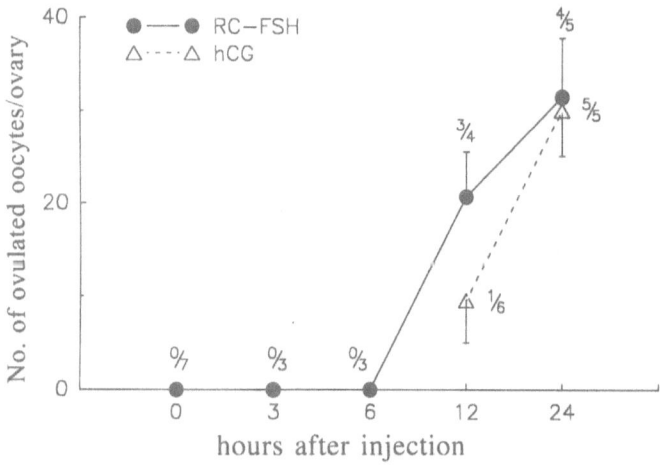

FIGURE 9.4. FSH treatment induces ovulation in hypophysectomized PMSG-primed rats. Immature PMSG-treated rats were injected with a single dose of recombinant FSH (RC/FSH) to induce ovulation. Number of ovulated oocytes in the oviduct was determined at different times after FSH treatment, whereas animals treated with hCG served as positive controls. Reprinted with permission from Endocrinology 1990;127:3023–28 © The Endocrine Society.

FSH as a Follicle Luteinizing Hormone

In addition to its role in follicle survival, growth, differentiation and rupture, FSH is also capable of inducing follicle luteinization (13). Ovulation and subsequent luteal tissue formation are preceded by midcycle surges of both LH and FSH. Although LH has been widely known as the LH, a potential role for FSH in the luteinization process is possible. We examined whether FSH alone is sufficient to induce normal corpus luteum formation. Immature hypophysectomized rats were implanted with an estrogen pellet. Two days later, a minipump releasing RCFSH was implanted to induce follicular growth. Forty-eight hours after FSH treatment, both the estrogen pellet and FSH minipump were removed and the rats were injected with a single dose of 40 IU RCFSH. Two days later, the animals were treated with ovine prolactin twice daily for 3 days to maintain luteal function. All rats that received a surge dose of RCFSH ovulated, whereas none of the control animals did. At 5 days after the gonadotropin surge, RCFSH increased ovarian weight compared with the controls. Serum progesterone levels were increased by almost 200-fold in RCFSH-treated animals, compared with those in the saline-treated rats (Fig. 9.5). Likewise, RCFSH induced a marked elevation of ovarian LH receptor content as reflected by hCG binding and increased the level of the ovarian cholesterol side chain cleavage enzyme mRNA. Accompanied by biochemical signs of luteinization, morphological features typical of luteinized ovaries were found in RCFSH-treated rats, showing the formation of large polyhedral lutein cells and small spindle-shaped lutein cells. These data suggested that FSH, like LH/hCG, is capable of inducing follicle luteinization in the present animal model system, providing a basis to formulate a new ovulation and luteinization protocol in patients.

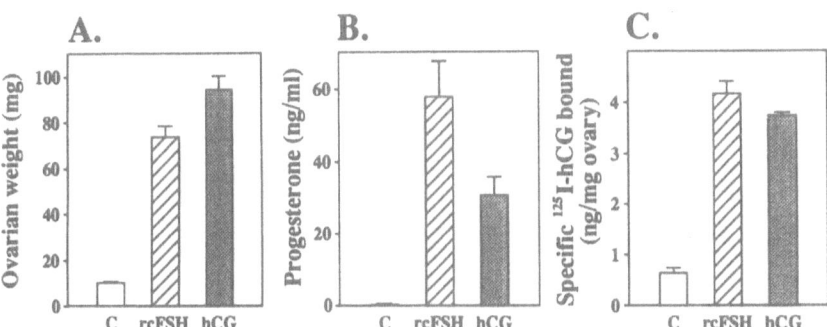

FIGURE 9.5. FSH treatment induces follicle luteinization in immature rats as reflected by increases in ovarian weight, serum progesterone levels, and ovarian LH receptor content. (A) Ovarian weight. (B) Serum progesterone. (C) Ovarian LH receptor content. Reprinted with permission from Endocrinology 1993;133:2875–80 © The Endocrine Society.

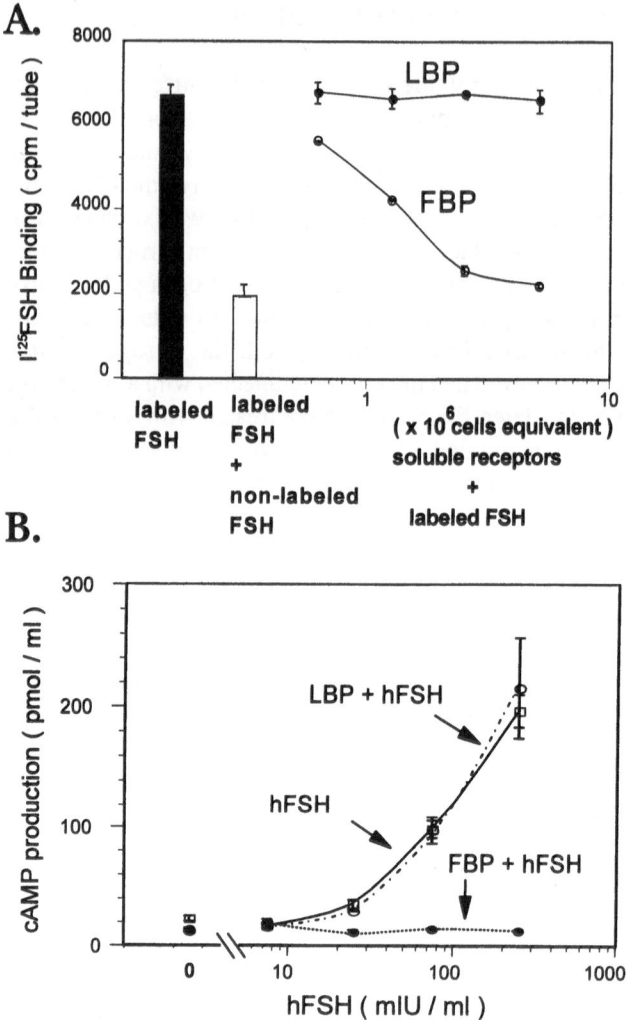

FIGURE 9.6. Soluble extracellular region of human FSH receptor (FBP) inhibits FSH binding to wild type receptors and blocks FSH-stimulation of cAMP production. (A) I^{125}FSH binding. (B) Cyclic AMP production. Reprinted with permission from Mol Endocrinol 1997;11:1659–68 © The Endocrine Society.

The Use of Recombinant FSH Receptor to Detect Bioactive FSH

To study the mechanism of FSH action in its target tissues, we have cloned the cDNA for human FSH receptor and analyzed its expression in gonadal tissues (14). Using cell lines that express recombinant FSH or LH receptors, one could set up sensitive in vitro bioassays for testing new gonadotropin agonists or antagonists, as well as for analysis of serum gonadotropins (15,16). The availability of these reagents further enhanced the understanding of the mechanism of gonadotropin actions mediated by specific receptors.

Derivation of Extracellular Region of FSH Receptor as a FSH Binding Protein to Neutralize Endogenous FSH Action

Because earlier studies indicated that the N-terminal extracellular (ecto-) domains of gonadotropin receptors confer ligand binding, we have attempted to express this region as soluble binding proteins for FSH (17). We fused the ectodomain of FSH or LH receptors to the single-transmembrane domain of CD8 and found that hybrid proteins anchored on the cell surface retained high-affinity ligand binding. Inclusion of a junctional thrombin cleavage site in the hybrids allowed generation of soluble receptor fragments that interfered with gonadotropin binding to specific receptors and blocked cAMP production stimulated by gonadotropins (Fig. 9.6). Cross-linking analyses confirmed the formation of high molecular weight complexes between receptor ectodomains and specific ligands. When administered to rats, the soluble FSH receptor fragment retarded testis growth and induced testis cell apoptosis (17). These findings demonstrate the feasibility of generating ligand-binding regions of FSH and LH receptors to selectively neutralize the actions of gonadotropins, thus allowing future design of novel contraceptives and management of different gonadal dysfunction. Future studies using this approach could allow further elucidation of the specific role of FSH in different physiological states in vivo.

References

1. Hsueh AJW, Bicsak TA, Jia XC, Dahl KD, Fauser BCJM, Galway AB, et al. Granulosa cells as hormone targets: the role of biologically active FSH in reproduction. Recent Prog Horm Res 1989;45:209–70.
2. Richards JS, Hedin L. Molecular aspects of hormone action in ovarian follicular development, ovulation, and luteinization. Ann Rev Physiol 1988;50:441–63.
3. Fauser BC, Van Heusden AM. Manipulation of human ovarian function: physiological concepts and clinical consequences. Endocrinol Rev 1997;18:71–106.
4. Chun SY, Eisenhauer KM, Minami S, Billig H, Perlas E, Hsueh AJW. Hormonal regulation of apoptosis in early antral follicles: follicle stimulating hormone as a major survival factor. Endocrinology 1996;137:1447–56.
5. Tapanainen JS, Tilly JL, Vihko KK, Hsueh AJW. Hormonal control of apoptotic cell death in the testis: gonadotropins and androgens as testicular cell survival factors. Mol Endocrinol 1993;7:643–50.
6. Hsueh AJW, Eisenhauer K, Chun SY, Hsu SY, Billig H. Gonadal cell apoptosis. Rec Prog Horm Res 1996;51:433–55.

7. Chun SY, Billig H, Tilly JL, Furuta I, Tsafriri A, Hsueh AJW. Gonadotropin suppression of apoptosis in cultured preovulatory follicles: mediatory role of endogenous insulin-like growth factor I. Endocrinology 1994;135:1845–53.

8. Chun SY, Eisenhauer KM, Kubo M, Hsueh AJW. Interleukin-1β suppresses apoptosis in rat ovarian follicles by increasing nitric oxide production. Endocrinology 1995;136:3120–7.

9. Furuta I, Porkka-Heiskanen T, Scarbrough K, Tapanainen J, Turek FW, Hsueh AJW. Photoperiod regulates testis cell apoptosis in Djungarian hamsters. Biol Reprod 1994;51:1315–21.

10. McGee E, Spears N, Minami S, Hsu SY, Chun SY, Billig H, et al. Preantral ovarian follicles in serum-free culture: suppression of apoptosis after activation of the cyclic guanosine 3',5'-monophosphate pathway and stimulation of growth and differentiation by follicle stimulating hormone. Endocrinology 1997;138:2417–24.

11. McGee EA, Perlas E, LaPolt PS, Tsafriri A, Hsueh AJW. Follicle stimulating hormone enhances the development of preantral follicles in juvenile rats. Biol Reprod 1997;57:990–98.

12. Galway AB, Lapolt PS, Tsafriri A, Dargan CM, Boime I, Hsueh AJW. Recombinant follicle stimulating hormone induces ovulation and tissue plasminogen activator expression in hypophysectomized rats. Endocrinology 1990;127:3023–28.

13. Tapanainen JS, Lapolt PS, Perlas E, Hsueh AJW. Induction of ovarian follicle luteinization by recombinant follicle stimulating hormone. Endocrinology 1993;133:2875–80.

14. Tilly JL, Aihara T, Nishimori K, Jia XC, Billig H, Kowalski KI, et al. Expression of recombinant human follicle stimulating hormone receptor: species-specific ligand binding, signal transduction, and identification of multiple ovarian messenger ribonucleic acid transcripts. Endocrinology 1992;131:799–806.

15. Jia XC, Perlas E, Su JG, Moran F, Lasley BL, Ny T, et al. Luminescence luteinizing early hormone/choriogonadotropin (LH/CG) bioassay: measurement of serum bioactive LH/CG during pregnancy in human and macaque. Biol Reprod 1993;49:1310–16.

16. Sugahara T, Sato A, Kudo M, Ben-Menahem D, Pixley MR, Hsueh AJW, et al. Expression of biologically active fusion genes encoding the common alpha subunit and the follicle stimulating hormone beta subunit. Role of a linker sequence. Biol Chem 1996;271:10445–48.

17. Osuga Y, Kudo M, Kaipia A, Kobilka B, Hsueh AJW. Derivation of functional antagonists using N-terminal extracellular domain of gonadotropin and thyrotropin receptors. Mol Endocrinol 1997;11:1659–68.

Part III

The Intraovarian Steroid Microenvironment

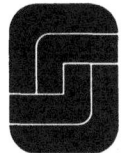

10

Progesterone: Lessons from the Progesterone Receptor Knockout

REBECCA L. ROBKER AND JOANNE S. RICHARDS

Early Studies

Progesterone has long been regarded as a pre-eminent hormone regulating female fertility, exerting diverse effects in ovarian, uterine, and mammary function to control implantation, pregnancy, and lactation (1). The major site of progesterone production is the ovary, where, in response to the leuteinizing hormone (LH) surge, production of this steroid increases in proestrous follicles and is followed by higher levels of progesterone secretion by corpora lutea during diestrous and pregnancy (2). A role for progesterone in ovulation was first demonstrated by Mori et al. (3), whose studies showed that injection of antiprogesterone antiserum reduced the number of ovulations in the PMSG, hCG-induced rat model. Furthermore, the inhibition could be reversed by a dose of progesterone, but not by estradiol. Studies by Snyder et al. (4) and Lipner and Greep (5) showed that inhibiting 3β-hydroxysteroid dehydrogenase (the enzyme that converts pregnenolone to progesterone) with either epostane (4) or cyanoketone (5) blocked ovulation in rats. Furthermore, the block in ovulation could be overcome by exogenous administration of progesterone (4).

Identification of a receptor for progesterone and cloning of the gene allowed further advances. The effects of progesterone are mediated by binding intracellular progesterone receptors (PR), of which there are two distinct isoforms, PR-A and PR-B (6), translated from a single gene. PR is expressed in the ovary, specifically in granulosa cells (7), where it is induced by the luteinizing hormone (LH) surge in vivo (7), and in vitro (8). The development of a specific PR antagonist RU486 (or mifepristone, reviewed in Ref. 9) allowed further delineation of progesterone-mediated effects in the ovary. Early studies by van der Schoot et al. (10) and Sanchez-Criado et al. (11) showed that ovulation failed to occur when RU486 was administered to cycling rats. Histological examination of the ovaries showed unruptured follicles exhibiting clear signs of luteinization. In this model, however, RU486 also blocked the LH surge (11,12), making it difficult to dissociate any intrinsic ovarian effects from those of disrupted LH secretion. Later, Loutradis et al. (13) administered RU486 to mice concurrent with surge levels of hCG. This regimen also completely blocked ovulation, whereas administration of the PR antagonist prior to hCG or 4 hours after hCG did not, indicating a direct effect of PR at the ovarian level.

Results from studies using the in vitro perfused rat ovary model, which enables isolation of the ovary from pituitary influences, have also supported a role for progesterone as a mediator of the ovulatory process. Brannstrom and Janson showed that inhibition of 3β-hydroxysteroid dehydrogenase with Compound A (14) decreased the number of LH-induced ovulations, an effect reversed by addition of progesterone but not testosterone to the perfusate.

The PR Knockout

The most compelling evidence delineating the specific role of progesterone (as opposed to indirect effects of estrogen or LH) in female reproduction has come from targeted deletion of the PR gene in mice (the PR knockout) by John Lydon, Bert O'Malley, and colleagues (15). Mice lacking PR develop normally to adulthood, but the ovaries, uterus, mammary gland, and brain of the homozygous females exhibit specific altered phenotypes. Based on these phenotypes, progesterone has been described as a "pleiotropic coordinator" of female reproductive events (15). The knockout females are completely infertile for several reasons: They fail to ovulate, exhibit an impaired lordosis response, lack uterine decidualization, and have limited mammary lobuloalveolar development (15). Histological analysis of the ovaries of PR knockouts showed that Graffian follicles develop, but they fail to rupture even in response to priming with PMSG and hCG. Granulosa cells responded to the LH surge despite the lack of ovulation, as evidenced by the cumulus expansion (15) and the expression in granulosa cells of specific biochemical markers of the luteal cell phenotype. For example, using these mice we have shown by in situ hybridization that cholesterol side-chain cleavage cytochrome P450, one marker of luteal cells, is expressed normally, at high levels in the unruptured follicles of PR knockouts (Fig. 10.1), those containing entrapped oocytes (arrowhead).

There have also been some conflicting data concening the role of progesterone in oocyte maturation or fertilization. One study (13) showed that treatment of mice with RU486 1 day after PMSG treatment did not affect ovulation rate; however, the treatment resulted in a 50% reduction in the number of two-cell embryos that progressed to the blastocyst stage, indicating a potential

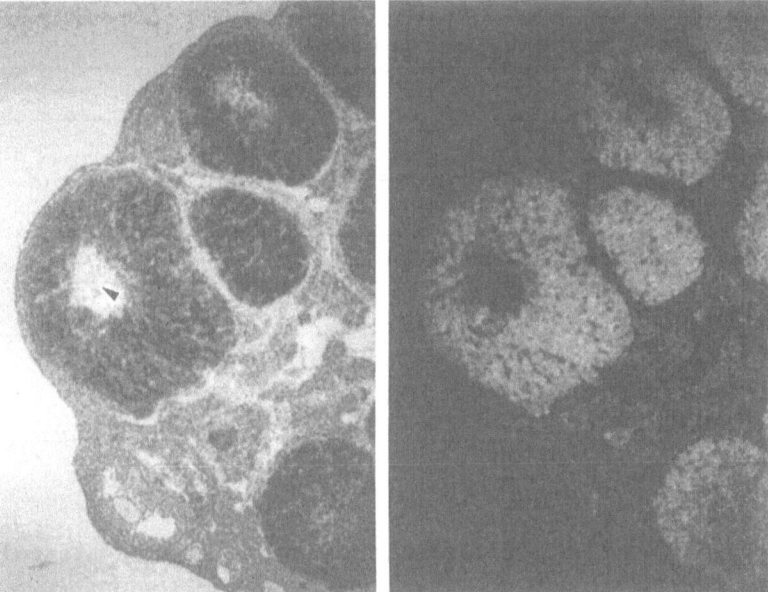

FIGURE 10.1. Luteinization in PR knockout mice. In situ hybridization using a radiolabeled antisense probe shows that although follicles of PR knockout mice do not rupture (left panel, brightfield), they do express high levels of the luteal cell marker cholesterol side-chain cleavage (right panel, dark field). Ovary is from PR knockout mouse 48 hours after hCG treatment; methods as in (31). Arrowhead indicates an unovulated oocyte.

PR-mediated process in either oocyte maturation or early embryonic development. Another study (16) used cyanoketone to inhibit 3β-hydroxysteroid dehydrogenase in an in vitro perfused rabbit ovary model. The results showed that cyanoketone treatment did not reduce the number of hCG- induced ovulations, but did impair the frequency of fertilization. The inhibition of oocyte fertilizability could be reversed by including estradiol in the perfusate, but not by including progesterone. Although steroids appear to have a role in oocyte maturation and/or competence for fertilization, there is, therefore discrepancy about the involvement of progesterone. Furthermore, because PR has only been shown to be expressed in granulosa cells in the rodent ovary (7), any role in the oocyte would presumably be mediated indirectly via products synthesized by and released from granulosa cells.

In order to determine specifically whether there is a role for PR in oocyte maturation, fertilization, or early development, in vitro fertilization experiments were performed in conjunction with Dr. John Eppig at Jackson Laboratories. Oocyte-cumulus complexes were isolated from either heterozygous or PR knockout PMSG-primed mice, matured in vitro (17) and then fertilized with wildtype

TABLE 10.1. In vitro fertilization of normal (PR+/–) and PR knockout (PR–/–) oocytes.

Oocytes fertilized in vitro which reached the two-cell stage

Oocyte genotype	PR+/–		PR–/–	
Experiment 1	90%	$n = 30$	89%	$n = 300$
Experiment 2	91%	$n = 43$	88%	$n = 265$
Experiment 3	59%	$n = 82$	92%	$n = 136$

Two-cell embryos that reached the blastocyst stage

Oocyte genotype	PR+/–		PR–/–	
Experiment 1	93%	$n = 27$	94%	$n = 267$
Experiment 2	79%	$n = 39$	86%	$n = 233$
Experiment 3	83%	$n = 48$	90%	$n = 135$

mouse sperm. The results of three separate experiments (Table 10.1) showed that oocytes from PR knockout (PR–/–) mice were fertilized and proceeded to the two-cell stage at the same frequency as heterozygotes. Development of two-cell embryos to blastocysts also occurred at the same frequency as normal, and when they were implanted into foster mothers they gave rise to normal pups. It does not appear, therefore, that PR plays an essential role at any point in oocyte maturation, fertilization, or early development.

Effects of Progesterone Action

In the pioneering studies by Rondell (18) progesterone was seen to exert very distinct effects on the follicle wall. When strips of porcine theca interna and externa were incubated together, addition of progesterone markedly increased the distensibiltiy of these follicle walls. Rondell proposed that the theca interna was the source of P stimulated follicle-weakening enzymes because the granulosa cell layers were removed in these cultures and since theca externa cultured alone did not exhibit enhanced distensibility in the presence of progesterone. Furthermore, the P-mediated production of enzymes required both transcription and translation of new products since either puromycin or actinomycin D blocked progesterone's effects on distensibility. Hence, Rondell proposed a two-step process of ovulation (18). (1) The LH surge acts on a steroid-secreting cell, causing it to produce progesterone. (2) Progesterone then acts on another cell type to affect either activation, synthesis, or secretion of an ovulatory enzyme that disrupts the collagen framework of the follicle wall, resulting in increased distensibility and culminating in ovulation.

An enormous amount of work (19) has contributed to current models of the ovulatory process since the early studies, the proteolytic enzymes that might be involved, and how progesterone might play a role in their regulation. In particular, studies (20) have shown that the collagenolysis that normally occurs at the time of ovulation could be blocked by inhibiting metalloproteinases including collagenase (with cysteine), serine proteases including plasminogen activator and plasmin (with caproic acid) or cyclooxygenase and lipoxygenase activity (with indomethacin and nordihydroguaiaretic acid respectively). These and many other studies (19) indicate that there are several candidate proteases that may be involved in the collagenolysis associated with ovulation. The role of progesterone in collagenolysis has also been analyzed extensively (19). For instance, studies have shown (21) that inhibition of progesterone action with RU486 blocked the collagenolysis and ovulation, and that the effect could be reversed by treatment with progesterone.

Candidate Proteases

In light of the cumulative studies examining the expression and activity of various proteases, it appears that the molecules most likely to trigger follicular rupture are matrix-metalloproteinases (MMPs), kallikreins, and plasminogen activators (19), all of which can activate collagenase. (Of course, the critical protease may also be currently unknown.) Our studies, therefore, have sought to determine whether progesterone is involved in the regulation of these candidate proteases by examining their expression and/or activity in the PR knockout mice.

The MMPs are a large group of serine proteases (reviewed in Refs. 22, 23) classified on the basis of substrate specificity. Members of the collagenase subclass, interstitial collagenase and neutrophil collagenase—are uniquely able to cleave fibrillar collagens type I, II, and III. In rodents MMP-13 appears to act as interstitial collagenase and is produced by fibroblasts and some additional cells. Neutrophil collagenase, MMP-8, has been detected in fibroblasts, usually in inflammatory conditions, as well as in neutrophils. Because both collagenases digest collagen I, which is the main component lending tensile strength to the follicle wall, and are expressed by fibroblasts, MMP-13 and MMP-8 are good candidates for putative ovulatory enzymes. Additional experiments will be necessary to determine whether they are regulated by PR—regulation that could take place at the level of protein synthesis, proenzyme activation, or secretion/localization of active collagenase. To add an additional layer of complexity, the activity of MMPs is inhibited by protease inhibitors such as the tissue inhibitor of metalloproteinases (TIMPs) and the serum inhibitor α2 macroglobulin. Progesterone, therefore, might modulate protease action by negatively regulating the levels or activity of inhibitors of proteases at the time of ovulation.

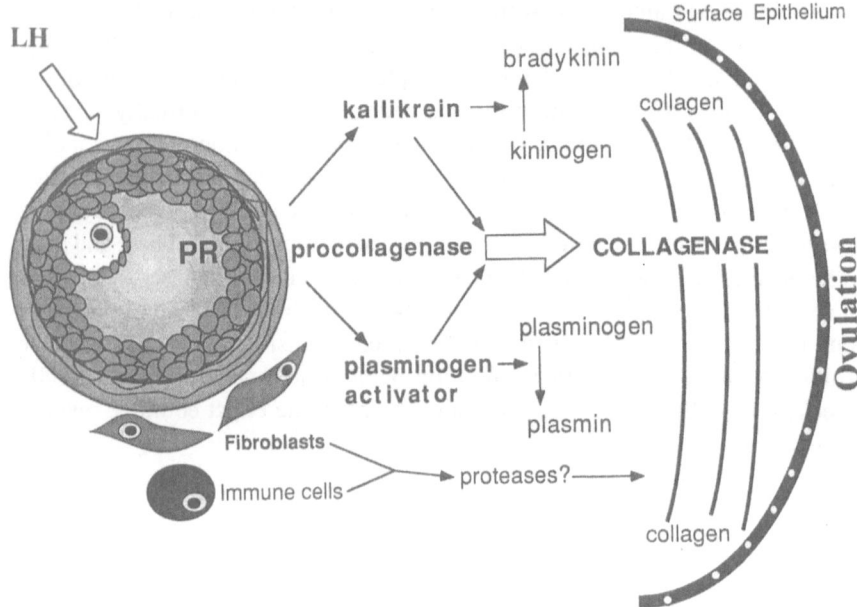

FIGURE 10.2. Potential modes of PR action during the process of ovulation. The LH surge induces the expression of PR in granulosa cells of follicles destined to ovulate. PR may then regulate the synthesis or secretion of proteases such as collagenases. PR may also regulate the activation of proteases by inducing the synthesis of molecules that trigger the activation of latent collagenase to the active form. Both kallikreins and plasminogen activator are able to cleave latent collagenase, as well as to catalyze the formation of additional bioactive peptides, bradykinin, and plasmin, respectively. PR might also somehow regulate the secretion of signaling molecules, which then act on surrounding theca cells, fibroblasts and immune cells to trigger their subsequent release of proteases or protease activators. As demonstrated by the PR knockout phenotype, downstream mediators of PR action ultimately result in degradation of the follicle wall and subsequent ovulation.

Kallikreins are another class of serine proteases that cleave plasma kininogens to form molecules (e.g., bradykinin). Kallikreins have been shown to increase at the time of ovulation (24), and progesterone may mediate this increase because epostane treatment blocks the increase in activity concurrent with inhibiting ovulation (25). The primary product of kallikrein activity, bradykinin, is known to be involved in vasodilation, vascular permeability, and prostaglandin synthesis. It has also been shown to stimulate LH-induced ovulations (26). Kallikreins are also known to activate procollagenase. It may be via activation of kallikreins, therefore, that progesterone induces collagenase activity. It may also be that progesterone might regulate kallikreins at the level of mRNA, protein synthesis, or activation of latent enzyme.

An additional protease known to activate procollagenase is plasminogen activator (PA). It also cleaves plasminogen to form plasmin that in turn activates procollagenase and stimulates downstream mediators of inflammation. Some studies (25) have shown PA activity to be inhibited by epostane, indicating potential regulation by progesterone. Furthermore, tissue plasminogen activator (tPA) is induced in granulosa cells of preovulatory follicles 12 hours after hCG treatment (27). Mice lacking tPA (28), however, remain completely fertile. tPA, therefore, may be just one of several enzymes with the redundant ability to activate procollagenase.

A confounding issue in the puzzle of the ovulatory process is that it has not been unequivocally determined what cell type is the source of the putative protease activity. The PR knockouts that appear to lack protease activity suggest that granulosa cells are the source because PR is expressed in granulosa cells. Rondell's model, however, suggests that the theca interna is the source, and the follicle wall cultures in his experiments were devoid of granulosa cells. Many other studies (reviewed in Ref. 29) suggest that infiltrating leukocytes may be the source of ovulatory proteases or at least signaling molecules (e.g., bradykinin, prostaglandins, or histamine). Fibroblasts are known to secrete an array of proteases, and their location within the theca externa makes them likely sources of proteases that must be localized to the ovarian surface. Furthermore, they exhibit very interesting cytoplasmic processes and multivesicular structures (30) near the time of ovulation. Any of these cell types may therefore be producing an ovulatory protease or an activator of the ovulatory protease (Fig. 10.2). The PR knockout provides an excellent model for analyzing this process because the ovary appears to be quite normal, except for the very specific failure to rupture. PR in granulosa cells may be producing procollagenase, which is then secreted and activated to form active collagenase which could then degrade the follicle wall. On the other hand, PR in granulosa cells may be regulating the synthesis or activation of kallikreins or plasminogen activator (or another enzyme), which then activates procollagenase (31). In addition, fibroblasts or immune cells may be the source of proteases that help cleave collagen directly, or they might secrete signaling molecules or cytokines that stimulate the surrounding cells (e.g., granulosa and theca) to secrete proteases or protease activators. A process as tightly regulated and precisely timed as ovulation will surely prove to be quite complex.

References

1. Graham JD, Clarke CL. Physiological action of progesterone in target tissues. Endocrinol Rev 1997;18:502–19.
2. Rothchild I. The regulation of the mammalian corpus luteum. Rec Prog Horm Res 1981;17:183–298.
3. Mori T, Suzuki A, Nishimura T, Kambegawa A. Inhibition of ovulation in immature rats by anti-progesterone antiserum. J Endocrinol 1977;73:185–86.
4. Snyder BW, Beecham GD, Schane HP. Inhibition of ovulation in rats with epostane, an inhibitor of 3b-hydroxysteroid dehydrogenase. Proc Soc Exp Biol Med 1984;176:238–42.

5. Lipner H, Greep RO. Inhibition of steroidogenesis at various sites in the biosynthetic pathway in relation to induced ovulation. Endocrinology 1971;88:602–7.
6. Conneely OM, Maxwell BL, Toft DO, Schrader WT, O'Malley BM. The A and B isoforms of the chicken progesterone receptor arise by alternate initiation of translation of a unique mRNA. Biochem Biophys Res Commun 1987;149:493–501.
7. Park O-K, Mayo KE. Transient expression of progesterone receptor messenger RNA in ovarian granulosa cells after the preovulatory luteinizing hormone surge. Mol Endocrinol 1991;5:967–78.
8. Natraj U, Richards JS. Hormonal regulation, localization, and functional activity of the progesterone receptor in granulosa cells of rat preovulatory follicles. Endocrinology 1993;133:761–69.
9. Baulieu E-E. Contragestation and other clinical applications of RU486, an antiprogesterone at the receptor. Science 1989;245:1351–57.
10. Van der Schoot P, Bakker GH, Klijn JGM. Effects of the progesterone antagonist RU486 on ovarian activity in the rat. Endocrinology 1987;121:1375–82.
11. Sanchez JE, Bellido C, Galiot F, Lopez FJ, Gaytan F. A possible mechanism of the anovulatory action of antiprogesterone RU486 in the rat. Biol Reprod 1990;42:877–86.
12. Rao IM, Mahesh VB. Role of progesterone in the modulation of the preovulatory surge of gonadotropins and ovulation in the pregnant mare's serum gonadotropin-primed immature rat and the adult rat. Biol Reprod 1986;35:1154–61.
13. Loutradis D, Bletsa R, Aravantinos L, Kallianidis K, Michalas S, Psychoyos A. Preovulatory effects of the progesterone antagonist mifepristone (RU486) in mice. Hum Reprod 1991;6:1238–40.
14. Brannstrom M, Janson PO. Progestrone is a mediator in the ovulatory process of the in vitro-perfused rat ovary. Biol Reprod 1989;40:1170–78.
15. Lydon JP, DeMayo FJ, Funk CR, Mani SK, Hughes AR, Montgomery CA Jr, et al. Mice lacking progesterone receptor exhibit pleiotropic reproductive abnormalities. Genes Dev 1995;9:2266–78.
16. Yoshimura Y, Hosoi Y, Bongiovanni AM, Santulli R, Atlas SJ, Wallach EE. Are ovarian steroids required for ovum maturation and fertilization? Effects of cyanoketone on the in vitro perfused rabbit ovary. Endocrinology 1987;120:2555–61.
17. Ho Yugong, Wigglesworth K, Eppig JJ, Schultz RM. Preimplantation development of mouse embryos in KSOM: augmentation by amino acids and analysis of gene expression. Mol Reprod Dev 1995;41:232–38.
18. Rondell P. Role of steroid synthesis in the process of ovulation. Biol Reprod 1974;10:199–215.
19. Espey LL, Lipner H. Ovulation. In: Knobil E, Neill JD, eds. The physiology of reproduction. Second ed. New York: Raven Press; 1994:725–80.
20. Reich R, Tsafriri A, Mechanic GL. The involvement of collagenolysis in ovulation in the rat. Endocrinology 1985;116:522–27.
21. Iwamasa J, Shibata S, Tanaka N, Matsuura K, Okamura H. The relationship between ovarian progesterone and proteolytic enzyme activity during ovulation in the gonadotropin-treated immature rat. Biol Reprod 1992;46:309–13.
22. Matrisian LM. The matrix-degrading metalloproteinases. BioEssays 1992;14:455–63.
23. McIntush EW, Smith MF. Matrix metalloproteinases and tissue inhibitors of metalloproteinases in ovarian function. Rev Reprod 1998;3:23–30.
24. Espey LL, Tanaka N, Winn V, Okamura H. Increase in ovarian kallikrein activity

during ovulation in the gonadotropin-primed immature rat. J Reprod Fertil 1989;87: 503–8.

25. Tanaka N, Espey LL, Stacy S, Okamura H. Epostane and indomethacin actions on ovarian kallikrein and plasminogen activator activities during ovulation in the gonadotropin-primed immature rat. Biol Reprod 1992;46:665–70.

26. Brannstrom M, Hellberg P. Bradykinin potentiates LH-induced follicular rupture in the rat ovary perfused in vitro. Hum Reprod 1989;4:475–81.

27. Shen X, Minoura H, Yoshida T, Toyoda N. Changes in ovarian expression of tissue-type plasminogen activator and plasminogen activator inhibitor type-1 messenger ribonucleic acids during ovulation in rat. Endocrine J 1997;44:341–48.

28. Carmeliet P, Schoonjans L, Kieckens L, Ream B, Degen J, Bronson R, et al. Physiological consequences of loss of plasminogen activator gene function in mice. Nature 1994;368:419–24.

29. Norman RJ, Brannstrom M. White cells and the ovary—incidental invaders or essential effectors? J Endocrinol 1994;140:333–36.

30. Espey LL. Ultrastructure of the ovulatory process. In: Familiari G, Makabe S, Motta PM, eds. Ultrastructure of the ovary. Boston: Kluwer Academic Publishers; 1991:143–59.

31. Robker RL, Richards JS. Hormone-induced proliferation and differentiation of granulosa cells: a coordinated balance of the cell cycle regulators cyclin D2 and p27Kip1. Mol Endocrinol 1998;12:924–40.

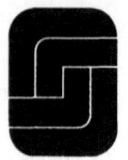

11

Intraovarian Control of Ovulation: Lessons from Steroid Ablation/ Replacement in Monkeys

RICHARD L. STOUFFER, DIANE M. DUFFY, TIMOTHY M. HAZZARD, THEODORE A. MOLSKNESS, MARY B. ZELINSKI-WOOTEN, AND CHARLES L. CHAFFIN

Introduction

An important action of estrogen secreted by the maturing follicle is to trigger the release of surge levels of the gonadotropic hormones, follicle stimulating hormone (FSH), and luteinizing hormone (LH) from the pituitary. The gonadotropin surge initiates a cascade of events within the follicle that promotes oocyte maturation, ovulation, and conversion of the follicle wall into a new endocrine structure, the corpus luteum. The latter process, termed *luteinization*, involves major changes in the structure–function of the tissue, including development of the molecular and cellular components required to produce large quantities of the steroid hormone progesterone. As the periovulatory interval proceeds, the luteinizing follicle switches from primarily an estrogen-secreting to a progesterone-secreting tissue. In some series, the corpus luteum is devoid of estrogen synthetic capacity, whereas in others (e.g., Old World macaques and women) significant production of estrogen (and its bioactive precursor, androgen) remains. Thus, the periovulatory follicle experiences remarkable changes in the steroid milieu as androgen and estrogen initially rise and then decline, and appreciable levels of progestins are achieved well before follicle rupture (1,2).

The dynamics of steroid secretion in the periovulatory follicle appear to be important for events both outside and within the ovary (3). For example, the early rise in circulating progesterone influences the strength–duration of the gonadotropin surge in rodents and primates. Likewise, preovulatory progestin plays a critical role in inducing reproductive behavior in some species. In the early

1970s (4,5), investigators first considered the hypothesis that ovarian steroido-genesis played an obligatory local role in the ovulatory process in rodent models. It was not until the development of more specific pharmacologic agents and gene knockout techniques, however, that significant information was obtained both in nonprimate (see Chap. 10) and primate species.

Use of a 3β-Hydroxysteroid Dehydrogenase Inhibitor to Examine the Role of Steroids in Ovulation

Our laboratory has used several techniques to examine steroid receptor mRNA and protein expression in the follicle (6) and corpus luteum (7) of the rhesus monkey throughout the menstrual cycle. These studies led to the discovery that appreciable levels of progesterone receptors were first detectable in the granulosa cell layer of the preovulatory follicle *after* the onset of the midcycle gonadotropin surge. This finding was confirmed using controlled ovarian stimulation (COS) cycles, which are analogous to PMSG-hCG treatment protocols in rodents. The advantages of COS cycles over monovular natural cycles include: 1) The multiple follicular development provides sufficient tissue for detailed experimentation, and 2) samples can be collected at specific timepoints prior to and after administration of the ovulatory gonadotropin (LH or CG) bolus. Our findings supported the hypothesis that the midcycle gonadotropin surge has two related effects that facilitate progesterone action in the mature follicle (7):

1. The expression of the cellular and molecular components necessary for progesterone production in the luteinizing follicle.

2. The expression of progesterone receptors that mediate local actions of the steroid in luteinizing granulosa cells.

Studies were therefore designed to determine whether steroids in general, and progesterone in particular, play key roles in the gonadotropin-initiated periovulatory events of oocyte maturation, follicle rupture, and luteal development in primates.

In Vivo Studies

Classical endocrine ablation–replacement techniques were employed in which an inhibitor of 3β-hydroxysteroid dehydrogenase (Trilostane, TRL, Sanofi Pharmaceutical, Inc., Malvern, PA), with or without progestin (R5020, Dupont/NEN) or androgen (5α-dihydrotestosterone propionate, DHT, Steraloids, Wilton, NH), was administered during the periovulatory interval in COS cycles of rhesus monkeys (8). All animals received exogenous gonadotropins (human [h] FSH ± LH, Serono Laboratories, Randolph, MA) to promote multiple follicular development, followed by a bolus of hCG (Serono Laboratories) to initiate periovulatory events. The monkeys received either no further treatment (control) or TRL with or without steroid replacement from the time of hCG treatment (0 hours) to 72 hours post-hCG.

Even though the COS protocol yielded similar numbers of large follicles and peak estrogen levels in all groups, there were marked differences in the ovulatory response (Table 11.1). All control (hCG alone) animals ovulated as evidenced by multiple ovulatory stigmata on the ovaries; oocytes could also be obtained by oviduct lavage. In contrast, TRL-treated animals demonstrated a complete absence of ovulation sites, and no oocytes were obtained by oviduct lavage. Progestin (R5020), but not androgen (DHT), replacement restored ovulation in all animals to a level that matched or exceeded that of control animals. Of the total number of oocytes collected per animal by either oviduct lavage or follicle aspiration, the percentage of mature (metaphase II) oocytes did not differ between groups. The in vitro fertilization rate, however, was high for oocytes from control animals, but markedly diminished by TRL treatment. It is noteworthy that R5020 replacement did not improve fertilizability, whereas DHT treatment partially restored the fertilization rate (Table 11.1).

There were also marked differences between groups in the luteal phases that followed hCG administration. Control animals exhibited the typical biphasic pattern of circulating progesterone, with levels increasing within 24 hours of hCG treatment, peaking at supraphysiologic (40–60 ng/ml) levels indicative of multiple corpora lutea by day 5 post-hCG, and then declining until menses at Day 14–15. During TRL treatment (Day 0–3 post-hCG), progesterone levels in the circulation (8) and follicular fluid (unpublished) remained at baseline as expected; however, levels remained profoundly suppressed throughout the luteal phase, with peak levels (1–5 ng/ml) no more than 10% of controls. Co-administration of R5020, but not DHT, with TRL increased progesterone above baseline by Day 4 post-hCG with levels not different from controls by Days 6–7.

The study supports the concept of a local role for steroids in periovulatory events in the primate follicle. Indeed, the evidence strongly suggests that

TABLE 11.1. Effects of steroid ablation (via trilostane, TRL) and replacement (progestin, R5020, or androgen, DHT) during the periovulatory interval of controlled ovarian stimulation cycles in macaques.

	Control	TRL	TRL + R5020	TRL + DHT
No. of ovulation sites	10 ± 3	0	22 ± 9	1 ± 1
% mature (MII) oocytes*	62 ± 23	74 ± 13	89 ± 14	71 ± 4
% fertilization in vitro*	87 ± 9	16 ± 2	0	42 ± 29

Means ± SEM with different superscripts within a row are significantly different ($p < 0.05$).
*Percentage of cohort from oviduct lavage and follicle aspiration 72 hours after administration of the ovulatory hCG stimulus. See Ref. 8 for details.

progesterone (or a bioactive progestin metabolite) is critical for ovulation, plus the function and/or development of the corpus luteum, but not for achievement of oocyte meiotic maturation. Our results extend those of others using steroid synthesis inhibitors or progesterone antagonists (9,10) in rodent models. Studies (11) on mice carrying the null mutation of the progesterone receptor gene (PRKO) have also indicated that mature preovulatory follicles in the ovary do not rupture, even upon exposure to an exogenous (hCG) ovulatory stimulus. Other observations (12) in PRKO mice that oocytes reinitiate meiosis, but follicles fail to develop histologic indices of luteinization after an hCG bolus, are also consistent with data obtained in our macaque studies. Thus, progesterone appears to have a common role, via a genomic receptor-mediated pathway, in the ovulatory and luteinization processes of the mature follicle, in mammalian species ranging from rodents to primates.

In Vitro Studies

The precise time-frame and mechanism(s) whereby progesterone exerts its influence during the periovulatory interval remains to be determined. These issues are confounded in primates by the lack of baseline data on the dynamics of periovulatory events in the 38-hour interval between onset of the midcycle gonadotropin surge and follicle rupture in macaques or humans. Studies were therefore initiated using COS cycles to elucidate the changes in the macaque follicle as monitored from follicular fluid and granulosa cells collected before (0 hours), 12, 24, and 36 hours following administration of an ovulatory bolus of hCG. Additional treatment groups were included to examine the effects of steroid ablation (Trilostane) and progestin replacement (R5020), as described earlier (8). Initial efforts (13) focused on studying the dynamics of steroid synthesis, for two reasons: (1) To determine if the changes in steroidogenesis during the periovulatory interval in COS cycles are similar to those in natural cycles, and (2) to consider the earliest timeframe when progesterone could be acting in the periovulatory follicle.

Progesterone levels were appreciable (nanograms per milliliter) in follicular fluid of large preovulatory follicles (≥4 mm diameter) prior to the ovulatory stimulus, but increased more than 180-fold within 12 horrs of hCG administration and remained at these high (micrograms per milliliter) levels through 36 hours (13). Frequent blood sampling indicated that serum progesterone concentrations increased significantly within 30 minutes of hCG administration and continued to rise for at least 18 hours. It is of note that serum and/or follicular fluid levels of androgen (androstenedione) and estrogen (estradiol and estrone) also increased modestly (two-fold) by 12 hours post-hCG, but then declined to or below pre-hCG levels, respectively. Similar to serum and follicular fluid levels, basal progesterone production by granulosa cells during acute (2-hour) incubations in chemically defined media in vitro increased dramatically after 12 hours of exposure to hCG in vivo. The addition of 1 µM pregnenolone, the immediate substrate for progestin synthesis, markedly increased progesterone levels to a comparable extent at 0, 12, and 36 hours. In contrast, the addition of 1 µM 25-hydroxycholesterol, a soluble cholesterol analog, significantly increased progesterone production after (12–36 hours), but *not* prior (0 hours) to the ovulatory hCG bolus. It is of note that the addition of cholesterol or low density lipoprotein (LDL) did not influence steroidogenesis at any timepoint.

We conclude that although the concentrations of serum steroids during the periovulatory interval are higher in COS cycles, the pattern of changes in circulating steroids is similar to that in natural cycles (1,2). These data, plus evidence that follicles will ovulate in an apparent timely manner [after 36, but before 72 hours; (8)], support the value of COS protocols in studying the dynamics and regulation of periovulatory events in primates. In addition, acquired information may be valuable to clinical *in vitro* fertilization programs [e.g., (14)]. The acquisition of robust progesterone synthetic activity, as well as progesterone receptor (13), within 12 hours of hCG administration, argues for an *early*, local role for a progesterone stimulus in periovulatory events. Initial evidence, based on granulosa cell incubations, suggests that the induction of P450 side chain cleavage activity, rather than 3β-hydroxysteroid dehydrogenase activity (which is already appreciable prior to the gonadotropin stimulus), is an important feature in the early rise in progesterone synthesis during follicle luteinization. Further studies are planned to examine mRNA expression for genes encoding components of the steroidogenic pathway, and whether they are regulated by gonadotropin and/or progesterone during the periovulatory interval.

Because ovulation and luteinization of the follicle involves extensive degradation and reorganization of the cell layers comprising the follicle wall (15), studies were initiated to characteize the protease systems, particularly the matrix metalloproteinases (MMPs) and their tissue inhibitors (TIMPs), in the periovulatory follicle of primates. Based on earlier reports on rabbits (4) and rats (16) that progesterone stimulates proteolytic activity in ovulatory follicles, we also hypothesized that one of the local actions of steroids was to regulate the expression of MMPs or their TIMPs. Using semi-quantitative RT-PCR assays, mRNAs for many (e.g., interstitial collagenase or MMP-1, gelatinases A and B or MMP-2 and -9, and matrilysin or MMP-7), but not all (stromelysin or MMP-3) MMPs were detectable in granulosa cells of preovulatory follicles (17). Likewise, mRNAs for TIMP-1 and -2 were also present; however, the patterns of expression varied between MMPs as well as TIMPs during the periovulatory interval (Table 11.2). For example, mRNA for interstitial collagenase was nondetectable prior to hCG administration (0 hours), but highly expressed by 12 hours post-hCG and thereafter. In contrast, gelatinase B mRNA remained low at 12–24 hours post-hCG, followed by a profound increase by 36 hours post-hCG. Matrilysin mRNA exhibited a triphasic pattern with peak levels at 12 and 36 hours separated by low levels comparable to pre-hCG expression at 24 hours post-hCG.

TABLE 11.2. Summary of the dynamics and influence of progestin on mRNA expression for MMPs/TIMPs in granulosa cells during the periovulatory interval of controlled ovarian stimulation cycles in macaques.

MMP/TIMP	Time of peak mRNA*	R5020 effect[†]
Interstitial collagenase	12 hr	+
Stromelysin	ND	NA
Matrilysin	12 and 36 hr	−
Gelatinase A	12 hr	None
Gelatinase B	36 hr	None
TIMP-1	12 hr	+
TIMP-2	36 hr	−

*mRNA levels were measured 0, 12, 24, and 36 hours after administration of the ovulatory hCG stimulus. See Ref. 17 for details.
[†]Comparison of data from trilostane and trilostane + R5020 treatment groups suggests that progestin either promotes (+), inhibits (−), or has no effect on expression of various MMP/TIMP mRNAs.
ND, nondetectable; NA, not applicable.

The influence of steroid depletion and progestin replacement also varied between the MMPs/TIMPs in macaque granulosa cells (Table 11.1). For example, trilostane treatment significantly suppressed mRNA levels for interstitial collagenase and TIMP-1 following the ovulatory hCG bolus, and this suppression was overcome by R5020 treatment. In other cases, such as for matrilysin and TIMP-2, trilostane treatment partially suppressed and addition of R5020 further reduced mRNA levels. In one instance, that of gelatinase B, trilostane treatment markedly inhibited mRNA expression, and co-administration of R5020 did not alter this effect. Finally, expression of gelatinase A mRNA in response to the hCG bolus was not altered by trilostane.

These data are the first to demonstrate that the ovulatory gonadotropin stimulus increases expression of several MMPs and their inhibitors within the primate follicle. Differences in the patterns of mRNA expression for various MMPs/TIMPs may relate to diverse roles for individual proteases and inhibitors in periovulatory events (e.g., follicle rupture versus luteinization or neovascularization of the follicle wall). Progesterone may promote ovulation and luteinization by stimulating MMP-1/TIMP-1 regulated disruption and remodeling of the periovulatory follicle; however, progesterone may also inhibit the expression of other protease systems (e.g., MMP-7/TIMP-2). Further studies are needed to determine if changes in mRNA expression correlate with enzyme-inhibitor protein or activity in the follicle, if the changes reflect activity in specific regions (e.g., putative rupture site) or compartments (granulosa vs. theca) of the follicle, actions of specific MMPs/TIMPs in periovulatory processes, and the role(s) of progesterone or other steroids in regulating protease activity in the primate follicle.

Do Other Steroids, in Addition to Progesterone, Have Roles in Periovulatory Events?

The preceding studies, which employ trilostane and R5020 treatment, strongly suggest that progestin replacement is *sufficient* to restore ovulation in rhesus monkeys. Indeed, progesterone action during the periovulatory interval could be critical for maintenance of granulosa cell/oocyte viability (18,19), perhaps in part by production of local growth or regulatory factors that promote the further differentiation and neovascularization (20,21) of the follicle wall. Although further efforts to unravel the apparent vital role(s) of progesterone in the ovulatory, luteinizing follicle are of a high priority, possible actions of other steroids in periovulatory events cannot be ruled out.

There are few reports to date of investigations that directly evaluate the role of androgens or estrogens in ovulation or luteinization. Mori and colleagues (22) observed that antisera to testosterone co-administered with the ovulatory hCG bolus markedly reduced the number of ovulations in PMSG-primed rats. In addition testosterone or DHT restored ovulations in this rodent model that were blocked by antisera to progesterone. In our studies on rhesus macaques (8), DHT failed to restore ovulation during steroid ablation via trilostane treatment; however, DHT treatment partially restored the fertilizability of oocytes and circulating progesterone levels during the late luteal phase. Further studies manipulating the androgen milieu or action in the periovulatory follicle are needed to elucidate the influence, if any, of this steroid on oocyte maturation, ovulation, and corpus luteum development.

Reports of targeted disruption of the estrogen receptor (ERα) and aromatase (Ar) genes, to produce mice devoid of estrogen actions or production (23,24), include evidence that the ovaries contained large (even cystic) antral follicles, but no corpora lutea. Likewise, women with aromatase deficiency have multiple follicular cysts on their ovaries (25). It remains to be determined, however, if the apparent arrest before ovulation is due in part to loss of estrogen action in the follicle, versus the failure of estrogen action in the hypothalamus–pituitary to elicit the midcycle gonadotropin surge. It is important to recognize that such knockout mouse models are devoid of steroid synthesis/actions throughout folliculogenesis. If future studies demonstrate that exogenous gonadotropin protocols (e.g., PMSG-hCG) produce subnormal numbers of ovulations, the experimental design should therefore demonstrate the normalcy of preovulatory follicles or the ability of acute steroid replacement to restore ovulatory events. Only then can one discern between lesions due to steroid action in the periovulatory follicle versus earlier in the growing, immature follicle. Further use of genetic and pharmacologic approaches to ablate or replace steroids or steroid action will provide complementary information on species differences, if any, in the ovulatory process, on chronic versus acute effects during follicular growth and maturation, and whether steroid effects are dependent or independent of specific receptor (e.g., ERα, ERβ, or nongenomic R) pathways.

Acknowledgments. The creative, skillful work of the many graduate students, postdoctoral fellows, clinical research fellows and staff scientists who contributed to this research endeavor in the author's laboratory is gratefully acknowledged. In addition, the collaboration and assistance of Dr. Robert Brenner and the Morphology Core Laboratory, Dr. David Hess and the Endocrine Services Core Laboratory, Drs. Don Wolf and Gerald Schatten and the Assisted Reproductive Technologies Core Laboratory, plus the animal care and surgical staffs at ORPRC contributed greatly to this research. A special thanks to Ms. Carol Gibbins for her assistance in preparation of this manuscript. Finally, this research would not have been possible without the generous contribution of human gonadotropins by Ares Advanced Technology, Inc., and Trilostane by Sanofi Pharmaceutical Inc. This research was supported by NIH HD20869, HD18185, and RR00163.

References

1. Weick RF, Dierschke DJ, Karsch FJ, Butler WR, Hotchkiss J, Knobil E. Periovulatory time courses of circulating gonadotropic and ovarian hormones in the rhesus monkey. Endocrinology 1973;93:1140–47.
2. Hoff JD, Quigley ME, Yen SSC. Hormonal dynamics at midcycle: a reevaluation. J Clin Endocrinol Metab 1983;57:792–96.
3. Yoshinaga K. Cyclic hormone secretion by the mammalian ovary. In: Jones R, ed. The vertebrate ovary. New York: Plenum Press; 1978:691–729.
4. Rondell P. Follicular processes in ovulation. Fed Proc 1970;29:1875–79.
5. Lipner H, Greep RO. Inhibition of steroidogenesis at various sites in the biosynthetic pathway in relation to induced ovulation. Endocrinology 1971;88:602–7.
6. Zelinski-Wooten MB, Stouffer RL. Steroid receptors and action in the primate follicle. Trends Endocrinol Metab 1996;7:177–83.
7. Stouffer RL, Duffy DM. Receptors for sex steroids in the primate corpus luteum. New insight into gonadotropin and steroid action. Trends Endocrinol Metab 1995;6:83–89.
8. Hibbert ML, Stouffer RL, Wolf DP, Zelinski-Wooten MF. Midcycle administration of a progesterone synthesis inhibitor prevents ovulation in primates. Proc Natl Acad Sci USA 1996;93:1897–901.
9. Brannstrom M, Janson PO. Progesterone is a mediator in the ovulatory process of the in vitro-perfused rat ovary. Biol Reprod 1989;40:1170–78.
10. Loutradis D, Bletsa R, Aravantinos L, Kallianidis K, Michalas S, Psychoyos A. Preovulatory effects of the progesterone antagonist mifepristone (RU486) in mice. Hum Reprod 1991;6:1238–40.
11. Lydon JP, DeMayo FJ, Funk CR, Mani SK, Hughes AR, Montgomery CA Jr, et al. Mice lacking progesterone receptor exhibit pleiotropic reproductive abnormalities. Genes Dev 1995;9:2266–78.
12. Lydon JP, DeMayo FJ, Conneely OM, O'Malley BW. Reproductive phenotypes of the progesterone receptor null mutant mouse. J Steroid Biochem Mol Biol 1996;56:67–77.
13. Chaffin CL, Hess DL, Stouffer RL. Dynamics of progesterone (P) and progesterone receptor (PR) expression in the primate follicle during the periovulatory interval. In: Annual Meeting of the Endocrine Society, New Orleans, Louisiana, June 24–27, 1998, Abstract P1-306.

14. Christenson LK, Stouffer RL. Follicle-stimulating hormone and luteinizing hormone/chorionic gonadotropin stimulation of vascular endothelial growth factor production by macaque granulosa cells from pre- and periovulatory follicles. J Clin Endocrinol Metab 1997;82:2135–42.

15. Espey LL. Current status of the hypothesis that mammalian ovulation is comparable to an inflammatory reaction. Biol Reprod 1994;50:233–38.

16. Iwamasa J, Shibata S, Tanaka N, Matsuura K, Okamura H. The relationship between ovarian progesterone and proteolytic enzyme activity during ovulation in the gonadotropin-treated immature rat. Biol Reprod 1992;46:309–13.

17. Chaffin CL, Stouffer RL. Progesterone (P) promotes the expression of matrix metalloproteinases (MMPs) and their inhibitors (TIMPs) in the primate periovulatory follicle. In: Thirty-first Annual Meeting of the Society for the Study of Reproduction, College Station, Texas, August 8–11, 1998. Abstract 126.

18. Chaffin CL, Stouffer RL. Dynamics and steroid regulation of oocyte maturation in macaque follicles during the periovulatory interval. In: Serono International Symposium on "Ovulation: evolving scientific and clinical concepts," Abstract, p.33. Salt Lake City, Utah, September 24–28, 1998.

19. Peluso JJ, Pappalardo A. Progesterone mediates its anti-mitogenic and anti-apoptotic actions in rat granulosa cells through a progesterone-binding protein with gamma aminobutyric acid$_A$ receptor-like features. Biol Reprod 1998;58:1131–37.

20. Hazzard TM, Molskness TA, Chaffin CL, Stouffer RL. Changes in expression of VEGF and angiopoietin-1 in the periovulatory follicle of the rhesus macaque. In: Serono International Symposium on "Ovulation: evolving scientific and clinical concepts," Abstract, p. 34. Salt Lake City, Utah, September 24–28, 1998.

21. Peluso JJ, Pappalardo A. Progesterone maintains large rat granulosa cell viability indirectly by stimulating small granulosa cells to synthesize basic fibroblast growth factor. Biol Reprod 1999;60:290–96.

22. Mori T, Suzuki A, Nishimura T, Kambegawa A. Evidence for androgen participation in induced ovulation in immature rats. Endocrinology 1977;101:623–26.

23. Lubahn DB, Moyer JS, Golding TS, Couse JF, Korach KS, Smithies O. Alteration of reproductive function but not prenatal sexual development after insertional disruption of the mouse estrogen receptor gene. Proc Natl Acad Sci USA 1993;90:11162–66.

24. Fisher CR, Graves KH, Parlow AF, Simpson ER. Characterization of mice deficient in aromatase (ArKO) because of targeted disruption of the cyp19 gene. Proc Natl Acad Sci USA 1998;95:6965–70.

25. Ito Y, Fisher CR, Conte FA, Grumbach MM, Simpson ER. Molecular basis of aromatase deficiency in an adult female with sexual infantilism and polycystic ovaries. Proc Natl Acad Sci USA 1993;90:11673–77.

Part IV

Putative Periovulatory Intraovarian Regulators

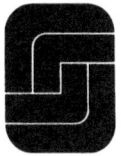

12

The Ovarian Renin Angiotensin System Viewed Through Ovarian Perfusion

C. Matthew Peterson, Masato M. Mikuni, and Mats Bränström

Introduction

In 1898, Tiegerstadt and Bergman noted that the crude saline extracts of the kidney had a powerful pressor activity, which they named *renin* (1). This discovery eventually lead to the understanding of the circulating renin angiotensin system (RAS) as a unique endocrine appendage with a clear role in blood pressure control. In the classical circulating RAS system, the JG cells secrete prorenin that is subsequently converted by endopeptidases to renin, a 347 amino acid (Fig. 12.1). Prorenin is secreted from the renal juxtaglomerular cells at 10 times the concentration of renin. Prorenin, which was originally considered a unique product of the kidney, has now been located in chorion, tumor cells, and blood vessels, as well as the adrenal gland, brain, testis, and ovary. In fact, these extrarenal sources, or tissue-based renin angiotensin systems, may account for up to 10% of the total plasma prorenin concentration.

In the circulating RAS the active cleavage product of prorenin is renin. Renin, an acid protease that cleaves the peptide bond between residues 10 and 11 of hepatically produced angiotensinogen, generates production of the decapeptide angiotensin I (Ang I). The precursor of Ang I, angiotensinogen, is routinely present in the circulation in concentrations that allow maximum velocity of Ang I production. In 1934, Goldblatt and colleagues clarified the fact that renin was actually the acid protease that initiated the formation of Ang I, and its subsequent products (2).

The peptide product of renin cleavage, now know as Ang I, was originally given two different names: angiotonin and hypertensin. From 1934 until 1958 the literature eratically used both names. In 1958, a nomenclature committee assigned it the name angiotensin. Ang I is a decapeptide with limited pharma-

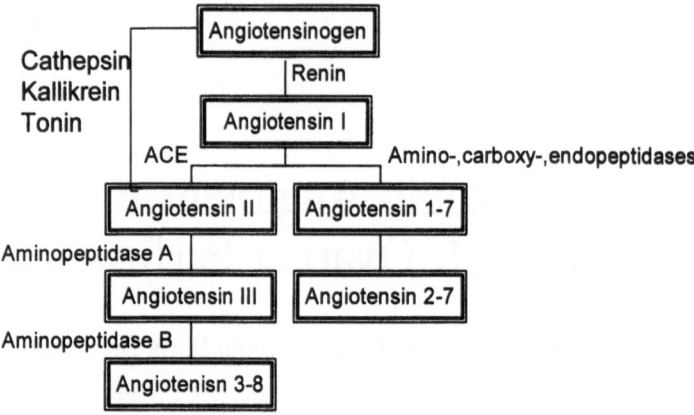

FIGURE 12.1. Schematic representation of the renin angiotensin system (RAS). Prorenin is secreted from the juxtaglomerular cells of the kidney. Renin is a proteolytic enzyme that generates the decapeptide angiotensin I (Ang I). Ang I is then cleaved through the angiotensin converting enzyme (ACE) to form the octapeptide angiotensin II (Ang II). Ang II modulates blood pressure by inducing vasoconstriction and stimulating the release of aldosterone. Tissue-based RAS systems independent of the circulating RAS have been recognized since the 1970s. Various classes of tissue enzymes capable of generating components of the renin angiotensin system are listed. The physiological activities of these peptides in various tissues are under investigation.

cological activity in the circulating RAS. It is further cleaved by a peptidyl dipeptidase know as angiotensin converting enzyme (ACE), to the octapeptide angiotensin II (Ang II). Ang II is the most potent pressor substance known, with an activity 40 times more potent than norepinephrine. Angiotensin II is the substance that possessed the pressor activity originally attributed by Tiegerstadt and Bergman to renin.

Sealey et al. initially highlighted the potential activities of a tissue-based RAS in the ovary (3). They recognized that prorenin concentrations rose dramatically during implantation, early pregnancy, and during corpus luteum formation. Subsequent studies in donor egg IVF cycles and catheterized monkey ovaries demonstrated that the major source of circulating prorenin in these cases was the ovary. Once bioactive peptides of the tissue-based RAS were discovered in the ovary investigators began to document multiple potential roles for these substances. Present knowledege suggests that the tissue-based ovarian RAS appears to possess autocrine, paracrine, and intracrine activities. Some of the physiological and pathophysiological activities of components of the tissue- based ovarian RAS include, respectively: steroidogenesis (4,5), angiogenesis (6–9), oocyte maturation (10–13), ovulation (12,14–19), and corpus luteum function (20–22); as well as ovarian hyperstimulation (23–24), polycystic ovary syndrome (25–28) , and ectopic pregnancy (29). These activities are summarized in Table 12.1.

TABLE 12.1. Summary of roles for components of the renin angiotensin system in normal and abnormal ovarian function.

• Angiogenesis	
1. Angiogenic factor in human follicular fluid	Frederick et al., 1984 (6)
2. Implantation of Ang II results in rabbit cornea neovascularization	Fernandez, 1985 (7)
3. Gonadotropin-stimulated porcine follicular fluid stimulates rabbit corneal neovascularization	Frederick et al., 1985 (8)
4. Ang II stimulates basic fibroblast growth factor in bovine luteal cells	Sterling et al., 1990 (9)
• Steroidogenesis (Conflicting data in various animal models and experimental conditions)	
1. In the presence of hCG, Ang II causes a concentration-dependent increase in P production in cultured granulosa cells and blocked by Saralasin	Morris, 1993 (4)
2. Ang II has no effect on P production in similar conditions	Rainey, 1993 (5)
• Oocyte Maturation	
1. Human follicular fluid prorenin levels correlate with follicular development, oocyte-cummulus complex maturity, and oocyte viability	Itskovitz et al., 1988 (10)
2. Saralasin (AT1/AT2) inhibits hCG stimulated GVBD in the rat	Palumbo et al., 1988 (11)
3. Saralasin reduces the stimulatory effect of hCG on maturation of ovulated oocytes without an effect on follicular oocytes in the rabbit	Yoshimura et al., 1992 (12)
4. Ang II increased GVBD in both follicular and ovulated oocytes in perfused rabbit ovaries	Kuo et al., 1993 (13)
• Ovulation	
1. Saralasin (AT1/AT2) inhibits ovulation in the rat in vivo and is reversed by Ang II	Pellicer et al., 1988 (14)
2. Inhibition of Ang II-and gonadotropin-induced ovulation in the rabbit ovarian perfusion model by Saralasin	Kuo et al., 1991 (15)
	Yoshimura et al., 1992 (12)
3. Saralasin inhibits ovulation in rat ovarian perfusion model and is reversed by Ang II	Peterson et al., 1993 (16)
4. ACE inhibition does not inhibit ovulation in the rat in vivo or in vitro	Peterson et al., 1993 (17)
5. AT2 antagonism does not inhibit ovulation in rat ovarian perfusion	Mikuni et al., 1998 (18)
6. AT1 + AT2 antagonism inhibits ovulation in rat ovarian perfusion	Mikuni et al., 1998 (18)
• Corpus Luteum Formation	
1. Cultured rat luteal cells express AT1 receptors in contrast to cultured rat granulose cells that have only AT2 receptors	Pucell et al., 1991 (20), 1993 (21)
2. Ang II induces a transient increase in cytosolic Ca 2+ concentration in rat luteal cells which is blocked by Losartan	Pepperell et al., 1993 (21)
3. Basic fibroblast growth factor (bFGF) mRNA is stimulated by Ang II and LH, which is inhibited by Saralasin	Sterling, 1990 (22)
• Pathophysiology	
1. Increased follicular fluid reninlike activity noted in OHSS	Haning, 1985 (23)
2. A direct correlation between plasma renin levels and the severity of OHSS	Navot et al., 1987 (24)
3. A direct correlation between prorenin and renin levels and bovine follicular atresia	Schultze et al., 1989 (25)
	Mukhopadhyay et al., 1991 (26)
4. PCOS patients show intense staining for renin and ANG II in all follicles in contrast to ovulatory women who stain only after luteinization	Palumbo et al., 1993 (27)
5. Low aromatase activity, hence estradiol levels, in PCOS women may be attributed to Ang II	Palumbo et al., 1988 (28)
6. Renin levels predict ectopic pregnancy	Meunier et al., 1991 (29)

Peptidyl Dipeptidase: A Link Between the Renin-Angiotensin and Kallikrein-Kinin System

The peptidyl dipeptidase, angiotensin converting enzyme (ACE, which converts Ang I to Ang II), is multifunctional. In addition to its role in converting Ang I to Ang II, it is also recognized in tissues as Kininase II. Kininase II is the enzyme responsible for the rapid degradation of bradykinin. More than two decades ago, Lawrence Espey elegantly detailed the inflammatorylike processes surrounding ovulation that include bradykinin and other similar molecules (30). The potential role of bradykinin in the ovulatory process has been documented in a number of studies. In 1976 McDonald and Perks noted that kininogen levels decreased nearly 50% in humans and rats at the time of ovulation (31). This decline was directly related to LH in subsequent investigations. Espey also confirmed an increase in kallikrein, the precursor of bradykinin, during ovulation in gonadotropin-primed immature rats (30). Bradykinin has been reported to induce ovulation in both the gonadotropin-primed perfused rat ovary as well as in the reflex ovulating rabbit (32,33). In considering the dual role of ACE activity in the tissue-based ovarian rennin–angiotensin and kallikrein–kinin systems, blockade of ACE activity in the isolated perfused rat ovary was initially investigated to determine the impact on ovulation (17). Additional studies followed that have further addressed the role of Ang II in rat ovarian function and are summarized in this chapter (16,18,19).

Isolated Rat Ovarian Perfusion Model

Isolated rat ovarian perfusion is a unique model that allows one to expose a cyclically ovulating ovary to various substances that may affect ovulation and its associated functions. This is done without exposure to other organs or organ systems that may dynamically interact with ovarian function. In this system, ovulation rates and other products (e.g., steroids, prostaglandins, cytokines, mRNA, or protein products) may be measured. This cyclically ovulating model occasionally provides results that conflict with those obtained in rabbit ovarian perfusion, which utilizes a reflex ovulating species.

In short, we utilized age, weight, litter, PMSG/hCG/IBMX lot, and experimental compound lot matched perfusions for isolated perfused rat ovay studies. We injected 26–27 day-old female Sprague-Dawley rats with 10–25 IU of PMSG (depending on the experiment). They were anesthetized 48 hours later and the right ovary was dissected and cannulated for perfusion. The ovary was then placed in the perfusion chamber and allowed to demonstrate adequate perfusion with flow rates of 0.8–1.3 ml/minute at a defined pressure before the test substance was added. Multiple ovaries may be perfused simultaneously (Fig. 12.2).

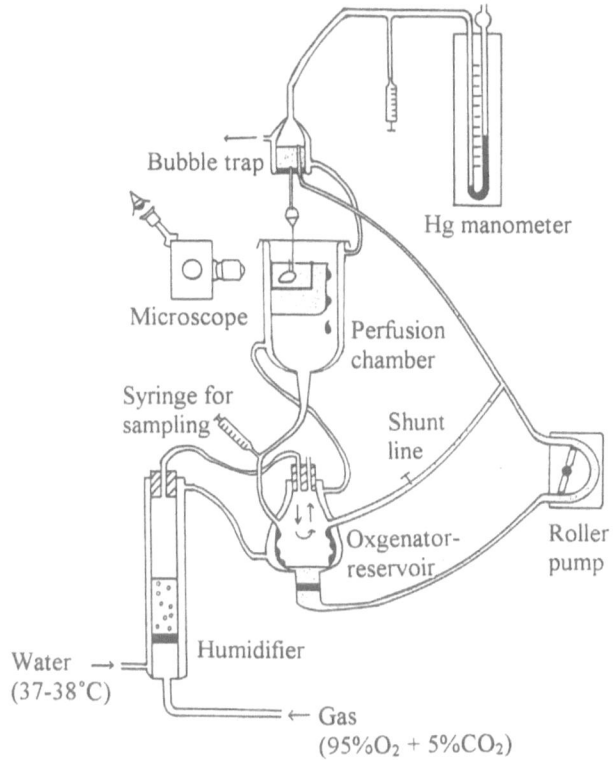

FIGURE 12.2. Schematic representation of the isolated rat ovarian perfusion apparatus.

Ovarian RAS Studies Utilizing the Isolated Rat Ovary Perfusion Model

ACE Inhibition

In initial experiments, Captopril, a potent dipeptidyl dipeptidase (ACE) inhibitor was evaluated both in vivo and using the isolated rat ovary perfusion model (17). First, homogenates of paired ovaries documented the ACE inhibitory activity of Captopril to be 26.5 nm (IC_{50}) which was consistent with the manufacturer's specifications. Endogenous ACE activity in the PMSG primed rat ovary was also found to be consistent with other tissues containing ACE. In vivo experiments, utilized three dosages designed to provide the ED_{50} of an anesthetized rat. Captopril was given prior to and during PMSG, as well as before and after hCG. In all of these regimens, Captopril demonstrated no evidence of inhibition (Table 12.2).

In isolated rat ovary perfusions, using 100 times the dose required to inhibit 100% of ACE activity, no inhibition was noted. In addition, a combina-

TABLE 12.2. Number of ovulations in vivo in captopril-treated rats.

| | Number of ovulations (mean ± SEM) | |
Regimen	Captopril group	Control group
Captopril (ip) (15 mg/kg/12 hours)	18 ± 1.5	16 ± 1.5
	(n = 5)	(n = 5)
Captopril (ip) (30 mg/kg/24 hours)	26 ± 3.2	26 ± 5.2
	(n = 11)	(n = 7)
Captopril (ip) (30 mg/kg/24 hours)	33 ± 3.0	33 ± 7.6
	(n = 10)	(n = 7)

Reprinted from Ref. 17, with permission from Elsevier Science.

tion of in vivo administration during PMSG stimulation combined with ACE inhibition in the perfusion chamber caused no inhibition. Finally, teprotide (BPP9a), another potent ACE inhibitor, caused no inhibition of ovulation (Fig. 12.3).

Nonselective Angiotensin II Inhibition with Saralasin

In 1988, Pellicer and Naftolin et al. demonstrated that the angiotensin II antagonist, saralasin, caused an inhibition of ovulation in rats stimulated with PMSG and hCG (14). Daud raised concerns regarding the report because

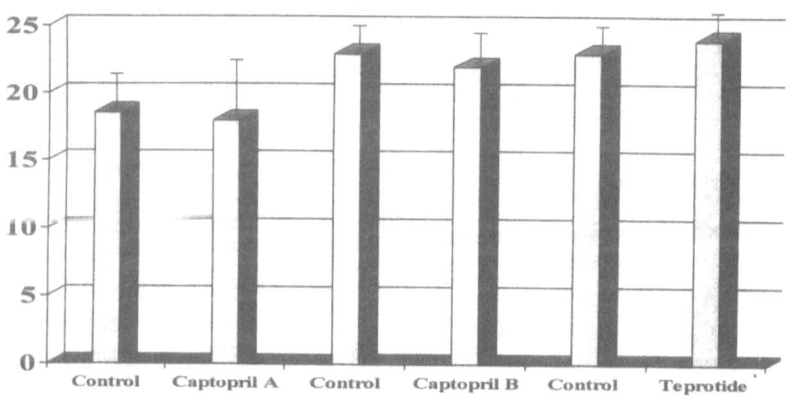

FIGURE 12.3. Number of ovulations in vitro in ACE inhibitor (Captopril and Teprotide [BPP9a]) treated perfusions demonstrated no effect. Control perfusions were performed with each set of experiments. Captopril A dose regimen utilized 30 µg/ml in the perfusate. Captopril B regimen utilized 30 µg/ml in the perfusate and 15 mg/kg /12 hour prior to and throughout PMSG stimulation. Teprotide (BPP 9a)-treated perfusions utilized 1 µg/ml in the perfusate. Reprinted from Ref. 17 with permission from Elsevier Science.

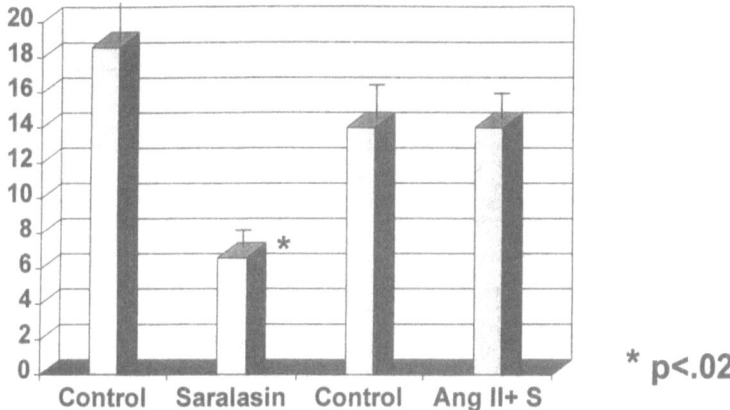

FIGURE 12.4. Saralasin, the nonspecific AT1 and AT2 inhibitor, inhibited ovulation that could be reversed by the addition of an equimolar amount of Angiotensin II. A dose–response curve for Saralasin demonstrated a progressive inhibition ovulation rate over a micro- to nanomolar range. From Ref. 16 with permission.

they could not reproduce the findings and had previously documented that Angiotensin II receptors are found in stroma, theca and lutein cells but that granulosa cells demonstrated little or no staining for Ang II until the immediate preovulatory period or when undergoing atresia (34). Hence, if Ang II played a significant role in ovulation, they expected more evidence of Ang II receptor activity in the purported tissue than immediately before ovulation.

Despite the discrepancy noted regarding Ang II, isolated rat ovarian perfusion studies found that saralasin significantly inhibited ovulation and this inhibition was reversed by the addition of an equimolar concentration of Angiotensin II (16) (Fig. 12.4).

The inhibition of ovulation by saralasin has been reconfirmed in additional experiments (18,19). Furthermore, Kuo et al., using the reflex ovulating rabbit ovary perfusion model, also noted inhibition of ovulation using saralasin (15). Thus, if Ang II was an important factor in the ovulatory process, the paradox of ligand and receptor disparity still required an explanation. A potential explanation came with the recognition of multiple subtypes of the angiotensin receptor, which are described in the following.

Angiotensin II Type 1 and 2 (AT1 and AT2) Receptors and Inhibitors

Angiotensin II receptors are functionally classified according to physio-chemical properties and binding affinities (35). AT1 receptors have a high

TABLE 12.3. Recognized AT1 and AT2 receptor antagonists.

AT1 selective	AT1/AT2	AT2 selective
DUP 753	Sar ^{1}Ile ^{8} AII	PD 123177
EXP3174	Sar^1 Ala^8 AII	PD 123319
DuP532	S-8308	CGP 42112A
L-158,809		

binding affinity for Losartan and a low affinity for PD 123319. On the other hand, AT2 receptors have the opposite characteristics. AT1 receptor binding affinities from highest to lowest are: saralasin > Ang II > Ang III >Ang I. AT1 receptors are inactivated by sulfhydryl reducing agents like dithiothreitol (DTT). They utilize calcium mobilization, inositidyl triphosphate, prostaglandins, and the reduction of adenyl cyclase as signal transduction mechanisms. AT2 receptors are enhanced and, in fact, were discovered by treatment with sulfydryl reducing reagents. They are not coupled to G proteins, and use prostaglandins and cGMP as signal transduction mechanisms. The binding affinities of AT2 receptors from highest to lowest are: Ang III >Ang II > Saralasin > Ang I. AT1 receptors, as noted, are found mainly in the follicular thecal cells and in atretic follicles. Pucell has documented the presence of AT2 receptors in follicular granulosa cells (20). A number of AT1 and AT2 receptor antagonists have been identified, which will expand our avenues of investigation. A number of the well-characterized AT1 and AT2 receptor antagonists are listed in Table 12.3.

Angiotensin II Mediated Responses

The majority of Ang II responses recognized as components of the classical renin angiotensin system are mediated through AT1 receptor. These effects include vasoconstriction, vascular contraction, nonvascular contraction, aldosterone secretion, catecholamine release, cell growth, protein synthesis; thymidine incorporation, drinking and vasopression release and the inhibition of renin release. It is probable that the AT2 receptor is activated secondary to the AT1 receptor in specific cell tissues (35). The AT2 receptor may then play a modulatory role on the AT1 receptor in biophysiological processes. Specific actions of the AT2 receptor are presently being defined.

Novel Angiotensin Receptors

Another potential explanation for the ligand–receptor paradox for Angiotensin II includes the discovery of additional novel Ang II receptors (36). A

TABLE 12.4. Novel angiotensin II receptors.

Occurrence	Response	Inhibitor	Insensitive
·Mas oncogene	Ca^{2+} Transients	D-Arg, D-Pro, D-Trp, Leu, Substance P	Losartan PD 123177
·Xenopus laevis oocytes	Ca^{2+} i	Saralasin CG 42112A	Losartan PD 123177
·Mycoplasma hyorhinis	Ang II binding	Ang I, aprotinin	Losartan CGP 42112A
·Neuroblastoma 2A	Ang II binding	Unknown	Losartan PD 123177

Reprinted in a modified form from Ref. 36, with permission.

second type of Ang II type 1 receptor named subtype 1B was identified in the rat pituitary. It has 74% sequence homology with Ang II subtype 1a. This receptor subtype is regulated to some extent by estrogen. This Ang II subtype 1b receptor is functionally the primary mediator of Ang II induced aldosterone, ACTH and prolactin secretion as well as drinking behaviors. Furthermore, there are numerous other binding sites or "novel receptors" in various tissues that are biochemically and or pharmacologically distinct from classical AT1 or AT2 receptors. For example, some bind Ang II with high affinity and selectivity, yet they are not blocked by Losartan (AT1) or PD 123177 (AT 2) (Table 12.4). The discovery of the Ang II receptor subtypes and additional novel receptors suggest that there are a multitude of potential receptor sites for Ang II.

Selective Angiotensin II Type I and II (AT1 and AT2) Inhibition Studies

To clarify the mode of action the results in the effects produced by the nonselective AT1 and AT2 inhibitor saralasin, additional ovarian perfusion studies were undertaken using saralasin and the selective inhibitors of AT1 (Losartan) and AT2 (PD 123319) (Fig. 12.5) (18,19). Comprehensive evaluations of the saralasin treated perfusions revealed reduced prostaglandin E2 (3 hours and 20 hours), and 6 keto PGF 1α (20 hours). The selective AT1 and AT2 receptor antagonists failed to inhibit ovulation when used separately. When both AT1 and AT2 receptor antagonists were added to the perfusion system, however, inhibition was noted. In this experiment the combination of 100 μM of the AT1 inhibitor, Losartan, combined with 10 μM of PD 123319, the AT2 receptor antagonist, resulted in an inhibition of ovulation. These findings suggest the necessity for dual receptor blockade to significantly affect ovulation (Fig. 12.6).

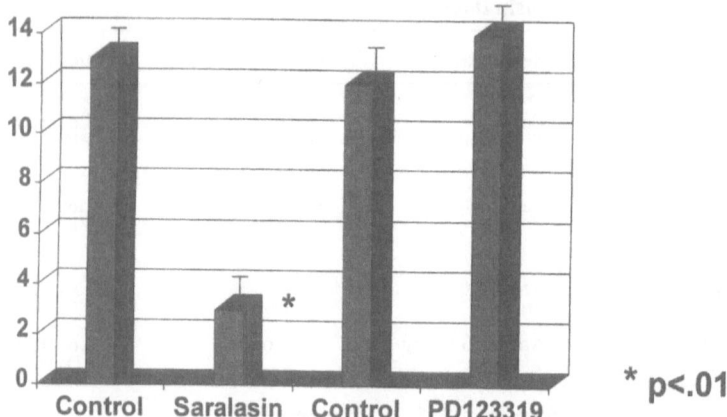

FIGURE 12.5. Saralasin, the nonspecific AT1 and AT2 inhibitor inhibited, but Angiotensin II type 2 receptor antagonist (PD 123319) did not inhibit ovulation in the perfused rat ovary. From Ref. 18 with permission.

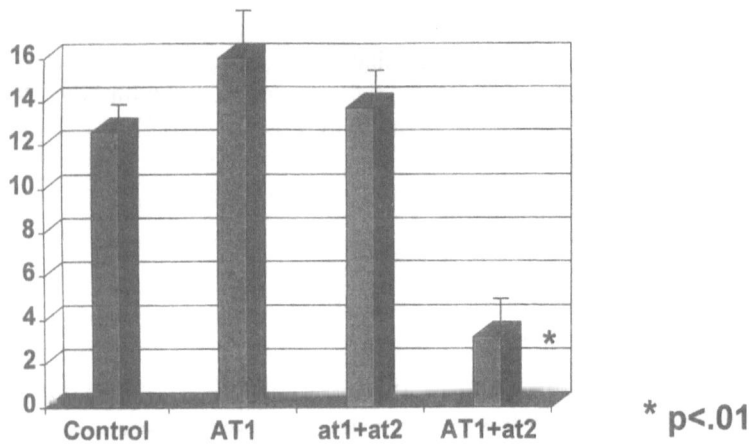

FIGURE 12.6. A combination of AT1 and AT2 receptor antagonists inhibited ovulation in the perfused rat ovary. AT1 represents Losartan, the selective AT1 inhibitor at 100 μm, which did not result in inhibition. AT1 symbolizes Losartan at 10 μm. AT1 combined with AT2, the selective AT2 inhibitor PD 123319, at 10 μm, did not inhibit ovulation. The combination of 100 μM of the AT1 antagonist, Losartan and PD123319, the AT2 receptor antagonist, at 10 μM (AT2) resulted in the inhibition of ovulation at a level similar to that produced by Saralasin. From Ref. 19 © European Society of Human Reproduction and Embryology. Reproduced by permission of Oxford University Press/ Human Reproduction.

Summary

From our viewpoint, using the rat ovarian perfusion model and anticipating future research endeavors, our results can be distilled into the following statements. First, the inhibition of ovulation associated with Ang II antagonism in isolated rat ovarian perfusion appears to be mediated through both AT1 and AT2 receptors acting in a tandem fashion. The signal transduction mechanisms and interactions between these two receptor pathways in the ovulatory process are yet unknown completely. Second, the number of possible receptor interactions for Ang II continues to expand as the discovery of additional receptor subtypes, isoforms and transcription factors occur. This is consistent with many other receptor superfamilies (37). Third, it is expected that the receptor subtypes and novel receptors will vary by tissue type, species, cycle stage, and experimental conditions. This fact will require specific evaluations for each tissue, species, cycle stage, and experimental model making extrapolation beyond any specific set of variables tenuous, if not invalid. Finally, Ang II and other peptides of the RAS (e.g., Ang I, Ang III, Ang 1-7, Ang 2-7, Ang 3-8) may originate from nonclassical tissue-based pathways and will invariably possess a host of possible receptor affinities and actions, which will also vary by tissue, cycle stage, species, and experimental conditions. Such will be the future projects designed to elucidate the function of various components of the RAS in the ovary.

References

1. Tiegerstedt R, Bergman PG. Niere und Kreislauf. Skand Arch Physiol 1898; 8:223.
2. Goldblatt H. Studies on experimental hypertension: production of persistent elevation of systolic blood pressure by means of renal ischemia. J Exp Med 1934;59: 347–79.
3. Itskowitz J, Sealey JE, Glorioso N, Laragh JH, Rosenwaks Z. The ovarian prorenin-angiotensin system. Ann NY Acad Sci 1988;541:179–89.
4. Morris RS, Paulson RJ. The ovarian renin angiotensin system: Recent advances and their relationship to assisted reproductive technologies. Assisted Reprod Rev 1993; 3:2–10.
5. Rainey WE, Bird JM, Byrd W, Carr BR. Effect of angiotensin II on human luteinized granulosa cells. Fertil Steril 1993;59:143–47.
6. Frederick JL, Shimanuki T, DiZerega GS. Initiation of angiogenesis by porcine follicular fluid. Am J Obstet Gynecol Science 1984;24:389–90.
7. Fernandez AL, Tarlatzis V, Rzaza PJ, Caride VJ, Laufer N, Negro-Villar AF, et al. Renin-like activity in ovarian follicular fluid. Fertil Steril 1985;44:219–23.
8. Frederick JL, Hoa N, Preston DS, et al. Initiation of angiogenesis by porcine follicular fluid. Am J Obstet Gynecol 1985;152:1073–78.
9. Sterling D, Magness RR, Stone R, Waterman MR, Simpson ER. Angiotensin II inhibits LH-stimulated cholesterol side chain cleavage expression and stimulates basic fi-

broblastic growth factor expression in bovine luteal cells in primary culture. J Biol Chem 1990;265:5–8.

10. Sealey JE, Glorioso N, Itskowitz J, Larah JH. Prorenin as a reproductive hormone. Am J Med 1986;81:1041–46.

11. Palumbo A, Pellicer A, DeCherney AH, Naftolin F. Angiotensin action in oocyte maturation in the rat. Thirty-fifth Annual Meeting, Society for Gynecological Investigation, Abstract 107. Baltimore, MD, 1988.

12. Yoshimura Y, Karube M, Koyama N, Shiokawa S, Nanno T, Nakamura Y. Angiotensin II directly induces follicular rupture and oocyte maturation in the rabbit. FEBS 1992;307:305–8.

13. Kuo T-D, Endo K, Dharmarajan AM, Miyazaki T, Atlas SJ, Wallach EE. Direct effect of angiotensin II on in vitro perfused rabbit ovary. J Reprod Fertil 1991;92: 469–74.

14. Pellicer A, Palumbo A, DeCherney AH, Naftolin F. Blocakage of ovulation by an angiotensin antagonist. Science 1988;240:1660–61.

15. Kuo T-C, Endo K, Dharmarajan AM, Miyazaki T, Atlas SJ, Wallach EE. Direct effect of angiotensin II on in-vitro perfused rabbit ovary. Reprod Fert 1991;92:469–72.

16. Peterson CM, Zhu C, Mukaida T, Butler TA, Woessner JJF, LeMaire WJ. The angiotensin II antagonist, saralasin, inhibits ovulation in the perfused rat ovary. Am J Obstet Gynecol 1993;168:242–45.

17. Peterson CM, Morioka N, Zhu C, Ryan JW, LeMaire WJ. Angiotensin-converting enzyme inhibitors have no effect on ovualtion and ovarian steroidogenesis in the perfused rat ovary. Reprod Toxicol 1993;7:131–35.

18. Mikuni M, Brannstrom M, Hellberg P, Peterson CA, Pall M, Edwin SS, Peterson CM. Saralasin-induced inhibition of ovualtion in the in vitro perfused rat ovary is not replicated by the angiotensin II type-2 receptor antagonist PD123319. Am J Obstet Gynecol 1998;179:35–40.

19. Mikuni M, Matousek M, Mitsube M, Peterson CM, Brannstrom M. I The combination of an angiotensin II type I (AT1) and a type 2 (AT2) receptor antagonist suppresses ovulation in the rat ovary perfused in vitro. Serono Symposium, Salt Lake City, 1999, invited presentation, and ESHRE, Goteborg, Sweden. Hum Reprod 1998;13:55, Abstract O-110.

20. Pucell AG, Hodges JC, Sen I, Bumpus FM, Husain A. Biochemical properties of the ovarian granulosa cell type 2-angiotensin II receptor. Endocrinology 1991;128: 1947–59.

21. Popperell JR, Nemeth G, Yamada Y, Naftolin F. The type 1 angiotensin II receptor mediates intracellular calcium mobilization in rat luteal cells. Endocrinology 1993;133:1678–84.

22. Sterling D, Magness RR, Stone R, Waterman MR, Simpson ER. Angiotensin II inhibits LH-stimulated cholesterol side chain cleavage expression and stimulates basic fibroblastic growth factor expression in bovine luteal cells in primary culture. J Biol Chem 1990;265:5–8.

23. Hanning EVJ, Strawn EY, Nolten WE. Pathophysiology of the ovarian hyperstimulation syndrome. Obstet Gynecol 1985;66:220.

24. Navot D, Margalioth EJ, Laufer N, Birkenfeld A, Relou A, Rosler A, et al. Direct correlation between plasma renin activity and severity of the ovarian hyperstimulation syndrome. Fertil Steril 1987;48(1):57–61.

25. Schultze D, Brunswig B, Mukhopadhyay AK. Renin and prorenin-like activities in bovine ovarian follicles. Endocrinology 1989;124:1389–98.
26. Mukhopadhyay AK, Holstein K, Szkudlinski M, Brunswig-Spickenheier B, Leidenberger FA. The relationship between prorenin levels in follicular fluid and follicular atresia in bovine ovaries. Endocrinology 1991;129:2367–72.
27. Palumbo A, Pourmotabbed G, Carcangiu ML, et al. Immunohistochemical localization of renin and angiotensin in the ovary: comparison between normal women and patients with histologically proven polycystic ovarian disease. Fertil Steril 1993;60:280–84.
28. Palumbo A, Alam M, Lightman A, DeCherney AH, Naftolin F. Angiotensin II affects in vitro steroidogeneisis by human granulosa-lutein cells. Seventieth Annual Meeting, Endocrine Society, Abstract 1075. New Orleans, LA, 1988.
29. Meunier K, Minot TM, Maria B, Guichad A, Zorn JR, Cedard L, Predictive value of the active renin assay for the diagnosis of ectopic pregnancy. Fertil Steril 1991;55:432–35.
30. Espey LL. Ovulation as an inflammatory reaction—a hypothesis. Biol Reprod 1980;22:73–106.
31. McDonald M, Perks AM. Plasma bradykininogen and reproductive cycles: studies during the oestrous cycle and pregnancy in the rat, and in the human menstrual cycle. Can J Zool 1976;54:941–47.
32. Hellberg P, Larson L, Olofsson J, Hedin L, Brannstrom M. Stimulatory effects of bradykinin on the ovulatory process in the in vitro-perfused rat ovary. Biol Reprod 1991;44:269–74.
33. Yoshimura Y, Espey L, Hosoi Y, Adachi T, Atlas SJ, Ghodgaonkar RB, et al. The effects of bradykinin on ovulation and prostaglandin production by the perfused rabbit ovary. Endocrinology 1988;122:2540–46.
34. Daud AJ, Bumpus FM, Husain A. Angiotensin II: does it have a direct obligate role in ovulation. Science 1989;243:870–71.
35. Katt KJ, Sandberg K, Balla T. Angiotensin II receptors and signal transduction mechanisms. In: Raizada MK, Phillips MI, Sumners C, eds. Cellular and molecular biology of the renin-angiotensin system. Boca Raton: CRC Press; 1993:307–56.
36. Chiu AT, Leung KH, Smith RD, Timmermans PBMWM. Defining angiotensin receptor subtypes. In: Raizada MK, Phillips MI, Sumners C, eds. Cellular and molecular biology of the renin-angiotensin system. Boca Raton: CRC Press; 1993:245–73.
37. Peterson CM. Estrogen and progesterone receptors: an overview from the year 2000. J Soc Gynecol Invest 2000;7(suppl. 1):53–57.

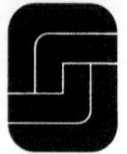

13

Ovarian Oxytocin:
Periovulatory Production and Effects

JOANN E. FORTUNE, CAROLYN M. KOMAR,
JOEL S. TABB, AND ANNE K. VOSS

Introduction

Oxytocin (OT) is most widely known for its role as a neuropeptide hormone
synthesized by hypothalamic cells for storage and release by the posterior pituitary gland to produce smooth muscle contraction during lactation and parturition. It is less widely known that the gonads secrete OT, and that OT in turn has
effects on gonadal cells. Although luteal oxytocin is believed to play a role in
luteolysis in cattle and sheep, it has been recognized that OT is also produced by
ovarian follicles and may regulate specific aspects of follicular function (for
review, see Ref. 1). OT has been detected in the follicular fluid of preovulatory
bovine, ovine, caprine, and human follicles (2–6). Experiments with cattle and
primates have shown that preovulatory follicles produce significant amounts of
OT only during the final stages of their differentiation, close to the time of ovulation (7–9), which suggests a role for OT in the ovulatory process and/or associated differentiative events (e.g., the transformation of follicular cells to luteal
cells). To study the regulation of OT production and secretion by ovarian follicles and its role in follicular function, we have used bovine preovulatory follicles obtained at specific stages of development during the follicular phase. In
this chapter we will review primarily the results of experiments with cattle conducted by our laboratory and others.

Secretion of Oxytocin by Ovarian Follicles

During the mid-1980s it was reported that bovine ovarian follicles contain
and secrete OT (2,10). To determine when during the course of their development preovulatory follicles begin to secrete OT, we isolated preovulatory
follicles at three different times during the follicular phase. In these and simi-

TABLE 13.1. OT production in vivo during development of bovine ovulatory follicles: OT mRNA and OT content in granulosa cells (GC), theca interna, and follicular fluid.

	Time during the follicular phase		
	Early	Mid	Late
OT in follicular fluid (pg/ml)	78 ± 21	61 ± 16	423 ± 96
OT in GC (pg/10^7 cells)	34 ± 13	29 ± 7	2034 ± 824
OT mRNA in GC	0.6 ± 0.6	0.3 ± 0.3	8.2 ± 3.5
OT mRNA in theca	0 ± 0	0 ± 0	0 ± 0

Data are means ± SEM ($n = 3 -9$ follicles). Preovulatory follicles were obtained in the early (24 hours after initiation of luteolysis), mid- (48 hours after initiation of luteolysis), or late (20 hours after onset of estrus) follicular phase. OT mRNA levels are based on northern blot analysis and expressed as arbitrary densitometry units (corrected for loading and transfer efficiency using values for 18 S rRNA).
Source: Regul Peptides, 45:257–261, Fortune JE, Voss AK, Oxytocin gene expression and action in bovine preovulatory follicles, from Ref. 39 © 1993, with permission from Elsevier Science.

lar experiments described in this chapter, luteolysis and a follicular phase were induced in Holstein heifers by injection of a luteolytic dose of prostaglandin F2α (PGF2α) during the luteal phase. With this model, a luteinizing hormone (LH) surge and the onset of estrous behavior begin about 48–72 hours after PGF2α injection and the preovulatory follicle ovulates about 30 hours after the LH surge. Preovulatory follicles were isolated 24 or 48 hours after PGF2α injection (i.e., in early or midfollicular phase) or 20 hours after the onset of estrous behavior. The follicular fluid was aspirated and theca and granulosa cells were separated and maintained in culture for 5 days.

As shown in Table 13.1, OT concentrations in granulosa cells and follicular fluid were low before the LH surge, but had increased dramatically by 20 hours after the onset of estrus (8). Likewise, the ability of granulosa cells to secrete OT during the first day of culture was negligible when cells were obtained before the LH surge, whereas cells isolated from periovulatory follicles 20 hours after the onset of estrus secreted large quantities of OT during the first day of culture (Fig. 13.1; 7). Regardless of the time of isolation of the preovulatory follicle, secretion of OT by granulosa cells increased during the course of culture (Fig. 13.1). For cells obtained before the LH surge/estrus the increase was linear from 48 to 120 hours of culture, but when granulosa cells were obtained after the LH surge the increase in OT secretion was linear for the first 72 hours of culture and then plateaued.

These experiments show that bovine granulosa cells synthesize and secrete OT in a developmentally regulated manner, beginning during the final day of preovulatory follicular development. Standing in contrast to the induction of OT secretion by granulosa cells at a specific time in follicular differentiation is the negligible secretion of OT by isolated theca interna, regardless of stage of follicular differentiation or time in culture (Fig. 13.1; 7). Jungclas

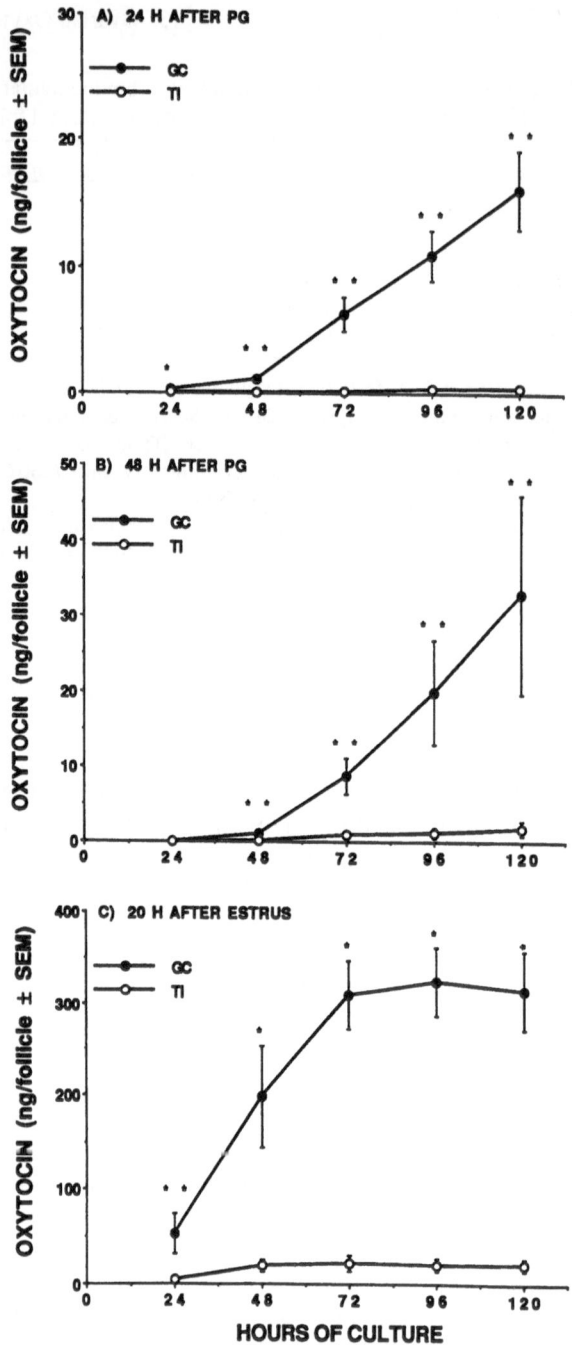

FIGURE 13.1. Comparison of OT secretion (ng/follicle ± SEM; n = 8 cultures, 2 from each of 4 follicles) by granulosa cells (GC) versus theca interna (TI) isolated at 24 or 48 hours after injection of PGF2α (PG) to induce luteolysis (panels A and B) or at 20 hours after onset of estrus (panel C), during 5 days of culture in defined medium. Within means for each culture type and time of media collection, $* = p < 0.05$, $** = p < 0.01$. From Voss AK, Fortune JE. Oxytocin secretion by bovine granulose cells. Endocrinology 1991;59:970–73. © The Endocrine Society, with permission.

and Luck (11) and Shukovski et al. (12), however, reported that co-culture with theca interna enhanced the secretion of OT by bovine granulosa cells. In our experiments, co-cultures of granulosa cells plus theca interna secreted more OT than granulosa cells alone when follicular cells were isolated before the LH surge, but not when they were isolated between the LH surge and ovulation (7).

To determine when after the LH surge bovine granulosa cells begin to upregulate OT production, we next used an experimental model in which luteolysis is induced on Day 7 of the estrous cycle (early–midluteal phase) to stimulate the development of the dominant follicle of the first follicular wave of the cycle to differentiate into a preovulatory follicle. Injection of a gonadotropin releasing hormone (GnRH) analogue 36 hours after PGF2α induces an endogenous LH surge that peaks about 2 hours after GnRH injection. Ovulation occurs about 24 hours after GnRH. Follicles were recovered at frequent intervals between GnRH injection and ovulation (at 0, 3.5, 6, 12, 18, or 24 hours), and follicular fluid and follicular cells were obtained. In organ cultures of follicle wall (theca interna with attached granulosa cells) OT secretion during the first 4 hours of culture was low when tissue was obtained at time 0 (time of GnRH injection), and was not significantly different from time 0 until 24 hours after GnRH, when OT secretion was about eightfold higher than at the other times of follicle isolation (Fig. 13.2A). In contrast, a significant rise in OT concentrations in the follicular fluid was first observed a little earlier, at 18 hours after GnRH (Fig. 13.2B).

Gonadotropins Induce OT Secretion

The dramatic increase in OT synthesis and secretion by granulosa cells after exposure to the gonadotropin surge in vivo suggests that the surge induces OT; indeed, the results of experiments in vitro support this suggestion. When granulosa cells were isolated at 24 or 48 hours after PGF2α (i.e., before the LH surge) addition of a high dose (300 ng/ml) of either LH or follicle stimulating hormone (FSH) to the culture medium increased OT secretion during 5 days of culture by about twofold (7). In contrast, neither gonadotropin stimulated granulosa cells obtained after the LH surge to increase OT secretion. Experiments with granulosa cells from preovulatory follicles isolated before the LH–FSH surge showed that the ability of LH and FSH to increase OT secretion is concentration-dependent. The lowest doses of LH or FSH that maximally stimulated OT secretion were also the lowest doses that stimulated progesterone and inhibited estradiol secretion by granulosa cells; in contrast, low doses of FSH stimulated estradiol, but not OT production by granulosa cells (13). These results in vitro lend support to the idea that a dramatic upregulation of OT is part of the panoply of changes induced in preovulatory follicles by the LH/FSH surge.

Our laboratory has begun to explore the responses of follicular cells to low versus high doses of gonadotropins to determine the signal transduction pathways that mediate the differential responses of follicular cells to low versus

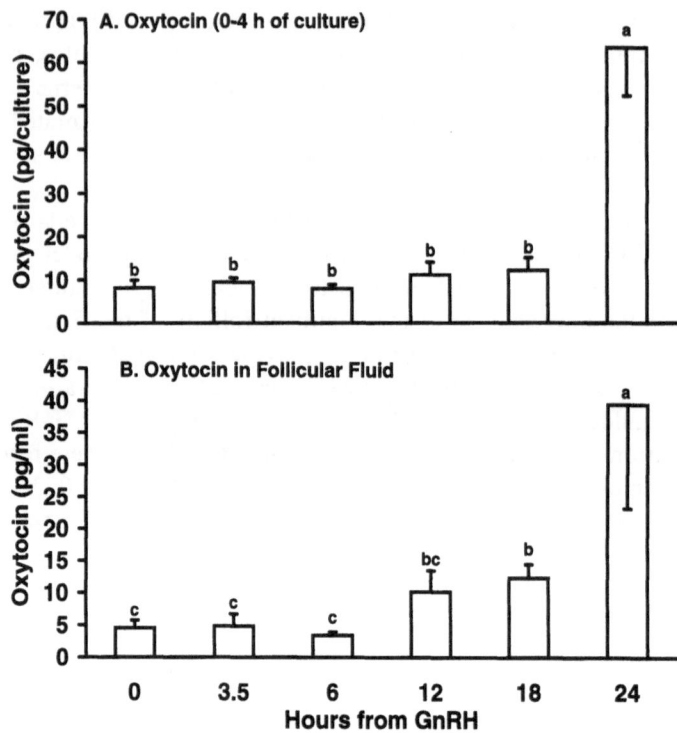

FIGURE 13.2. (A) The secretion of OT during the first 4 hours of culture by granulosa cells obtained from periovulatory follicles at various times after injection of Holstein heifers with GnRH to induce an LH surge (which peaks about 2 hours after GnRH injection). (B) Concentrations of OT in follicular fluid obtained from the same periovulatory follicles. Means ± SEM; $n = 3$ follicles per time in vivo. Within each panel, bars with no common superscripts are different ($p < 0.05$).

high concentrations of LH and FSH. Granulosa cells from preovulatory follicles obtained 24 hours after a luteolytic injection of PGF2α were cultured with low (1 or 2 ng/ml) or high (100 ng/ml) doses of ovine FSH (NIH S17), with graded doses of the cyclic AMP analogue, 8-bromo-cyclic AMP, which activates the protein kinase A (PKA) signaling pathway or with the phorbol ester TPA, which activates the protein kinase C intracellular signalling pathway. Figure 13.3, which depicts OT secretion during the third day of culture, shows that OT was maximally stimulated by 100 ng/ml FSH. High doses of 8-bromo-cyclic AMP partially mimicked the stimulatory effect of LH on OT secretion in a dose-dependent fashion, whereas TPA completely replicated the effects of FSH. The effects of 8-bromo-cyclic AMP in our experiments are consistent with the results of Meidan et al. (14), who observed an increase in OT in cultured bovine granulosa cells in response to 10 M forskolin, which

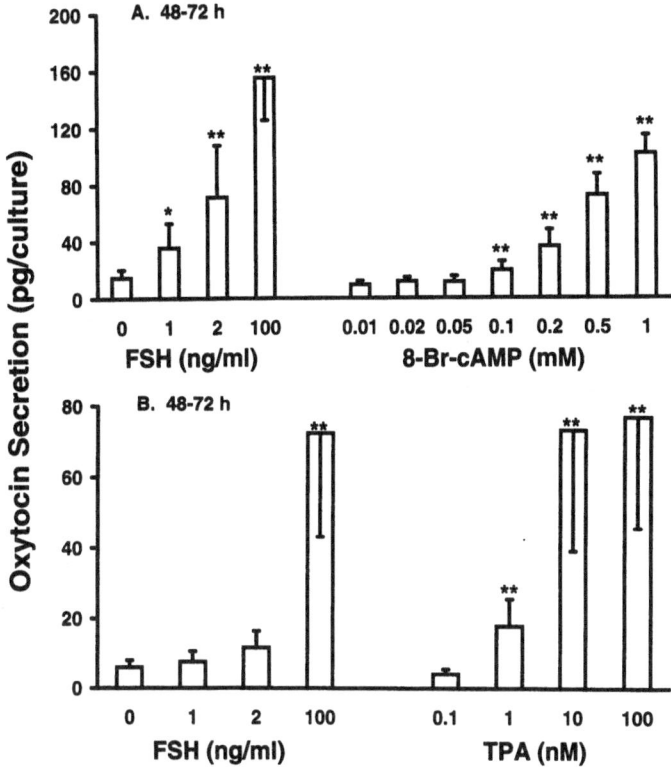

FIGURE 13.3. Effects of graded doses of the cyclic AMP analogue 8-bromo cyclic AMP or the phorbol ester TPA, a stimulator of the PKC pathway, on OT secretion by granulosa cells obtained from bovine preovulatory follicles before the LH surge. Means ± SEM; $n = 8$ cultures, 2 from each of 4 preovulatory follicles, $* = p < 0.05$, $** = p < 0.01$.

presumably activates the PKA pathway. Our results, however suggest that engagement of the PKC signaling pathway in response to a luteinizing dose of gonadotropin is necessary and sufficient for maximal OT secretion.

Expression of Messenger RNA (mRNA) for OT/neurophysin-I

During the development of ruminant corpora lutea, maximal expression of the OT/neurophysin-I (NP-I) gene, in terms of levels of mRNA, was observed 4–10 days in advance of maximal content of the peptide in luteal tissue (15,16). To determine if a similar discontinuity in synthesis of mRNA for OT and its translation into the peptide occurs in bovine ovarian follicles, we first measured mRNA for OT/NP-I by northern analysis in follicular cells obtained in the early (24 hours after PGF2α injection), mid- (48 hours after PGF2α), or late (20 hours after onset of estrus) follicular phase. OT/NP-I mRNA was not detected in theca cells at any of the three stages of preovulatory follicular differentiation (Table 13.1). In contrast, although mRNA for OT/NP-I was barely detectable in granulosa cells collected before the LH surge, by 20 hours after the onset of estrus a strong signal for the mRNA was present (Table 13.1).

When granulosa cells were obtained from preovulatory follicles before the LH surge, levels of mRNA for OT/NP-I increased dramatically with time in culture (8). Exposure in vitro to a luteinizing dose of LH (300 ng/ml) induced further increases in OT mRNA (2.5-fold greater than control cultures at 72 hours). The increases in mRNA for OT/NP-I, over time in culture and in response to LH, closely parallelled increases in OT secretion into the culture medium observed in the same cultures of granulosa cells (8). Synthesis of OT mRNA and peptide therefore appear to be closely coordinated in preovulatory follicles, in contrast to reports that suggested a delayed translation of OT/NP-I mRNA in the ruminant corpus luteum (15,16).

Modulation of OT Secretion by Insulin, Activin-A, Steroids, and Other Factors

Although gonadotropins, specifically the gonadotropin surge in vivo, appear to be the major regulators of OT production by bovine granulosa cells, other hormones and metabolic regulators can modulate its production. Insulin and insulinlike growth factor (17,18), adrenal steroids (19), and catecholamines and ascorbic acid (20, 21) enhance OT secretion by bovine granulosa cells in vitro. In contrast, activin-A inhibits both OT and progesterone secretion (22).

Because the follicular fluid is rich in steroid hormones and because their concentrations within follicular fluid are developmentally regulated (e.g., see Ref. 23), it seemed possible that steroids could modulate OT production by granulosa cells that are bathed in follicular fluid. Our laboratory examined the effects of graded doses of estradiol, testosterone, and progesterone (1 ng– 10 µg/ml) on the secretion of OT by granulosa cells obtained from preovulatory follicles during the early follicular phase (24 hours after the initiation of luteolysis) and cultured with or without a luteinizing dose of FSH (24). Estradiol had a biphasic effect. The two lowest doses of estradiol (1 and 10 ng/ml) significantly stimulated OT secretion, particularly during Days 4–5 of culture. In contrast, high doses of estradiol (1 or 10 µg/ml) dramatically decreased OT secretion. Because the estradiol concentration in follicular fluid from preovulatory follicles obtained before the LH surge is about 1.5 µg/ml, we hypothesize that an environment high in estradiol may inhibit granulosa cells from producing OT before the LH surge (i.e., it may prevent them from spontaneously luteinizing). In the presence of a luteinizing dose of FSH (100 ng/ml), only the highest dose of estradiol (10 µg/ml) inhibited OT secretion;

this effect is unlikely to be physiological because the dose is many times higher than are the concentrations of estradiol in follicular fluid after the LH surge. The effects of testosterone on OT secretion were consistent with the hypothesis that testosterone exerted effects by acting as a precursor for estradiol, but that hypothesis requires direct testing (e.g., culture of granulosa cells with a nonaromatizable androgen). Progesterone, at concentrations similar to those in follicular fluid, increased OT secretion during Days 4–5 of culture in the absence of FSH. In the presence of a luteinizing dose of FSH, progesterone was without effect, except at 10 µg/ml, which is well above the physiological range. Lioutas et al. (25) provided support for the hypothesis that progesterone upregulates OT by showing that progesterone receptor antagonists inhibit the upregulation of OT gene expression (mRNA and protein secretion) in granulosa cells luteinizing in vitro in response to forskolin.

Effects of OT on Preovulatory Follicles

Effects on Steroidogenesis

From the preceding discussion it is clear that preovulatory follicles, at least in some species, produce OT and that its production is developmentally regulated. OT mRNA is synthesized and OT is produced and secreted only during the final hours of differentiation of the periovulatory follicle. What is the role of this nonapeptide during the periovulatory period? The timing of the upregulation of OT suggests that it may play a role in the cascade of changes that leads to ovulation or that it might be important for transformation of follicular cells into luteal cells. Our laboratory has explored potential effects of OT on steroid production by follicular cells. Our initial experiments showed that OT stimulates a dose-dependent increase in progesterone secretion by granulosa cells obtained from preovulatory follicles isolated before the LH surge (26). The stimulatory effect of OT on progesterone secretion by granulosa cells was blocked completely, and in a dose-dependent manner, by an antagonist specific for OT (26). When culture medium contained a luteinizing dose of FSH, however, progesterone secretion was increased, as expected, but the addition of OT had no effect on FSH-stimulated secretion. OT had no effect on estradiol secretion in the absence or presence of a luteinizing dose of FSH (300 ng/ml). It also failed to affect the secretion of androstenedione or progesterone by theca interna cultured in control medium or with a luteinizing concentration of LH (300 ng/ml).

The next series of experiments determined that, once granulosa cells had been exposed to the LH surge in vivo, progesterone secretion in vitro was no longer stimulated either by OT or by treatment with a high dose (300 ng/ml) of LH or FSH in the medium (27). Taken together, these data suggested a specific effect of OT to stimulate progesterone secretion during the periovulatory period. It remains to be elucidated how this is affected and how important it is. OT could be an essential intermediary in the upregulation of progesterone secretion that is stimulated by the LH/FSH surge. On the other hand, LH and FSH could stimulate an increase in progesterone production by granulosa cells by more than one pathway: One that involves OT and another(s) that is independent of OT. In the latter scenario OT would play a facilitative or "fail-safe" role to insure the upregulation of progesterone secretion after the gonadotropin surge. In the experiments in which we isolated granulosa cells from periovulatory follicles at 0, 3.5, 6, 12, 18, or 24 hours after the LH surge, the upregulation of OT and progesterone occurred coincidently (data for progesterone not shown). This finding supports a connection between the two hormones, but does not help to determine which is upregulated first. Lioutas et al. (25) reported that a progesterone receptor blocker inhibits bovine granulosa cells from producing OT in response to forskolin, which implyies that upregulation of progesterone secretion is necessary for the increase in OT production by luteinizing granulosa cells.

To begin to explore the molecular mechanisms by which OT increases progesterone secretion by granulosa cells, we measured levels of mRNA for two enzymes involved in progesterone biosynthesis, cytochrome P450 side chain cleavage enzyme (P450scc) and 3β-hydroxysteroid dehydrogenase (3β-HSD) in granulosa cells cultured with or without 100 ng/ml OT (28). A small increase in mRNA for the two steroidogenic enzymes was observed, but the increase in progesterone secretion was proportionately greater. In the same experiments granulosa cells were cultured with low doses of FSH (1 and 2 ng/ml) that had previously been shown to increase estradiol secretion in vitro above untreated controls. In these experiments OT decreased both basal (contrary to our earlier experiment using a different culture medium) and FSH-stimulated estradiol secretion; however, no effects on levels of mRNA for cytochrome P450 aromatase could be detected by RNase protection assay (28). These experiments suggested that OT exerts its autocrine effects on granulosa cells by mechanisms in addition to effects on levels of mRNA.

Effects on Cumulus Expansion

There is evidence that OT may play a role in cumulus expansion in cattle. Okuda et al. (29) reported that OT stimulates cumulus expansion, in a dose-dependent manner, in bovine cumulus-oocyte complexes aspirated from small (3–5 mm) antral follicles. This effect was inhibited by an OT antagonist and by anti-OT serum.

Follicular Receptors for OT

OT presumably exerts effects on follicular cells via the seven transmembrane domain OT receptor typical of other OT target tissues. Although Einspanier et al. (9) detected immunoreactivity for OT receptor in the basal layer of granulosa cells and a few theca interna cells of marmoset preovulatory follicles before the LH surge and in all granulosa cells after injection of human chorionic gonadotropin (hCG) to induce an LH surge, there is no information about the pattern of OT receptor expression during the periovulatory period in cattle. Okuda et al. (29) have detected mRNA for OT receptor (by RT-PCR) and OT binding to granulosa cells from both small (3–5 mm) and large antral bovine follicles obtained at an abattoir. It is surprising that they reported a lower level of OT receptor expression in large, preovulatory-size follicles than that in small antral follicles. The relationship between OT secretion and expression of OT receptor in preovulatory follicles at carefully timed stages of development remains to be determined.

Comparative Aspects of Follicular OT Secretion and Action

The preceding sections were focused primarily on the production of OT and its effects on bovine preovulatory follicles; however, it is of interest to know whether the postulated role of OT as an autocrine–paracrine modulator during the final stage of follicular differentiation extends to other species. OT has been detected in follicular fluid from primates (6), sheep (4), and goats (5), as well as cattle. In addition to cattle, its production and effects have been most extensively studied in primate species. Einspanier et al. (9) reported that although OT and its receptor can be detected by immunohistochemistry in antral follicles of marmoset monkeys before the LH surge, injection of hCG greatly increases expression of both the peptide and its receptor. OT was secreted by granulosa cells collected during aspiration of human preovulatory follicles for in vitro fertilization (30) and treatment of aspirated granulosa cells with OT-decreased FSH-stimulated estradiol production, but only if the cells came from women who became pregnant after IVF (31).

Ovulation was stimulated in mice by i.p. injection of OT on the morning of proestrus, but it is not clear whether OT's action was on the anterior pituitary-hypothalamus or directly on the ovary (32). Intrabursal injection of rats with an antiserum against OT inhibited ovulation by about 50% (33), which suggests that OT may play a direct role in stimulating ovulation in rodents. A 10-fold higher ovarian content of OT in estrous ovaries compared with other cycle stages, in the absence of similar fluctuations in plasma, suggests that the rat ovary synthesizes OT (34). Mutant mice lacking two exons that code for parts of the NP-1 portion of the OT/NP-1 preprohormone (35), or lacking exon 1, which codes for OT peptide (36), are fertile, which suggests that, at least in mice, OT is not essential for follicular development or ovulation. Although homozygous mutant mice lacked processed OT in the hypothalamus or posterior pituitary, the ovaries of mutant mice were not examined for processed OT. In experiments with granulosa and theca cells isolated from rat preovulatory follicles on the morning of proestrous, we have thus far been unable to detect either OT secretion or effects of OT on steroidogenesis (Fortune, Chen, and Patel, unpublished data). Our laboratory was unable to detect

OT in follicular fluid collected from equine preovulatory follicles during the early, mid-, and late follicular phase, and equine granulosa cells did not secrete OT in vitro (37). These results are consistent with a previous report by Stevenson et al. (38), who failed to detect OT in equine CL or follicles collected at various times during the estrous cycle.

Conclusions

The data available thus far suggest that in some species (ruminants and primates) upregulation of follicular OT is part of the cascade of changes triggered by the LH–FSH surge, whereas in other species the nonapeptide either does not play a role in periovulatory events or evidence for a role is limited. OT has effects on steroid production by ruminant and primate granulosa cells, particularly a stimulatory effect on progesterone secretion, and can induce cumulus expansion in cattle. It remains to be determined whether OT plays a direct role in the ovulatory process or other periovulatory events.

Acknowledgments. The unpublished data presented in this chapter were generated with funding from the NIH (HD-14584) and the USDA (No. 96-35203-3450).

References

1. Ivell R. The physiology of ovarian oxytocin. Reprod Med Rev 1999;7:11–25.
2. Schams D, Kruip TAM, Koll R. Oxytocin determination in steroid producing tissues and in vitro production in ovarian follicles. Acta Endocrinol 1985;109:530–36.
3. Wathes DC, Swann RW, Pickering BT. Variations in oxytocin, vasopressin and neurophysin concentrations in the bovine ovary during the oestrous cycle and pregnancy. J Reprod Fertil 1984;71:551–57.
4. Wathes DC, Guldenaar SEF, Swann RW, Webb R, Porter DG, Pickering BT. A combined radioimmunoassay and immunocytochemical study of ovarian oxytocin production during the periovulatory period in the ewe. J Reprod Fertil 1986;78:167–83.
5. Kiehm DJ, Walters DL, Daniel SAJ, Armstrong DT. Preovulatory biosynthesis and granulosa cell secretion of immunoreactive oxytocin by goat ovaries. J Reprod Fertil 1989;87:485–93.
6. Schaeffer JM, Liu J, Hsueh AJW, Yen SSC. Presence of oxytocin and arginine vasopressin in human ovary, oviduct, and follicular fluid. J Clin Endocrinol Metab 1984;59:970–73.
7. Voss AK, Fortune JE. Oxytocin secretion by bovine granulosa cells: effects of stage of follicular development, gonadotropins, and coculture with theca interna. Endocrinology 1991;128:1991–99.
8. Voss AK, Fortune JE. Oxytocin/neurophysin-I messenger ribonucleic acid in bovine granulosa cells increases after the luteinizing hormone (LH) surge and is stimulated by LH *in vitro*. Endocrinology 1992;131:2755–62.
9. Einspanier A, Jurdzinski A, Hodges JK. A local oxytocin system is part of the lutein-

ization process in the preovulatory follicle of the marmoset monkey (*Callithrix jacchus*). Biol Reprod 1997;57:16–26.

10. Geenen V, Legros JJ, Hazee-Hagelstein MT, Louis-Kohn F, Lecomte-Yerna MJ, Demoulin A, et al. Release of immunoreactive oxytocin and neurophysin I by cultured luteinizing bovine granulosa cells. Acta Endocrinol 1985;110:263–70.

11. Jungclas B, Luck MR. Evidence for granulosa-theca interaction in the secretion of oxytocin by bovine ovarian tissue. J Endocrinol 1986;109:R1–R4.

12. Shukovski L, Fortune JE, Findlay JK. Oxytocin and progesterone secretion by bovine granulosa cells of individual preovulatory follicles cultured in serum-free medium. Mol Cell Endocrinol 1990; 69:17–24.

13. Berndtson AK, Vincent SE, Fortune JE. Low and high concentrations of gonadotropins differentially regulate hormone production by theca interna and granulosa cells from bovine preovulatory follicles. Biol Reprod 1995;52:1334–42.

14. Meidan R, Altstein M, Girsh E. Biosynthesis and release of oxytocin by granulosa cells derived from preovulatory bovine follicles: effects of forskolin and insulin-like growth factor-I. Biol Reprod 1992;46:715–20.

15. Jones DSC, Flint APF. Concentrations of oxytocin-neurophysin prohormone mRNA in corpora lutea of sheep during the oestrous cycle and in early pregnancy. J Endocrinol 1988;117:409–14.

16. Ivell R, Brackett KH, Fields MJ, Richter D. Ovulation triggers oxytocin gene expression in the bovine ovary. FEBS 1985;190:263–67.

17. Holtorf A-P, Furuya K, Ivell R, McArdle CA. Oxytocin production and oxytocin messenger ribonucleic acid levels in bovine granulosa cells are regulated by insulin and insulin-like growth factor-I: dependence on developmental status of the ovarian follicle. Endocrinology 1989;125:2612–20.

18. Schams D, Koll R, Li CH. Insulin-like growth factor-I stimulates oxytocin and progesterone production by bovine granulosa cells in culture. J Endocrinol 1988;116: 97–100.

19. Luck MR. Enhanced secretion of oxytocin from bovine granulosa cells treated with adrenal steroids. J Reprod Fertil 1988;83:901–7.

20. Luck MR, Jungclas B. Catecholamines and ascorbic acid as stimulators of bovine ovarian oxytocin secretion. J Endocrinol 1987;114:423–30.

21. Luck MR, Jungclas B. The time-course of oxytocin secretion from cultured bovine granulosa cells, stimulated by ascorbate and catecholamines. J Endocrinol 1988;116:247–58.

22. Shukovski L, Findlay JK. Activin-A inhibits oxytocin and progesterone production by preovulatory bovine granulosa cells *in vitro*. Endocrinology 1990;126:2222–24.

23. Fortune JE, Hansel W. Concentrations of steroids and gonadotropins in follicular fluid from normal heifers and heifers primed for superovulation. Biol Reprod 1985;32:1069–79.

24. Voss AK, Fortune JE. Estradiol-17β has a biphasic effect on oxytocin secretion by bovine granulosa cells. Biol Reprod 1993;48:1404–9.

25. Lioutas C, Einspanier A, Kascheike B, Walther N, Ivell R. An autocrine progesterone positive feedback loop mediates oxytocin upregulation in bovine granulosa cells during luteinization. Endocrinology 1997;138:5059–62.

26. Aladin Chandrasekher Y, Fortune JE. Effects of oxytocin on steroidogenesis by bovine theca and granulosa cells. Endocrinology 1990;127:926–33.

27. Voss AK, Fortune JE. Oxytocin stimulates progesterone production by bovine granu-

losa cells isolated before, but not after, the luteinizing hormone surge. Mol Cell Endocrinol 1991;78:17–24.

28. Berndtson AK, Weaver CJ, Fortune JE. Differential effects of oxytocin on steroid production by bovine granulosa cells. Mol Cell Endocrinol 1996;116:191–98.

29. Okuda K, Uenoyama Y, Fujita Y, Iga K, Sakamoto K, Kimura T. Functional oxytocin receptors in bovine granulosa cells. Biol Reprod 1997;56:625–31.

30. Plevrakis I, Clamagirand C, Pontonnier G. Oxytocin biosynthesis in serum-free cultures of human granulosa cells. J Endocrinol 1990;124:R5–R8.

31. Clamagirand C, Plevrakis I, Bussenot I, Parinaud J, Vieitez G, Grandjean H. The effect of oxytocin on oestradiol-17β and testosterone secretion by cultured human granulosa cells. Hum Reprod 1991;6:774–78.

32. Robinson G, Evans JJ, Forster ME. Oxytocin can affect follicular development in the adult mouse. Acta Endocrinol 1985; 108:273–76.

33. Viggiano M, Franchi AM, Zicari JL, Rettori V, Gimeno MAF, Kozlowski GP, et al. The involvement of oxytocin in ovulation and in the outputs of cyclo-oxygenase and 5-lipoxygenase products from isolated rat ovaries. Prostaglandins 1989;37:367–78.

34. Ho M-L, Lee J-N. Ovarian and circulating levels of oxytocin and arginine vasopressin during the estrous cycle in the rat. Acta Endocrinol 1992;126:530–34.

35. Young WS III, Shepard E, Amico J, Hennighausen L, Wagner KU, LaMarca ME, et al. Deficiency in mouse oxytocin prevents milk ejection, but not fertility or parturition. J Neuroendocrinol 1996; 8:847–53.

36. Nishimori K, Young LJ, Guo Q, Wang Z, Insel TR, Matzuk MM. Oxytocin is required for nursing but is not essential for parturition or reproductive behavior. Proc Natl Acad Sci USA 1996; 93:11699–704.

37. Stock AE, Emeny RT, Sirois J, Fortune JE. Oxytocin in mares: lack of evidence for oxytocin production by or action on preovulatory follicles. Domest Anim Endocrinol 1995;12:133–42.

38. Stevenson KR, Parkinson TJ, Wathes DC. Measurement of oxytocin concentrations in plasma and ovarian extracts during the oestrous cycle of mares. J Reprod Fertil 1991; 93:437–41.

39. Fortune JE, Voss AK. Oxytocin gene expression and action in bovine preovulatory follicles. Reg Peptides 1993;45:257–61.

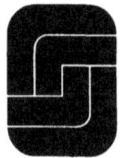

14

Neurotrophins and the Ovulatory Process: A Role for NGF and trkA?

GREGORY A. DISSEN, ARTUR MAYERHOFER, AND SERGIO R. OJEDA

It has become abundantly clear that the ovary is controlled by two systems that act in concert: The pituitary gonadotropins which reach the gland via the blood stream, and an intraovarian complex of regulatory factors, which are produced by the ovary and act in various paracrine, autocrine, and juxtacrine manners. One such factor is nerve growth factor (NGF), which belongs to a family of related target-derived proteins known as *neurotrophins* (NTs), which are required for the survival and development of discrete neuronal populations in the central and peripheral nervous systems (1,2). Five NTs have been identified, of which NGF is the best known (1). The rest of the family consists of brain-derived neurotrophic factor (BDNF) (3), neurotrophin-3 (NT-3) (4–6), neurotrophin-4/5 (NT-4/5) (7,8), and neurotrophin-6 (NT-6) (9). Select members of the neurotrophin family are required for the survival of different and overlapping neuronal populations in both the central and peripheral nervous system.

Although initial observations led to the conclusion that the biological actions of neurotrophins are restricted to the nervous system (10,11), evidence now suggests that they can also affect nonneuronal cells; particularly NGF. There are two different receptors for NGF, both of which are membrane-spanning molecules. One, which displays rapid dissociation kinetics and contains a short intracellular domain devoid of classical signaling motifs, is known as low affinity NGF receptor or p75^{NTR} (12). The other, with a slow dissociation rate and endowed with tyrosine kinase activity, is known as trkA (13). Although p75^{NTR} binds all NTs, with a similar low affinity (11,12), the trkA receptor binds NGF preferentially and with high affinity (14,15). The p75^{NTR} enhances the actions of trkA following NGF binding (16,17), but also has an independent role in programmed cell death. Binding of NGF to p75^{NTR} promotes cell death in the developing nervous system (18) and also activates the translocation of the antiapoptotic transcription activator NF-κB to the cell nucleus (19). In contrast, the trkA receptor has been shown to mediate the trophic/differentiating effects of NGF exclusively. Binding of NGF to the trkA receptor results in activation of the receptor's tyrosine kinase, which sets in motion a signaling pathway similar to that activated by other receptor tyrosine kinases (20–22).

The ovary contains four of the known neurotrophins (NGF, BDNF, NT-3 and NT-4/5) (7,23–27), and the receptors for each of them (p75^{NTR}, trkA, trkB and trkC) (28–32). Our laboratory has been examining, first, the expression of NTs and their receptors in the ovary and, second, the possible roles that these molecules may play in ovarian function. Select NTs and their receptors are expressed during key phases in the natural history of ovarian development, which suggests their involvement in the regulatory control of these phases. For example, expression of the NT-4/5 and trkB genes increases at the time of definitive ovarian histogenesis (27), and expression of the gene encoding NGF and its trkA receptor become markedly elevated in periovulatory follicles during the hours preceding the first ovulation at puberty (26). This periovulatory expression will be the focus of this chapter.

The Role of NGF and TrkA in Ovulation

Ovulation resembles an inflammatory reaction that is initiated by hormonal stimulation rather than by injury. The inflammatorylike changes that lead to ovulation result in the rupture of a healthy antral follicle(s) to allow release of the oocyte(s) for fertilization. Inflammation is driven by numerous factors, including interleukins, prostaglandins, vasoactive agents, and proteases. All of these have been found to be produced by follicular cells during the periovulatory period (33). A connection between NGF and inflammation was first suggested by the rapid activation of NGF synthesis and NGF-dependent processes that follows injury to the peripheral nervous system (34). In fact, NGF appears to be the only NT involved in inflammatory processes (19), both because its levels are upregulated in inflammation, and because cells of the immune system activated by inflammation are able to release NGF (19). In the ovary, trkA and NGF gene expression increase following the gonadotropin surge and preceding the ovulatory rupture of the follicle (26). The timing and magnitude of the NGF–trkA gene activation suggests that NGF-initiated trkA-mediated responses are integral components of ovulation; virtually no trkA mRNA can be detected either before the preovulatory LH surge (morning of proestrus) or a few hours after ovulation (i.e., on the morning of the first estrus). In contrast, more than a 100-fold increase in mRNA levels occurs shortly after the LH surge (26). Immunohistochemistry and hybridization histochemistry studies showed that NGF and trkA are synthesized by thecal cells of large antral follicles and interstitial cells (26).

TrkA gene activation in nonneural cells of the ovarian follicle at the time when the follicle is undergoing biochemical and cytological differentiation to become a new structure, the corpus luteum, suggests that ligand-mediated activation of trkA receptors contributes to these acute differentiating events. Supporting this view is the finding that selective inhibition of NGF biological actions by intrabursal administration of either an NGF antiserum or the trk-kinase blocker K-252a inhibited ovulation, as evidenced by the reduced number of corpora lutea detected in the treated ovary compared with that in the contralateral gland (26). Although the inhibitory effect of K-252a on ovulation may have not been entirely specific, immunoneutralization of NGF appeared to be exclusively related to the ability of the antiserum to obliterate the biological effect of NGF. Exposure of PC-12 cells to this antiserum prevented NGF-induced neurite extension. In contrast, the antiserum did not prevent the biological actions of BDNF or NT-4/5 on PC12 cells expressing trkB receptors (26) despite recognizing antigenic determinants in BDNF, NT-3, and NT-4/5.

The similarities between ovulation and inflammation are further exemplified by the effectiveness of IL-1β in increasing NGF and trkA mRNA levels in ovarian cells and the ability of both NGF antibodies and K-252a to reduce the increase in prostaglandin E_2 (PGE_2) elicited by the cytokine. Thus, NGF may mediate at least some of the actions of IL-1β in the preovulatory ovary (26). An involvement of NGF and its trkA receptor in the biochemical cascade that leads to ovulation is further suggested by the ability of trkA receptor activation to increase phospholipase Cγ activity (35–38), and to increase PGE_2 formation in other cell systems (39). Thecal cells placed in monolayer culture and transfected with a trkA cDNA, to express the trkA receptor in a preovulatorylike fashion, respond to NGF with a rapid increase in PGE_2 release (40). The LH-like hormone hCG also stimulates PGE_2 release, but it requires a period of at least 8 hours of hormonal treatment to do so. Although trkA receptor mRNA levels increase 3–6 hours after hCG treatment, NGF mRNA content is maintained at a high level during culture, which suggests that an active trkA is needed to mediate at least part of the stimulatory effect of hCG on PGE_2 release (40).

Interruption of cell–cell communication between thecal cells and weakening of the collagenous matrix within the follicular wall are critical events in the process leading to ovulatory rupture (33). The cells of the theca externa begin to dissociate within just a few hours after the gonadotropin surge, and this process is markedly accelerated near the actual time of ovulation (41). Dissociation of the cells of the theca externa is accompanied by elevated collagenolytic and protease enzyme activity, and by edema and dissociation of the theca interna (41–44). Although it is clear that these complex events are critical for ovulation to take place, the factors that set in motion the cellular dissociation of the follicular theca have not been identified. The increase in trkA gene expression that occurs before ovulation suggests that the NGF–trkA complex may be one of the factors involved in the initiation of this process. To test this hypothesis, we examined the ability of NGF to disrupt gap junctional communication in cultured thecal cells.

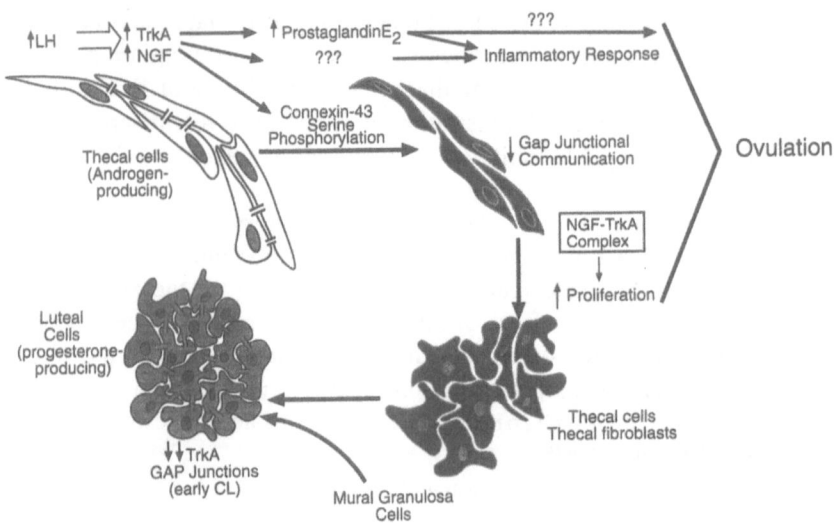

FIGURE 14.1. Postulated role of NGF and the high affinity trkA receptor in ovulation.

Loss in gap junctional communication among follicular cells is one of the initial events preceding ovulation (45). Gap junctions are small channels formed between cell membranes of juxtaposed cells that permit the exchange of ions, second messengers, and small metabolites among neighboring cells (46,47). Both granulosa and thecal cells of developing follicles form independent functional syncytia via gap-junctional intercellular coupling (48–50). The preovulatory surge of LH disrupts gap junctional communication between follicular granulosa cells (51), first causing an increase in the phosphorylation of connexin-43 (Cx43) (51), the predominant protein constituent of gap junctions in the ovary (50,52–54), and a later decrease in Cx43 protein levels (51,54). A similar effect of LH on Cx43 in thecal cells has not been described. Double hybridization histochemical experiments in rat ovaries demonstrate the presence of trkA mRNA in Cx43-expressing cells of the theca externa (55). When bovine thecal cells transiently transfected with trkA cDNA to endow them with trkA receptors were exposed to NGF, there was a rapid phosphorylation of Cx43 at serine residues (55). Dye transfer experiments confirmed that there was a decrease in transfer via gap junctions in trkA receptor-expressing thecal cells following treatment with NGF. Serine phosphorylation of connexin molecules is considered to be one of the initial steps in the sequence of events leading to gap junctional disruption in several cell types (47,56), including ovarian cells (54).

Following disruption of cell–cell contacts, both structural and communicative, fibroblastlike thecal cells switch from a quiescent to an active, proliferative condition (33). It can be inferred that NGF stimulates at least part of this process by the finding that transfection and expression of trkA receptors in cells of mesenchymal origin (e.g., fibroblasts) results in proliferative responses (17,57). Direct evidence for this view was obtained using purified bovine thecal cells transiently expressing trkA receptors. Upon exposure to NGF, but not BDNF or NT-4/5, thecal cells that express the trkA receptor responded with a significant increase in their rate of proliferation (40). Thus, NGF may play a role both in disrupting the communication between thecal cells before ovulation, as well as in stimulating the increase in proliferative activity that accompanies and follows follicular rupture.

Summary

Our current concept of the involvement of NGF and its high affinity receptor in the ovulatory process is shown in Figure 14.1. Expression of the NGF and the trkA genes is dramatically unregulated in the follicular wall at the time of the gonadotropin surge, prior to the ovulatory rupture. NGF then acts on responsive thecal cells to induce cellular changes associated with ovulation (e.g., release of PGE_2, serine phosphorylation of Cx43, a decrease in gap junctional communication, and cell proliferation). Our results suggest that NGF contributes to that cascade of events that lead to the rupture of the follicular wall at ovulation and subsequent corpus luteum formation.

Acknowledgments. This work was supported by NIH grants HD24870, P30 Population Center Grant HD18185, and RR00163 for the operation of the ORPRC.

References

1. Levi-Montalcini R. The nerve growth factor 35 years later. Science 1987;237:1154–62.
2. Snider WD. Functions of the neurotrophins during nervous system development: what the knockouts are teaching us. Cell 1994;77:627–38.
3. Leibrock J, Lottspeich F, Hohn A, Hofer M, Hengerer B, Masiakowski P, et al. Molecular cloning and expression of brain-derived neurotrophic factor. Nature 1989;341:149–52.
4. Maisonpierre PC, Belluscio L, Squinto S, Ip NY, Furth ME, Lindsay RM, et al. Neurotrophin-3: a neurotrophic factor related to NGF and BDNF. Science 1990; 247:1446–51.
5. Hohn A, Leibrock J, Bailey K, Barde Y-A. Identification and characterization of a novel member of the nerve growth factor/brain-derived neurotrophic factor family. Nature 1990;344:339–41.
6. Rosenthal A, Goeddel DV, Nguyen T, Lewis M, Shih A, Laramee GR, et al. Primary structure and biological activity of a novel human neurotrophic factor. Neuron 1990;4:767–73.

7. Berkemeier LR, Winslow JW, Kaplan DR, Nikolics K, Goeddel DV, Rosenthal A. Neurotrophin-5: a novel neurotrophic factor that activates trk and trkB. Neuron 1991;7:857–66.
8. Ip NY, Ibañez CF, Nye SH, McClain J, Jones PF, Gies DR, et al. Mammalian neurotrophin-4: structure, chromosomal localization, tissue distribution, and receptor specificity. Proc Natl Acad Sci USA 1992;89:3060–64.
9. Götz R, Köster R, Lottspeich F, Schartl M, Thoenen H. Neurotrophin-6 is a new member of the nerve growth factor family. Nature 1994;372:266–69.
10. Raffioni S, Bradshaw RA, Buxser SE. The receptors for nerve growth factor and other neurotrophins. Ann Rev Biochem 1993;62:823–50.
11. Thoenen H. The changing scene of neurotrophic factors. Trend Neurosci 1991;14: 165–70.
12. Meakin SO, Shooter EM. The nerve growth factor family of receptors. Trend Neurosci 1992;15:323–31.
13. Barbacid M, Lamballe F, Pulido D, Klein R. The *trk* family of tyrosine protein kinase receptors. Biochim Biophys Acta 1991;1072:115–27.
14. Kaplan DR, Hempstead BL, Martin-Zanca D, Chao MV, Parada LF. The *trk* proto-oncogene product: a signal transducing receptor for nerve growth factor. Science 1991;252:554–58.
15. Klein R, Jing S, Nanduri V, O'Rourke E, Barbacid M. The *trk* proto-oncogene encodes a receptor for nerve growth factor. Cell 1991;65:189–97.
16. Benedetti M, Levi A, Chao MV. Differential expression of nerve growth factor receptors leads to altered binding affinity and neurotrophin responsiveness. Proc Natl Acad Sci USA 1993;90:7859–63.
17. Hantzopoulos PA, Suri C, Glass DJ, Goldfard MP, Yancopoulos GD. The low affinity NGF receptor, p75, can collaborate with each of the trks to potentiate functional responses to the neurotrophins. Neuron 1994;13:187–201.
18. Dechant G, Barde Y-A. Signalling through the neurotrophin receptor p75^NTR. Curr Opin Neurobiol 1997;7:413–18.
19. Carter BD, Kaltschmidt C, Kaltschmidt B, Offenhäuser N, Böhm-Matthaei R, Baeuerle PA, et al. Selective activation of NF-κB by nerve growth factor through the neurotrophin receptor p75. Science 1996;272:542–45.
20. Martin-Zanca D, Oskam R, Mitra G, Copeland T, Barbacid M. Molecular and biochemical characterization of the human *trk* proto-oncogene. Mol Cell Biol 1989;9:24–33.
21. Kaplan DR, Martin-Zanca D, Parada LF. Tyrosine phosphorylation and tyrosine kinase activity of the *trk* proto-oncogene product induced by NGF. Nature 1991;350:158–60.
22. Szeberényi J, Erhardt P. Cellular components of nerve growth factor signaling. Biochim Biophys Acta 1994;1222:187–202.
23. Ernfors P, Wetmore C, Olson L, Persson H. Identification of cells in rat brain and peripheral tissues expressing mRNA for members of the nerve growth factor family. Neuron 1990;5:511–26.
24. Hallböök F, Ibañez CF, Persson H. Evolutionary studies of the nerve growth factor family reveal a novel member abundantly expressed in Xenopus ovary. Neuron 1991;6:845–58.
25. Lara HE, Hill DF, Katz KH, Ojeda SR. The gene encoding nerve growth factor is expressed in the immature rat ovary: effect of denervation and hormonal treatment. Endocrinology 1990;126:357–63.
26. Dissen GA, Hill DF, Costa ME, Dees WL, Lara HE, Ojeda SR. A role for *trk*A

nerve growth factor receptors in mammalian ovulation. Endocrinology 1996;137:198–209.

27. Dissen GA, Hirshfield AN, Malamed S, Ojeda SR. Expression of neurotrophins and their receptors in the mammalian ovary is developmentally regulated: changes at the time of folliculogenesis. Endocrinology 1995;136:4681–92.

28. Klein R, Parada LF, Coulier F, Barbacid M. *trk*B, a novel tyrosine protein kinase receptor expressed during mouse neural development. EMBO J 1989;8:3701–9.

29. Lamballe F, Klein R, Barbacid M. *trk*C, a new member of the *trk* family of tyrosine protein kinases, is a receptor for neurotrophin-3. Cell 1991;66:967–79.

30. Dissen GA, Hill DF, Costa ME, Ma YJ, Ojeda SR. Nerve growth factor receptors in the peripubertal rat ovary. Mol Endocrinol 1991;5:1642–50.

31. Amano O, Abe H, Kondo H. Ultrastructural study on a variety of non-neural cells immunoreactive for nerve growth factor receptor in developing rats. Acta Anat 1991;141:212–19.

32. Wheeler EF, Bothwell M. Spatiotemporal patterns of expression of NGF and the low-affinity NGF receptor in rat embryos suggest functional roles in tissue morphogenesis and myogenesis. J Neurosci 1992;12:930–45.

33. Espey LL, Lipner H. Ovulation. In: Knobil E, Neill JD, eds. Physiology of reproduction, Second edition. New York: Raven Press; 1994:725–80.

34. Lindholm D, Heumann R, Meyer M, Thoenen H. Interleukin-1 regulates synthesis of nerve growth factor in non-neuronal cells of rat sciatic nerve. Nature 1987;330:658–9.

35. Ohmichi M, Decker SJ, Pang L, Saltiel AR. Nerve growth factor binds to the 140 kd *trk* proto-oncogene product and stimulates its association with the *src* homology domain of phospholipase C gamma 1. Biochem Biophys Res Commun 1991;179:217–23.

36. Vetter ML, Martin-Zanca D, Parada LF, Bishop JM, Kaplan DR. Nerve growth factor rapidly stimulates tyrosine phosphorylation of phospholipase C-gamma 1 by a kinase activity associated with the product of the *trk* protooncogene. Proc Natl Acad Sci USA 1991;88:5650–54.

37. Stephens RM, Loeb DM, Copeland TD, Pawson T, Greene LA, Kaplan DR. Trk receptors use redundant signal transduction pathways involving SHC and PLC-gamma 1 to mediate NGF responses. Neuron 1994;12:691–705.

38. Kim U-H, Fink D Jr, Kim HS, Park DJ, Contreras ML, Guroff G, et al. Nerve growth factor stimulates phosphorylation of phospholipase C-gamma in PC12 cells. J Biol Chem 1991;266:1359–62.

39. Kaplan MD, Olschowka JA, O'Banion MK. Cyclooxygenase-1 behaves as a delayed response gene in PC12 cells differentiated by nerve growth factor. J Biol Chem 1997;272:18534–37.

40. Dissen GA, Mayerhofer A, Parrot JA, Hill DF, Skinner MK, Ojeda SR. Neurotrophins and ovarian function: activation of *trk*A receptors causes periovulatory-like changes in thecal cell activity. Proceedings of the Tenth International Congresss on Endocrinology 1996; 578 (abstract).

41. Bjersing L, Cajander S. Ovulation and the mechanism of follicle rupture. Cell Tissue Res 1974;153:15–30.

42. Reich R, Daphna-Iken D, Chun SY, Popliker M, Slager R, Adelmann-Grill BC, et al. Preovulatory changes in ovarian expression of collagenases and tissue metalloproteinase inhibitor messenger ribonucleic acid: role of eicosanoids. Endocrinology 1991; 129:1869–75.

43. Curry TE Jr, Mann JS, Estes RS, Jones PBC. α2-Macroglobulin and tissue inhibitor of metalloproteinases: collagenase inhibitors in human preovulatory ovaries. Endocrinology 1990;127:63–68.
44. Curry TE Jr, Dean DD, Sanders SL, Pedigo NG, Jones PBC. The role of ovarian proteases and their inhibitors in ovulation. Steroids 1989;54:501–21.
45. Dekel N. Regulation of oocyte maturation by cell to cell communication. In: Piva F, Bardin CW, Forti G, Motta M, eds. Cell to cell communication in endocrinology. New York: Raven Press; 1988;181–94.
46. Dermitzel R, Spray DC. Gap junctions in the brain: where, what type, how many and why? Trend Neurosci 1993;16:186–92.
47. Bennett MVL, Barrio LC, Bargiello TA, Spray DC, Hertzberg E, Sáez JC. Gap junctions: new tools, new answers, new questions. Neuron 1991;6:305–20.
48. Amsterdam A, Rotmensch S. Structure-function relationships during granulosa cell differentiation. Endocr Rev 1987;8:309–37.
49. Erickson GF, Magoffin DA, Dyer CA, Hofeditz C. The ovarian androgen producing cells: a review of structure/function relationships. Endocr Rev 1985;6:371–99.
50. Mayerhofer A, Garfield RE. Immunocytochemical analysis of the expression of gap junction protein connexin 43 in the rat ovary. Mol Reprod Dev 1995;41:331–38.
51. Granot I, Dekel N. Phosphorylation and expression of connexin-43 ovarian gap junction protein are regulated by luteininzing hormone. J Biol Chem 1994;269:30502–9.
52. Beyer EC, Paul DL, Goodenough DA. Connexin 43: a protein from rat heart homologous to gap junction protein from liver. J Cell Biol 1987;105:2621–29.
53. Risek B, Guthrie S, Kumar N, Gilula NB. Modulation of gap junction transcript and protein expression during pregnancy in the rat. J Cell Biol 1990;110:269–82.
54. Wiesen JF, Midgley AR Jr. Changes in expression of connexin 43 gap junction messenger ribonucleic acid and protein during ovarian follicular growth. Endocrinology 1993;133:741–46.
55. Mayerhofer A, Dissen GA, Parrott JA, Hill DF, Mayerhofer D, Garfield RE, et al. Involvement of nerve growth factor in the ovulatory cascade: TrkA receptor activation inhibits gap-junctional communication between thecal cells. Endocrinology 1996;137:5662–70.
56. Lau AF, Kanemitsu MY, Kurata WE, Danesh S, Boynton AL. Epidermal growth factor disrupts gap-junctional communication and induces phosphorylation of connexin43 on serine. Mol Biol Cell 1992;3:865–74.
57. Cordon-Cardo C, Tapley P, Jing S, Nanduri V, O'Rourke E, Lamballe F, et al. The trk tyrosine protein kinase mediates the mitogenic properties of nerve growth factor and neurotrophin-3. Cell 1991;66:173–83.

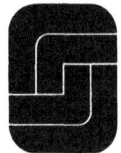

15

Cooperative Roles for the Angiopoietins and Vascular Endothelial Growth Factor in Ovarian Angiogenesis

STANLEY J. WIEGAND, PATRICIA BOLAND, AND GEORGE D. YANCOPOULOS

Angiogenesis is characterized by the initiation of blood vessel growth from an existing vascular plexus and the subsequent elaboration and remodeling of the newly generated vessels to form a definitive vasculature. The process of angiogenesis is governed by the complex interplay of numerous regulatory factors. Among these, vascular endothelial growth factor (VEGF) is the best known and most thoroughly studied of the pro-angiogenic factors (1). A second family of vascular endothelium specific growth factors has been discovered (2–4). This chapter provides a brief introduction to the biology of the angiopoietins and their receptors, and reviews findings that indicate that VEGF and the angiopoietins play critical and complementary roles in the regulation of ovarian angiogenesis.

VEGF, the Angiopoietins, and Their Receptors

VEGF is relatively unique among proangiogenic growth factors in terms of its specificity for the vascular endothelium (1). This specificity of action is attributable to the restricted distribution of the VEGF receptors, Flt-1 and Flk-1/KDR, which are expressed predominantly by vascular endothelial cells and endothelial cell precursors. VEGF can induce endothelial cell differentiation, proliferation and migration, as well as the formation of new blood vessels. The angiopoietins, like VEGF, act specifically on endothelial cells and their precursors as a consequence of the restricted distribution of their receptors, the Ties, to these cell types. The Ties are receptor tyrosine kinases, as are the receptors for VEGF. All known angiopoietins bind to Tie2/Tek, but it is still unclear as to whether they also utilize the closely related receptor, Tie1.

The angiopoietins are unusual among growth and regulatory factors because the family contains both receptor activators as well as naturally occurring receptor antagonists (2–4). For example, when angiopoietin-1 (Ang1) binds to Tie2, the tyrosine residues within the intracellular domain of the receptor become phosphorylated (2). This, in turn, initiates a signaling cascade within the affected cell. Although angiopoietin-2 (Ang2) also binds to Tie2 on endothelial cells, these receptors and downstream signaling molecules are not activated. Furthermore, by binding competitively to Tie2, Ang2 can block its activation by Ang1. The discovery of Ang2 provided the first example of a naturally occurring ligand antagonist for a vertebrate tyrosine kinase receptor (3). The existence of this naturally occurring antagonist immediately suggested that blockade of Tie2 function might itself play an important role in vascular remodeling. Studies have indeed shown that VEGF and the angiopoietins act in a coordinated and complementary manner during angiogenesis. Their respective actions have been particularly well defined in the course of embryonic development and cyclic remodeling of the female reproductive tract.

The Interplay of VEGF and the Angiopoietins During Embryonic Angiogenesis

Gene knockout studies have demonstrated that VEGF and its receptors are absolutely required for the earliest stages of vascular development in the embryo. When both alleles of Flk-1/KDR (5) or Flt-1 (6) are inactivated, mouse embryos exhibit gross abnormalities in endothelial cell differentiation and vasculogenesis and die between Days 8 and 9 of gestation. Mice lacking even a single VEGF allele (7,8) do not survive beyond embryonic Day 12. In contrast, the early stages of VEGF-dependent vascular development appear to occur normally in embryos that lack either Ang1 (9) or its Tie2 receptor (10,11). Subsequent development of the primitive vasculature is severely disrupted, however, leading to embryonic lethality between embryonic Days 11 and 12. It is now well established that Ang1 and Tie2 play key roles in mediating the interactions of vacular endothelial cells with the surrounding extracellular matrix and supporting cells (e.g., smooth muscle) (12,13). In the absence of optimized extracellular interactions, primitive vessels fail to undergo normal remodeling and also appear to be at risk for regression (14,15). Thus, even though VEGF plays an essential role in the formation of the primordial vascular system, Ang1 acts later in development to promote the survival and differentiation of the newly formed vasculature (3). Consistent with the notion that Ang2 acts as a natural antagonist for Ang1–Tie2 interactions, transgenic overexpression of Ang2 during embryogenesis produces a lethal phenotype reminiscent of that seen in embryos lacking either Ang1 or Tie2 (3).

In contrast to embryos and young animals, the vascular system in adults is remarkably stable and undergoes significant growth or remodeling only under certain physiological or pathophysiological conditions; for example, co-incident with cyclic changes in the female reproductive tract, during wound healing and in association with the growth of solid tumors. It is interesting that both VEGF and Ang1 continue to be expressed in many adult tissues following the cessation of active angiogenesis (1,9), which suggests that these proangiogenic factors may also play important roles in maintaining the integrity or in regulating the function of mature vascular networks. In contrast, Ang2 is expressed at high levels only in those tissues that are uniquely subject to ongoing vascular remodeling: the uterus, placenta and ovary (3).

VEGF, the Angiopoietins, and Ovarian Angiogenesis

The stereotypic pattern of vascular remodeling that occurs in the uterus and ovary over the course of the reproductive cycle has been well characterized (16), making these tissues particularly suited to the study of mechanisms that regulate angiogenesis and vascular regression. Indeed, in situ hybridization studies in the ovary provided the first clear evidence that VEGF acts as a mediator of physiological angiogenesis in mature rodents and primates (17–20). To further elucidate the roles of Ang1 and Ang2 in angiogenesis we therefore elected to evaluate their expression in the ovary (3). In addition to examining ovaries of adult rats, ovaries obtained from immature animals were evaluated at selected times following administration of pregnant mare serum gonadotrophin (PMSG). Adjacent frozen sections were processed for localization of VEGF, Ang1 and Ang2 mRNAs by in situ hybridization, and the ovarian vasculature was visualized in corresponding sections by immunostaining with an antibody against rat endothelial cell antigen (RECA), which is a universal marker of vascular endothelial cells (21).

Expression Patterns of VEGF, Ang1, and Ang2 in the Ovary

The vasculature of ovarian follicles comprises two concentric rings of blood vessels within the theca: an inner plexus immediately subjacent to the basement membrane separating the theca interna and the stratum granulosum, and an outer vascular plexus at the interface of the theca interna and theca externa. This circumferential vascular network expands as the follicle grows, but remains confined to the thecal layers (Fig. 15.1). As described previously (19), VEGF is expressed at low to moderate levels in the ovarian stroma and by the thecal cells of small follicles. Ang1 is also expressed at low levels by the interstitial tissue of the ovary, with moderately higher levels apparent in the theca of small and intermediate follicles (3). Ang2 mRNA is expressed at moderate to high levels by a subset of blood vessels within the ovarian stroma.

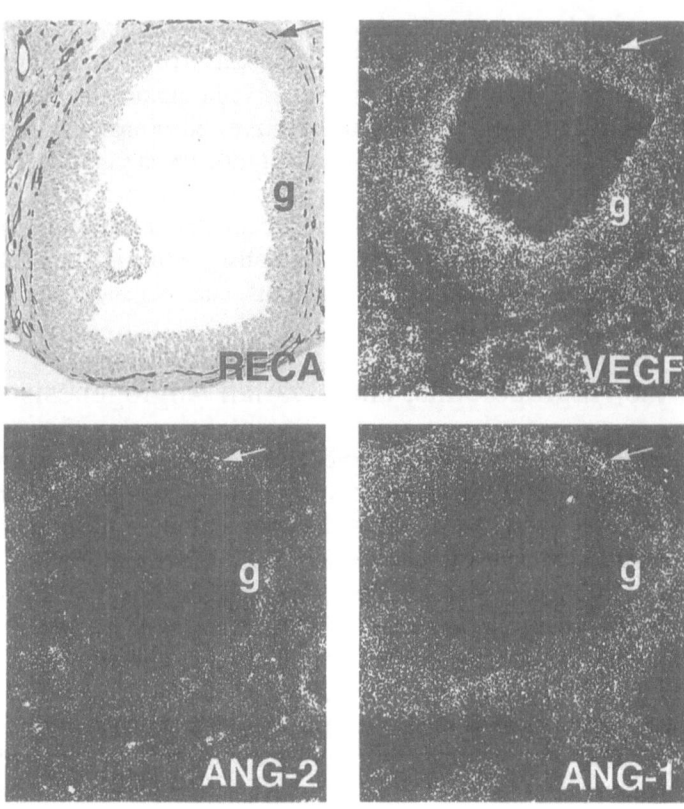

FIGURE 15.1. Preovulatory follicles in ovaries taken from prepubertal rats 56 hours after treatment with PMSG. The micrograph at the upper left shows a section stained for rat endothelial cell antigen (RECA). The vasculature of the preovulatory follicle is confined to the theca. The remaining micrographs illustrate adjacent sections taken from an equivalent specimen and hybridized for detection of VEGF, Ang1, and Ang2 mRNAs. Note that even though VEGF expression is highest in the granulosa layer (g), Ang1 mRNA is expressed primarily in the theca. Ang2 is expressed only by blood vessels present in the theca and ovarian stroma. The arrow indicates the approximate boundary between the theca and granulosa layers.

Unlike VEGF and Ang1, however, Ang2 is not expressed in preantral follicles, or in vesicular follicles of small or intermediate size (3).

The expression patterns of VEGF and Ang2 change dramatically immediately prior to and following ovulation. As antral follicles increase in size, VEGF mRNA becomes apparent in the granulosa as well as the theca, initially in cells that surround the oocyte (19). As the follicle matures, VEGF expression continues to increase in the cumulus and surrounding regions. In preovulatory follicles (Fig. 15.1), VEGF is expressed at high to moderate levels throughout the inner portion of granulosa layer, and at distinctly lower levels within the theca and contiguous outer part of the stratum granulosum. Ang2 mRNA first becomes apparent in follicles near the time of ovulation, when intense, focal expression of Ang2 is specifically associated with blood vessels in the thecal layers. In contrast, Ang1 mRNA continues to be expressed diffusely in the theca as follicles grow to the preovulatory stage, and there is little or no expression in the stratum granulosum.

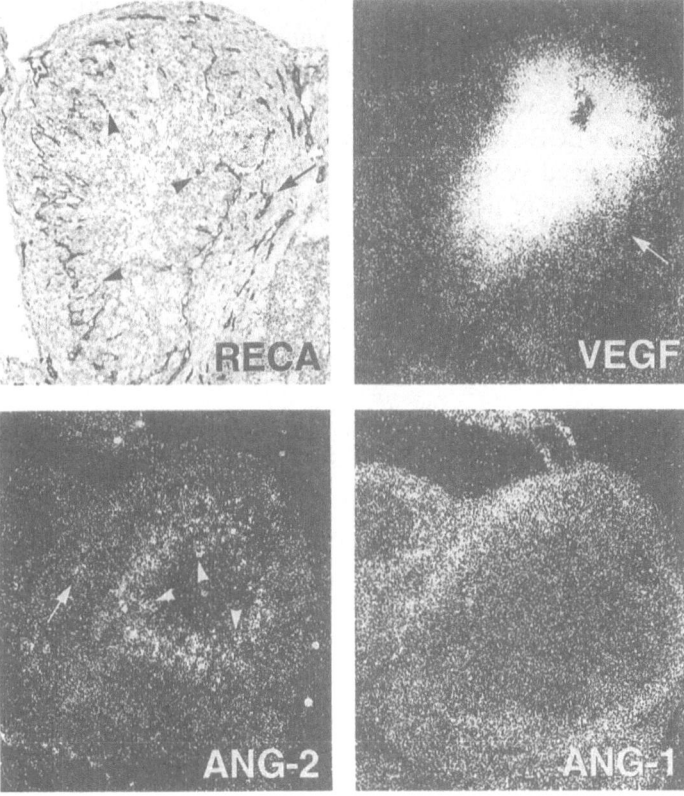

FIGURE 15.2. Developing corpora lutea; 72 hours following PMSG treatment (approximately 8 hours after ovulation). Figure format and abbreviations are the same as for Figure 15.1. Arrowheads delimit the front of new vessels growing into the developing corpus luteum from the extant thecal vasculature (arrow). At this time, the center for the newly forming corpus luteum is avascular and cells in this region have not yet undergone luteinization. Ang2 expression is highest in the growing front of blood vessels in the pericentral region of the corpus luteum. VEGF mRNA is expressed at highest levels in the central and pericentral regions of the developing corpus luteum, although Ang1 is expressed at highest levels peripherally.

Shortly after ovulation, the basement membrane that separates the theca and granulosa regresses, and new vessels begin to extend from the original circumferential thecal network into the rapidly differentiating cell mass that forms the developing corpus luteum (Fig. 15.2). VEGF mRNA is expressed at very high levels, particularly at the center of the developing corpus luteum, which has not yet been vascularized. VEGF expression decreases rather abruptly toward the periphery of the forming corpus luteum, and is especially low in regions that correspond to the original thecal layers. The pattern of Ang1 expression is virtually a mirror image of that seen for VEGF. The highest levels of Ang1 mRNA are found peripherally, with little or no detectable expression of Ang1 evident at the center of the developing corpus luteum. At this early stage of luteal development, punctate Ang2 mRNA expression is particularly apparent within the pericentral region of the developing corpus luteum, over the growing front of blood vessels, partially overlapping the field of intense VEGF expression. Ang2 mRNA also continues to be expressed by occasional blood vessels at the periphery of the developing corpus luteum, in the vicinity of the original thecal vasculature.

Approximately 36 hours after ovulation, the process of luteinization is essentially complete (Fig. 15.3). There is again a marked change in the ex-

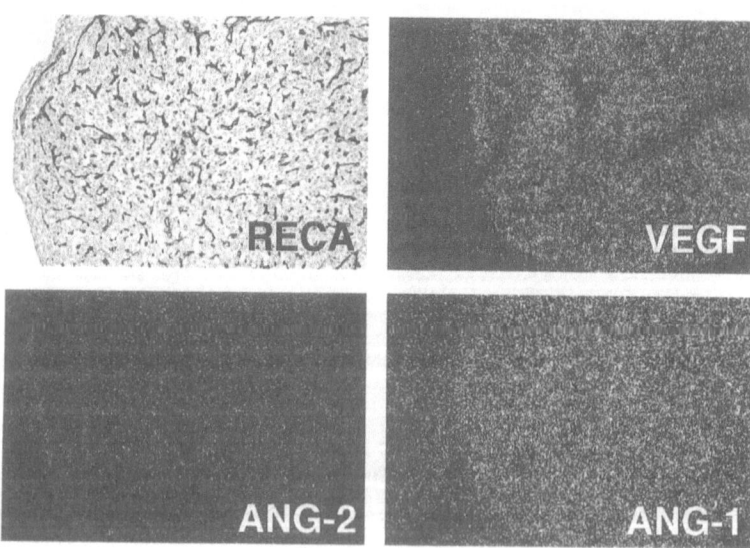

FIGURE 15.3. Functionally mature corpora lutea, approximately 4.5 days following PMSG treatment. Figure format and abbreviations as for Figure 15.1. Luteinization is complete and the corpus luteum is well vascularized. VEGF and Ang1 mRNAs are both expressed uniformly throughout the body of the corpus luteum, but Ang2 expression is dramatically downregulated.

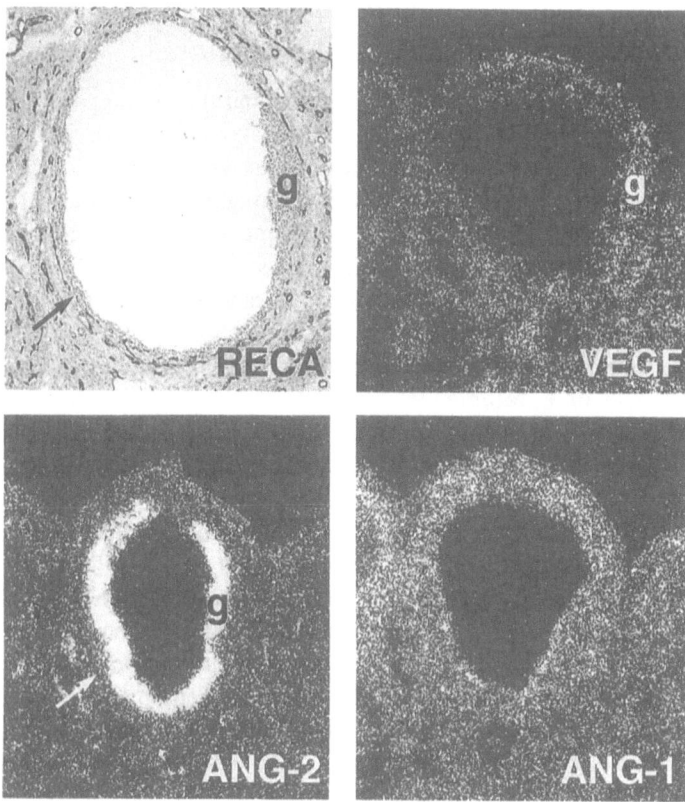

FIGURE 15.4. Atretic follicles; 72–96 hours after PMSG treatment; format and abbreviations as for Figure 15.1. Ang2 is dramatically upregulated in the stratum granulosum of regressing follicles, coincident with dissolution of the thecal vasculature. Ang1 mRNA is expressed at moderate levels in both the theca and granulosa, whereas VEGF is expressed only at very low levels.

pression of VEGF and the angiopoietins that is coincident with the functional maturation of the corpus luteum and its vasculature. At this stage, VEGF and Ang1 mRNAs are expressed uniformly and at moderate levels throughout the luteinized tissue, although Ang2 mRNA is no longer detectable within the corpus luteum. It is interesting that the pattern of angiopoietin and VEGF expression in atretic follicles is completely distinct from that of either preovulatory follicles, or ovulated follicles that have undergone luteinization (Fig. 15.4). VEGF mRNA is expressed only at low levels in atretic follicles, whereas Ang1 is expressed at moderate levels in both the theca and granulosa layers. Ang2 is expressed at remarkably high levels in the stratum granulosum of atretic follicles.

The Roles of the Angiopoietins in the
Cyclic Remodeling of Ovarian Vasculature

The preceding observations strongly suggest that the angiogpoietins act co-operatively with VEGF in the process of ovarian angiogenesis. Ang1 mRNA is abundant in the functionally mature corpus luteum, but, unlike VEGF, it is not expressed at high levels in early stages of luteal development. These observations are consistent with those made in gene knockout studies, and they support the notion that VEGF plays a pivotal role in the earliest phases of angiogenesis, whereas Ang1 acts somewhat later in the process. Ferrara and colleagues have provided unequivocal proof that VEGF is essential for the initiation of luteal angiogenesis in rats (22). In these experiments, administration of a soluble, truncated VEGF receptor (Flt-1) blocked neovascularization of the corpus luteum following gonadotropin-induced ovulation. Ang2 is highly expressed by thecal and luteal blood vessels immediately preceding and during luteal angiogenesis. This observation suggests that, like VEGF, Ang2 plays an important role in neovascularization of the corpus luteum; however, Ang2 is also expressed at very high levels in atretic follicles and involuting corpora lutea (not illustrated), which are conditions that are characterized by vascular regression (16,23). In considering this apparent paradox, it is important to note that there are two important features that distinguish Ang2 expression in the contexts of angiogenesis and vascular regression. In angiogenic environments, Ang2 is expressed by blood vessels, probably endothelial cells themselves, and VEGF mRNA is expressed at high levels in the surrounding tissues. In contrast, in environments characterized by vascular regression Ang2, is expressed at high levels by parenchymal cells and VEGF is down-regulated. Similarly distinct patterns of VEGF and Ang2 expression have been described in relation to angiogenesis and vascular regression in the bovine ovary (24).

On the basis of the above observations, we have proposed that Ang2 plays an important facilitative role in diverse aspects of vascular remodeling (3); specifically, high local levels of Ang2 are thought to abrogate a constitutive survival signal mediated by Ang1 activation of Tie2. In the absence of a compensatory increase in the expression of other endothelial cell survival factors (e.g., VEGF) overexpression of Ang2 results in endothelial cell detachment, apoptosis, and ultimately regression of the affected vessels. On the other hand, coincident expression of high levels of VEGF would prevent apoptosis of the affected endothelial cells. In this circumstance, neutralization of Ang1–Tie2-mediated interactions between endothelial cells and the surrounding stroma would serve only to "destabilize" the existing vasculature. This would in turn enhance VEGF-mediated endothelial cell mobilization and proliferation, thus facilitating initiation of a robust angiogenic response from an extant vascular network. Subsequent downregulation of Ang2 and concomitant upregulation of Ang1 expression in the surrounding tissue would be essential for the differentiation and stabilization of the newly formed vascular network.

Discussion

Although the preceding schema for coordinate action of VEGF and the angiopoietins is based on observations made in the embryo and the ovary, it may well apply to a broad range of normal and pathological conditions where vascular remodeling is a prominent feature. For example, in the adult, Ang2 is normally expressed at high levels, together with VEGF and Ang1, only in tissues that undergo physiological vascular remodeling; specifically, the ovary, uterus and placenta. Although the precise pattern of angiopoietin expression has not yet been examined in relation to vascular proliferation and regression in the uterus and placenta, it is likely that the expression patterns and functional that obtain in the ovary will be recapitulated. This is certainly the case for VEGF, which has been shown to promote both angiogenesis and vascular permeability in the uterus (25–27). Moreover, VEGF appears to mediate these same effects in a wide variety of pathological conditions in which abnormal angiogenesis and/or increased vascular permeability are hallmarks (e.g., tumors, rheumatoid arthritis, diabetic retinopathy and age-related macular degeneration) (1). Although the data is currently quite limited, it appears that the angiopoietins will also be shown to reprise their physiological roles in a variety of pathological conditions. For example, it has been reported that VEGF and the angiopoietins affect the remodeling of tumor vasculature in much the same manner as they regulate the remodeling of blood vessels in the ovary (28–30).

Therapeutic Opportunities in Reproductive Disorders

Given that cyclic angiogenesis and vascular regression are prominent features of the normal ovary and uterus, it is not surprising that abnormal blood vessel growth and/or vascular dysfunction have been found to characterize many pathological conditions that affect these organs. These vascular abnormalities are thought to be caused or perpetuated by the dysregulated expression of one or more angiogenic or antiangiogenic factors, most prominently VEGF. For example, abnormal angiogenesis is characteristic of polycystic ovary disease, endometriosis, and endometrial carcinoma. In each case VEGF is overexpressed in the affected tissue (20,31–33). Overexpression of VEGF is also thought to play a pathogenic role in the establishment of vascular hyperpermeability in preeclampsia (34) and ovarian hyperstimulation syndrome (35,36). A number of strategies have been devised to inhibit the action of endogenous VEGF in various pathological conditions, including administration of neutralizing antibodies or soluble, truncated VEGF receptors (1). On the other hand, specific kinase inhibitors are being developed , that block ligand-mediated activation of the VEGF receptors (37). Even though each of these approaches has shown some success in inhibiting the growth of various cancers in experimental animals, anti-VEGF therapies to date have, for the most part, not been tested in the context of reproductive disorders. One study, however, found that administration of a VEGF-neutralizing antibody can inhibit the growth of human ovarian carcinoma cells transplanted into nude mice, and completely block the formation of malignant ascites (38). These findings suggest that anti-VEGF therapies may soon find applications for the treatment of the various reproductive disorders in which VEGF is over-expressed.

To date, the role of angiopoietins in the pathogenesis of reproductive disorders has been little studied. Thus, their potential therapeutic utility, or that of agents that neutralize their activity, is more speculative. Administration of a soluble form of Tie2, however, has been reported to inhibit the growth and metastases of mammary carcinoma and melanoma in mice (39). Whether this effect is mediated through neutralization of Ang1 and/or Ang2 is presently unclear. It has also been reported that transgenic overexpression of Ang1 results in the development of blood vessels that are resistant to vascular leak caused by application of various inflammatory agents, including VEGF (40). Thus, Ang1 itself may effectively ameliorate pathogenic vascular hyperpermeability. Given the advances being made, it is likely that an increased understanding of the biology of VEGF, the angiopoietins, and other angiogenic factors will lead to the development of novel therapies for the treatment of diseases in which aberrant angiogenesis or vascular dysfunction contribute significantly to the pathology.

References

1. Ferrara N, Davis-Smyth T. The biology of vascular endothelial growth factor. Endocrinol Rev 1997;18:4–25.
2. Davis S, Aldrich TH, Jones PF, Acheson A, Compton D, Vivek J, et al. Isolation of Angiopoietin-1, a ligand for the TIE2 receptor, by secretion-trap expression cloning. Cell 1996;87:1161–69.
3. Maisonpierre PC, Suri C, Jones PF, Bartunkova S, Wiegand SJ, Radziejewski C, et al. Angiopoietin-2, a natural antagonist for Tie2 that disrupts in vivo angiogenesis. Science 1997;277:55–60.
4. Valenzuela DM, Griffiths JA, Rojas J, Aldrich T, Jones PF, Zhou H, et al. Angiogpoietins 3 and 4: diverging gene counterparts in mice and humans. Proc Natl Acad Sci USA 1999;96:1904–9.
5. Shalaby F, Rossant J, Yamaguchi TP, Gertsenstein M., Wu XF, Breitman, MI., et al. Failure of blood-island formation and vasculogenesis in Flk-1-deficient mice. Nature 1995;376:62-66.
6. Fong G-H, Fossant J, Gertsenstein M, Breitman M. Role of Flt-1 receptor tyrosine kinase in regulation of assembly of vascular endothelium. Nature 1995;376:66–67.
7. Ferrara N, Carver-Moore K, Chen H, Dowd M, Lu L, O'Shea KS, et al. Heterozygous embryonic lethality induced by targeted inactivation of the VEGF gene. Nature 1996;380:439–42.
8. Carmeliet P, Ferreira V, Breier G, Pollefeyt S, Kieckens L, Gertsenstein M, et al. Abnormal blood vessel development and lethality in embryos lacking a single VEGF allele. Nature 1996;380:435–39.
9. Suri C, Jones PF, Patan S, Bartunkova S, Maisonpierre PC, Davis S, et al. Requisite role of Angiopoietin-1, a ligand for the Tie2 receptor, during embryonic angiogenesis. Cell 1996;87:1171–80.

10. Dumont, DJ, Gradwohl G, Fong GH, Puri MC, Gertsenstein M, Auerbach A, et al. Dominant-negative and targeted null mutations in the endothelial receptor tyrosine kinase, tek, reveal a critical role in vasculogenesis of the embryo. Gene Dev 1994;8:1897–909.

11. Sato TN, Tozawa Y, Deutsch U, Wolburg-Buchholz K, Fujiwara Y, Gendron-Maguire M, et al. Distinct roles of the receptor tyrosine kinases Tie-1 and Tie-2 in blood vessel formation. Nature 1995;376:70–74.

12. Patan S. TIE1 and TIE2 receptor tyrosine kinases inversely regulate embryonic angiogenesis by the mechanism of intussusceptive microvascular growth. Microvasc Res 1998;56:1–21.

13. Lindahl P, Hellstrom M, Kalen M, Betsholtz C. Endothelial-perivascular cell signaling in vascular development: lessons from knockout mice. Curr Opin Lipidol 1998;9:407–11.

14. Koblizek TI, Weiss C, Yancopoulos GD, Deutsch U, Risau W. Angiogpoietin-1 induces sprouting angiogenesis in vitro. Curr Biol 1998;8:529–32.

15. Papapetropoulos A, Garcia-Cardena G, Dengler TJ, Maisonpierre PC, Yancopoulos GD, Sessa WC. Direct actions of angiopoietin-1 on human endothelium: evidence for network stabilization, cell survival, and interaction with other angiogenic growth factors. Lab Invest 1999;79:213–23.

16. Reynolds LP, Killeas SD, Redmer DA. Angiogenesis in the female reproductive system. FASEB J 1992;6:886–92.

17. Phillips HS, Hains J, Leung DW, Ferrara N. Vascular endothelial growth factor is expressed in rat corpus luteum. Endocrinology 1990;127:965–68.

18. Ravindranath N, Little-Ihrig L, Phillips HS, Ferrara N, Zeleznick AJ. Vascular endothelial growth factor mRNA expression in the primate ovary. Endocrinology 1992;131:254–60.

19. Shweiki D, Itin A, Neufeld G, Gitay-Goren H, Keshet E. Patterns of expression of vascular endothelial growth factor (VEGF) and VEGF receptors in mice suggest a role in hormonally regulated angiogenesis. J Clin Invest 1993;91:2235–43.

20. Kamat BR, Brown LF, Manseau EJ, Senger DR, Dvorak HF. Expression of vascular permeability factor/vascular growth factor by human granulosa and theca lutein cells. Role in corpus luteum development. Am J Pathol 1995;146:157–65.

21. Duijvestijn AM, van Goor H, Klatter F, Majoor GD, van Bussel E, van Breda Vriesman PJ. Antibodies defining rat endothelial cells: RECA-1, a pan-endothelial cell-specific monoclonal antibody. Lab Invest 1992;66:459–66.

22. Ferrara N, Chen H, Davis-Smyth T, Gerber HP, Nguyen TN, Peers D, et al. Vascular endothelial growth factor is essential for corpus luteum angiogenesis. Nat Med 1998;4:336–40.

23. Modlich U, Kaup FJ, Augustin HG. Cyclic angiogenesis and blood vessel regression in the ovary: blood vessel regression during luteolysis involves endothelial detachment and vessel occlusion. Lab Invest 1996;74:771–80.

24. Goede V, Schmidt T, Kimmina S, Kozian D, Augustin HG. Analysis of blood vessel maturation processes during cyclic ovarian angiogenesis. Lab Invest 1998;78:1385–94.

25. Cullinan-Bove K, Koos RD. Vascular endothelial growth factor/vascular permeability factor expression in the rat uterus: rapid stimulation by estrogen correlates with estrogen-induced increases in uterine capillary permeability and growth. Endocrinology 1993;133:829–37.

26. Chakraborty I, Das SK, Dey SK. Differential expression of vascular endothelial growth

factor and its receptor mRNAs in the mouse uterus around the time of implantation. J Endocrinol 1995;147:339–52.

27. Das SK, Chakraborty I, Wang J, Dey SK, Hoffman LH. Expression of vascular endothelial growth factor (VEGF) and VEGF-Receptor messenger ribonucleic acids in the peri-implantation rabbit uterus. Biol Reprod 1997;56:1390–99.

28. Holash J, Maisonpierre PC, Compton D, Boland P, Alexander CR, Zagzag D, et al. Vessel cooption, regression and growth in tumors mediated by angiopoietins and VEGF. Science 1999;284:1994–98.

29. Zagzag D, Hooper A, Friedlander DR, Chan W, Holash J, Wiegand, SJ, et al. In situ expression of angiopoietins in astrocytomas identifies angiopoietin-2 as an early marker of tumor angiogenesis. Exp Neurol 1999;159:391–400.

30. Siemeister G, Schirner M, Weindel K, Reusch P, Menrad A, Marme D, et al. Two independent mechanisms essential for tumor angiogenesis: inhibition of human melanoma xenograft growth by interfering with either the vascular endothelial growth factor receptor pathway or the Tie-2 pathway. Cancer Res 1999;59:3185–91.

31. Shifren JL, Tseng JF, Zaloudek CJ, Ryan IP, Meng YG, Ferrara N, et al. Ovarian steroid regulation of VEGF in the human endometrium: implications for angiogenesis during the menstural cycle and in the pathogenesis of endometriosis. J Clin Endocrinol Metab 1996;81:3112–18.

32. Donnez J, Smoes P, Gillerot S, Casanas-Roux F, Nisolle M. Vascular endothelial growth factor (VEGF) in endometriosis. Hum Reprod 1998;13:1686–90.

33. Guidi AJ, Abu-Jawdeh G, Tognazzi K, Dvorak HF, Brown LF. Expression of vascular permeability factor (vascular endothelial growth factor) and its receptors in endometrial carcinoma. Cancer 1996;78:454–60.

34. Baker PN, Krasnow J, Roberts JM, Yeo KT. Elevated serum levels of vascular endothelial growth factor in patients with preeclampsia. Obstet Gynecol 1995;86:815–21.

35. McClure N, Healy DL, Rogers PAW, Sullivan J, Beaton L, Haning RV Jr, et al. Vascular endothelial growth factor as capillary permeability agent in ovarian hyperstimulation syndrome. Lancet 1994:344:235–36.

36. Levin ER, Rosen GF, Cassidenti DL, Yee B, Meldrum D, Wisot A, et al. Role of vascular endothelial cell growth factor in ovarian hyperstimulation syndrome. J Clin Invest 1998;102:1978–85.

37. Fong TAT, Shawver LK, Sun L, Tang C, App H, Powell TJ, et al. SU5416 is a potent and selective inhibitor of the vascular endothelial growth factor receptor (Flk-1/KDR) that inhibits tyrosine kinase catalysis, tumor vascularization, and growth of multiple tumor types. Cancer Res 1999;59:99–106.

38. Mesiano S, Ferrara N, Jaffe RB. Role of vascular endothelial growth factor in ovarian cancer: inhibition of ascites formation by immunoneutralization. Am J Pathol 1998;153:1249–56.

39. Lin P, Buxton JA, Acheson A, Radziejewski C, Maisonpierre PC, Yancopoulos GD, et al. Antiangiogenic gene therapy targeting the endothelium-specific receptor tyrosine kinase Tie2. Proc Natl Acad Sci USA 1998;95:8829–34.

40. Thurston G, Suri C, Smith K, McClain J, Sato TN, Yancopoulos GD, et al. Leakage-resistant blood vessels in mice transgenically overexpressing Angiopoietin-1. Science 1999;286:2511–14.

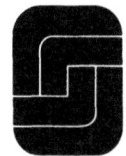

16

Visualization of the Periovulatory Follicle: Morphological and Vascular Events

Ulf J. Zackrisson, Masato M. Mikuni, and Mats Brännström

Introduction

The rapid development of molecular biology methods have led to a considerable increase in the understanding of ovarian physiology. In parallel, several in vitro techniques have been utilized to investigate the morphological and vascular changes during the ovulatory process. Although there has been a comparative development of technical equipment to capture dynamic morphology changes, there are very few in vivo observations regarding morphological changes that occur during the ovulatory process. This is most likely due to the technical difficulties involved in following a delicate prolonged physiological process that occurs intraabdominally. In this chapter we will discuss observations of changes in and around the follicle during ovulation as seen during in vitro perfusion (1,2) and in vivo (3) in relation to earlier studies in this field.

Morphological Changes and Dynamics of Ovulation

Ovulation involves the process whereby the fertilizable oocyte is released from the interior of the follicle to the exterior surface of the ovary. The most prominent feature of this process is the rupture of the follicle wall. The follicle wall consists of five layers (Fig 16.1). The outermost layer is the *surface epithelium*, consisting of a single cell layer of cuboidally formed cells, which are formed as a continuation of the peritoneal sheet that covers the inside of the abdominal cavity. The second layer from the exterior is the *tunica albu-*

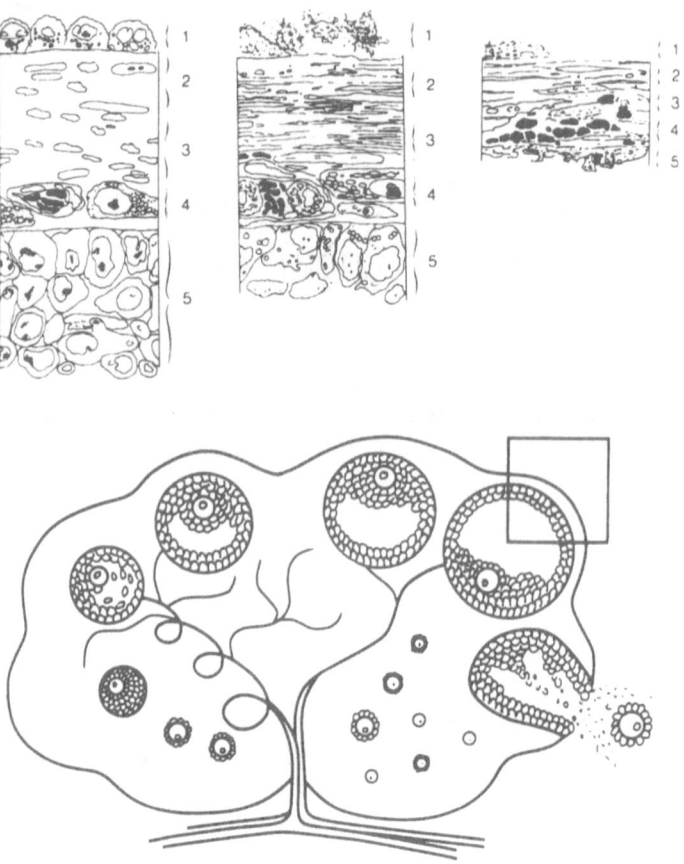

FIGURE 16.1. Schematic figure of the rat ovary illustrating the vascular system and follicles of various developmental stages. At the top, gradual morphological changes of the follicle wall prior to ovulation are illustrated. 1) surface epithelium; 2) tunica albuginea; 3) theca externa; 4) theca interna; 5) stratum granulosum.

ginea, mainly formed by collagen fibers (collagen I, III) and fibroblasts. This capsular structure surrounds the entire ovary. The third layer, named *theca externa*, delinates the outermost part of the follicle and is composed of connective tissue (collagen I, III) with fibroblasts and theca cells. Interior to the theca externa is a layer of secretory theca cells, called *theca interna*. The innermost cell layer is the stratum granulosum, including the cumulus mass around the oocyte. Two basal laminas, a lattice-type network of collagen IV intertwined with a network of laminin, are seen within the follicular wall. The outer is located between the germinal epithelium and the tunica albuginea; the inner is located between the theca interna and the stratum granulosum.

The preovulatory LH surge induces an array of morphological changes in the follicle caused by a biochemical cascade involving a number of inflammatory mediators (e.g., eicosanoids, tissue degrading enzymes, and cytokines) (4). The structural changes induce a gradual weakening of the follicle wall. Luteinization of the steroidogenic cells of the follicle and oocyte maturation take place parallel to this.

Weakening and thinning of the follicular wall, together with increased volume, causes the apical part of the follicle to bulge over the ovarian surface with an increased transluscency (2). These findings are substantiated by other in vitro findings of decreased tensile strength of the follicular connective tissue prior to ovulation (5) with an increased distensibility of the follicular wall (6). The weakening of the follicle wall has been explained by the action of proteolytic enzymes (7) with degradation of the collagen rich cell layers of the follicular wall. Furthermore, electron microscopic demonstrations of accumulating multivesicular bodies within cells of the follicle wall (8) supports increased levels of enzymatic activity prior to ovulation.

In vivo observations during early stages of the ovulatory process show uniform morphological changes with increased transparency of the follicle wall, detachment of germinal epithelium over the apex with subsequent appearence of a textured stigma (9,10). These observations are in line with electron microscopy studies (11,12) as well as recordings of the perfused rabbit and rat ovary (1,2). We have observed that during the subsequent later stages of the ovulatory process (3), the morphological changes on the apex can be quite different between ovulations (Fig. 16.2). In some cases, the apex and the stigma change in shape to form a cone and no leakage of follicular fluid prior to the extrusion is seen. In other cases, a highly viscous mass is gradually formed over the stigma without the typical cone formation. A similar viscous mass was seen in vitro (2), where a meshlike structure consisting of a sticky transluscent material would capture cells extruded from the interior of the follicle.

The extrusion (Fig. 16.3) is a relatively slow process that varies in time (2–12 minutes) with an intermittent extrusion of cumulus cells (2,3,9). In most cases a modest but variable bleeding is observed in the follicular wall and into the antrum, although some ovulations occur without any visible bleeding (3). It is not known what major forces generate the follicular rupture. In early studies it was thought that an increase in intrafollicular pressure was responsible for the rupture of the follicle. In line with this, contractile activity of the follicle was suggested to be an integral part of the process of extrusion (12). Reports have identified myoidlike filaments in the tissue of the follicular wall (13,14) and also cytoplasmatic filaments in follicular fibroblast tissue (15). It is interesting that artificial increase of intravascular pressure does not cause follicular rupture in the sow (16), and that micromanometric measurements of intrafollicular pressure in the rabbit ovary demonstrated constant pressure levels with a rapid drop immediatly prior to the onset of rupture (17). Previous studies have also documented that ovulation occurs

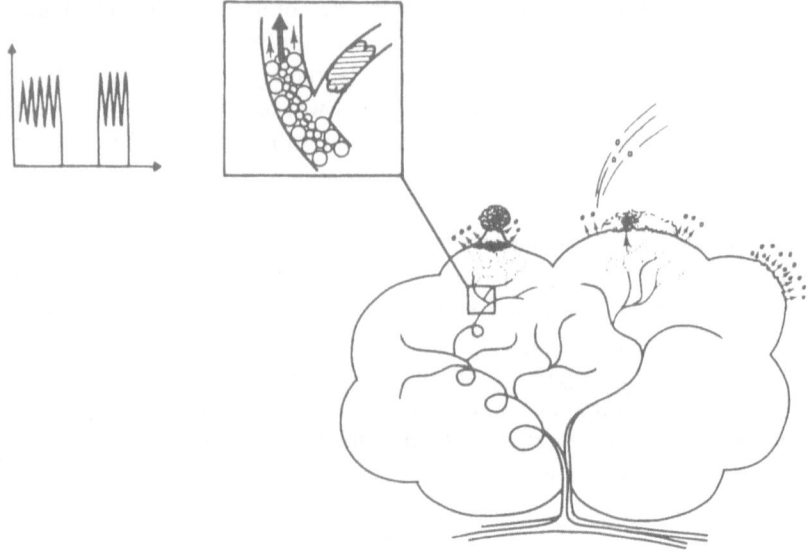

FIGURE 16.2. Schematic illustration of the morphological and vascular changes that ocur during the ovulatory process as observed by intravital microscopy of the rat ovary. To the right, the general finding of detachment of germinal epithelium is illustrated. In the middle of the ovarian surface, a gelatinous mass captures the extruded cumulus cells/oocyte. A cone-shaped ovulation is seen to the left of the ovary. The inserts illustrate blood flow velocity variations (vasomotion) with a period of longer stagnation of blood flow velocity. Margination of leukocytes and microembolus formation are illustrated in the right insert.

without obvious contractions of the follicle (2,18). Taken together, contractile activity does not seem to be a major force during the ovulatory process.

Another interesting intravital microscopy observation is the leakage of a low viscous fluid through the porous stigma (19). This leakage disappeared when the ovarian circulation was inhibited. It was demonstrated in the rabbit perfused ovary (1) that the extrusion of the cumulus mass was temporarily interrupted when the perfusion was stopped for 10 minutes. After resumption of perfusion, the extrusion was completed without any further obvious delay. Transmission electron microscopy studies of the rabbit ovary have demonstrated highly permeable capillaries at the follicular base at the time of ovulation (20,21) with leakage of resin and carbon particles to interstitium. In addition, the latter study showed that indomethacin treatment reduced the ovulation rate with a concomitant decreased permeability at the base of the follicle. It is possible that transudation of plasma into the base of the follicular antrum is important for the cumulus mass to penetrate the porous apex and that the escape of follicular fluid inhibits elevation of the intrafollicular pressure prior to the extrusion. Additional data on this subject may be achieved

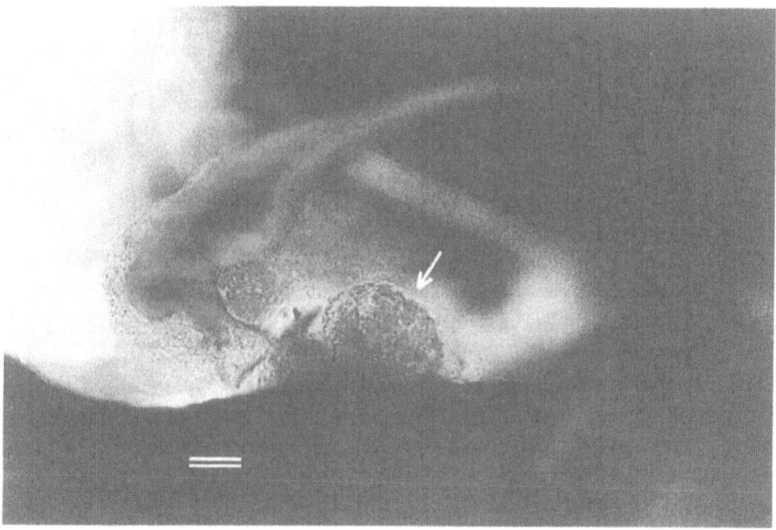

FIGURE 16.3. Photography taken during intravital microscopy of the rat ovary, showing an ovulation. The cumulus mass (arrow) is attached to the follicular surface by a gelatinous mass after the oocyte extrusion. Within the gelatinous mass, the oocyte/cumulus complex is trapped. A blood clot is seen at the left above the gelatinous mass.

in future studies if micromanometric measurements of the follicular pressure are combined with in vivo microscopy observations.

Vascular Changes During the Ovulatory Process and Corpus Luteum Formation

The ovarian tissue is one of the most vascularized tissues of the body. In the rat, the right ovarian artery usually arises from the aorta, whereas the left ovarian artery arises from the left renal artery. The ovarian arteries on both sides run in close proximity and caudal to the kidneys. Close to the ovary, the ovarian artery on each side anastomose with respective uterine artery, whereafter a common branch enters the hilus of the ovary. After division into primary-, secondary-, and tertiary spiral arteries the follicles in the cortical area are supplied through surrounding meshlike vascular wreaths that are located in the theca interna (22,23). During ovulation, an increase in ovarian blood volume (24), increased blood flow (25), increased permeability (21), and redistribution of blood flow from the apex to the base of the follicle in the human (26) have been demonstrated. An avascular area is formed at the apex prior to the extrusion (9). This avascular area has been suggested to be caused

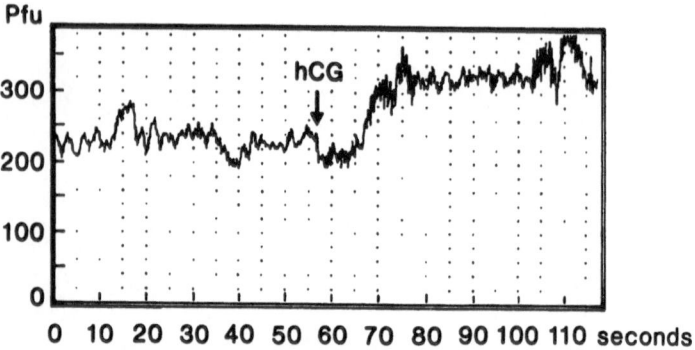

FIGURE 16.4. Rat ovarian blood flow, recorded by laser Doppler. Blood flow is expressed as arbitrary perfusion units (Pfu; *y*-axis); time is shown in seconds (*x*-axis). Arrow indicates administration of 15 IU hCG, resulting in a rapid and marked increase in ovarian blood flow.

by formations of microthrombi in vessels of this segment (27). Identical vascular changes can be induced by prostaglandins (28). During intravital microscopy of the rat ovary, microemboli formations were evident in the apical vessels 6–8 hours after hCG injection, causing a progressive reduction of blood flow in this segment (3).

Further evidence for the importance of blood flow changes are the transmigration of white blood cells into the perifollicular tissue (29) and the importance of leukocytes for optimal ovulatory response (30). Transmigration of leukocytes is indirectly supported by our in vivo observations of slowly rolling leukocytes adjacent to the vascular endothelium in apical blood vessels (3).

By investigating the in vivo short-term dynamics of ovarian blood flow by the means of intravital microscopy and laser Doppler flowmetry, we have been able to demonstrate regular short-term variations of blood flow velocity (vasomotion) in this organ for the first time, with intense activity late in the ovulatory phase and in the corpus luteum (19). These short-term variations of blood flow may be essential for edema formation (31), transmigration of blood cells (29), and hormonal exchange.

It has been discussed what mechanisms are involved and how sudden the LH-induced increase in ovarian blood flow takes place. In the rabbit, ovarian blood flow increases within 2 min after hCG injection (25), suggesting an LH-induced release of preformed mediators such as histamine. In preliminary experiments, utilizing laser Doppler flowmetry, we found a 45% increase of ovarian blood flow with onset as rapid as 12 seconds after hCG injection (Fig. 16.4).

Postovulatory Events

In vitro (2) and in vivo studies (19) have shown that the extruded cumulus complex remains attached to the surface of the rat ovary for at least 2 hours and that a fibrinlike sheet is formed over the rupture site. The oocyte–cumulus mass is then captured by the fimbria apparatus, after which it enters the oviduct for preparation for fertilization and further transport to the uterus for implantation. The transport through the entire oviduct does not occur at a uniform speed because the released oocytes are arrested for a considerable time in the ampullary region. The relative time that the oocytes are present in the ampulla varies between species. In the rat, this time is about one third of the total time of about 88 hours in which they are contained within the oviduct (32). The driving forces for oocyte–embryo transport are cooperatively generated by ciliary movement (33) and contractions caused by the smooth muscle tissue of the oviduct. In intravital microscopy experiments (19), we could observe the oocytes–cumulus masses through the extended and transparent wall of the oviductal ampulla. The cumulus masses moved back and forth in parallell with the contractions of the ampulla. The frequency of the ampullary contractions was increased from 9–10 to 14–16 contractions per minute from a time prior to follicular rupture to postovulation. The contractions were multifocal, meeting at the central part with the highest frequency at the uterine end of the ampulla. This oviductal motility is controlled by several mediators [e.g., catecholamines (34), ovarian steroids (35), prostaglandins (36) and peptidergic transmittors (37)].

During the ampullary contractions, the cumulus cells became detached from the oocyte and separated by another flow between the contractions (19). A study with human material has suggested a current of oviductal fluid into the less cilated mucosal crypts in an ovarian direction (38). In vivo observations in the rat showed a slow current of denuded cells moving in direction toward the uterus (19).

Conclusions

The morphology of the early ovulatory process is uniform with increased transparency of the follicular apex, and detachment of germinal epithelium, resulting in increasingly textured surface of the stigma. In later stages, the ovulations are heterogenous with clearly notable differences between ovulations. There is either leakage of follicular fluid for several hours before rupture with formation of a gelatinous mass over the apex, or formation of a cone-shaped apex, without any visible follicular fluid leakage before rupture. The extrusion is a relatively slow process with intermittent passage of cumulus masses varying in size. Variable degrees of bleeding occur during the ovulatory process. After completed extrusion, the oocyte is attached to the ovarian surface. The oviduct shows contractility variations, and the oocytes in the ampulla are progressively denuded.

Vascular changes of the ovulatory process include an initially increased blood flow to the ovarian tissue, regular variations of blood flow velocity in ovarian tissue, and formation of microemboli in apical vessels, resulting in an avascular area around the stigma.

Acknowledgments. The research in this chapter was supported by grants from The Swedish Medical council (11607 to M. B.), Medical Faculty of Göteborg University, the Reasearch Foundations of Hjalmar Svensson, Medical Society of Göteborg, Sahlgrens Hospital, and the Swedish Society for Medical Research.

References

1. Löfman CO, Janson PO, Källfelt B, Ahren K, LeMaire WJ. The study of ovulation in the perfused rabbit ovary: photographic and cinematographic observations. Biol Reprod 1982;3:467–73.
2. Löfman CO, Brännström M, Holmes PV, Janson PO. Ovulation in the isolated perfused rat ovary as documented by intravital microscopy. Steroids 1989;54:481–90.
3. Brännström M, Löfman CO, Mikuni M, Janson PO, Zackrisson U. Morphological and vascular changes during ovulation in vivo in the rat. Biol Reprod 1997;56(suppl. 1):178.
4. Brännström M, Mikuni M, Peterson C. Ovulation-associated intraovarian events. In: Filicori M, Flamgini C, eds. The ovary: regulation, dysfunction and treatment. Amsterdam: Elsevier Science BV; 1996:113–23.
5. Espey LL. Ultrastructure of the apex of the rabbit Graafian follicle during the ovulatory process. Am J Physiol 1967;212:1397–401.
6. Rondell P. Follicular pressure and distensibility in ovulation. Am J Physiol 1964; 207:590–94.
7. Morales T, Woessner LJ, Marsh J, LeMaire W. Collagen, collagenase and collagenolytic activity in rat Graafian follicles during follicular growth and ovulation. Acta Biochem Biophys 1983;756:119–22.
8. Bjersing L, Cajander S. Ovulation and the mechanism of follicular rupture. V. Ultrastructure of tunica albuginea and theca externa of rabbit ovarian follicle prior to induced ovulation. Cell Tiss Res 1975;153:15–30.
9. Blandau R. Ovulation in the living albino rat. Fertil Steril 1955;6:391–401.
10. Bjersing L, Cajander S. Ovulation and the mechanism of follicular rupture. II. Scanning electron microscopy of rabbit germinal epithelium prior to induced ovulation. Cell Tiss Res 1975;149:301–12.
11. Bjersing L, Cajander S. Ovulation and the mechanism of follicular rupture. III. Transmission electron microscopy of rabbit germinal epithelium prior to induced ovulation. Cell Tiss Res 1975,149:313–27.
12. Talbot P, Chancon R. In vitro ovulation of hamster oocytes depends on contraction of follicular smooth muscle cells. J Exp Zool 1982;224:409–15.
13. Amenta F, Allen D, Didio L, Motta P. A transmission electron study of smooth muscle cells in the ovary of rabbits, cats and mice. J Submicrosc Cytol 1979;11:39–51.
14. Self D, Schroeder P, Gown A. Hamster thecal cells express muscle characteristics. Biol Reprod 1988;39:119–30.
15. Gabbiani G, Badonnel M-C. Contractile elements during inflammation. Agents Actions 1976;6:277–84.
16. Guttmacher M, Guttmacher A. Morphological and physiological studies of the musculature of the mature Graafian follicle of the sow. John Hopkins Hosp Bull 1921;32:394–99.

17. Espey LL, Lipner H. Measurement of the intrafollicular pressure in the rabbit ovary. Am J Physiol 1963;205:1067–72.
18. Kobayashi Y, Kitai H, Santulli R, Wright K, Wallach E. Influence of calcium and magnesium deprivation on ovum maturation in the perfused rabbit ovary. Biol Reprod 1984;31:287–95.
19. Zackrisson U. Intra-ovarian events of ovulation: vascular mechanisms and morphological alterations in the rat and the human. Göteborgs University, Sweden (Thesis), 1997:6–94.
20. Okuda Y, Okamura H, Kanzaki H, Tanenaka A, Morimoto K, Nishimura T. An ultrastructural study of capillary permeability of rabbit follicles during the ovulatory process. Acta Obstet Gynaecol Jpn 1980;7: 859–67.
21. Okuda Y, Okamura H, Kanzaki H, Tanenaka A, Morimoto K. Capillary permeability of rabbit ovarian follicles prior to ovulation. J Anat 1983;269:263–69.
22. Basset D. The changes in the vascular pattern of the ovary of the albino rat during the estrous cycle. Am J Anat 1943;73:251–91.
23. Murakami T, Ikebuchi Y, Ohtsuka A, Kikuta A, Taguchi T, Ohtani O. The vascular wreath of the rat ovarian follicle, with special reference to its changes in ovulation and luteinization: a scanning electron microscopic study of corrosion casts. Arch Histol Cytol 1988;51:299–313.
24. Tanaka N, Espey LL, Okamura H. Increase in ovarian blood volume in the gonadotrophin-primed rat. Biol Reprod 1989;40:762–68.
25. Janson PO. Effects of the luteinizing hormone on blood flow in the follicular rabbit ovary, as measured by radioactive microspheres. Acta Endocrinol 1975;79:122–33.
26. Brännström M. Zackrisson U, Hagström H-G, Josefsson B, Hellberg P, Granberg S, et al. Preovulatory changes of blood flow in different regions of the human follicle. Fertil Steril 1998;69:435–42.
27. Okamura H. Vascular role in the mechanism of ovulation. In: Ichinoe K, Segal SJ, Mastrioanni I, eds. Ovarian function in benignant and malignant disease. Serono Symposia Publications, New York: Raven Press; 1988;48:191–200.
28. Yoshimura Y, Dharmarajan AM, Gips S, Adachi T, Hosoi Y, Atlas SJ, et al. Effects of prostacyclin on ovulation and microvasculature of the in vitro perfused rabbit ovary. Am J Obstet Gynecol 1988;159:977–82.
29. Brännström M, Mayerhofer G, Robertson S. Localisation of leukocyte subsets in the rat ovary during the periovulatory period. Biol Reprod 1993;48:277–86.
30. Hellberg P, Thomsen P, Janson PO, Brännström M. Leukocyte supplementation increases the luteinizing hormone-induced ovulation rate in the in vitro perfused rat ovary. Biol Reprod 1991;44:791–97.
31. Espey LL. Ovulation as an inflammatory reaction. Biol Reprod 1980;22:72–106.
32. Croxatto H, Ortiz M, Frocedello M, Fuentealba B, Noe G, Moore G, et al. Hormonal control of ovum transport through the rat oviduct. Arch Biol Med Exp 1991;24: 403–10.
33. Harper M. The mechanism involved in newly ovulated eggs through the ampulla of the rabbit fallopian tube. J Reprod Fertil 1961;2:522–24.
34. Owman C, Falck B, Jahansson E. Autonomic nerves and related amine receptors mediating the motor activity in the oviduct of the monkey and man. Histochemical, chemical and pharmacological study. In: Harper MJK, Pauerstein CJ, Adams CE, Couthino EM, Croxatto HB, Paton DM, eds. Ovum transport and fertility regulation. Copenhagen: Scriptor; 1976:256–75.
35. Forcedello M, de la Cerda M, Croxatto HB. Effectiveness of different estrogen pulses

in plasma for accelerating ovum transport and their relation to estradiol levels in the rat oviduct. Endocrinology 1986;119:1189–94.

36. Lindblom B, Wilhelmsson L, Wiquist N. The action of prostacyclin (PGI$_2$) on the contractility of the isolated circular and longitudinal muscle layers of the human oviduct. Prostaglandins 1979;17: 99–104.

37. Alm P, Alumets D, Håkansson R. Vasoactive intestinal polypeptide nerves in the human female genital tract. Am J Obstet Gynecol 1980;136:449–51.

38. Blake J, Vann P, Winet H. A model for ovum transport. Theoret Biol 1983;102:145–66.

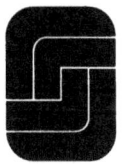

17

Inhibins, Activins, and Estrogens: Roles in the Ovulatory Sequence

JOCK K. FINDLAY, ANN E. DRUMMOND, ANNA J. BAILLIE,
MITZILEE DYSON, ANITA DHAR, KARA J. ALLEN, KARA L. BRITT,
VICTORIA A. COX, MARGARET E.E. JONES, AND EVAN R. SIMPSON

Introduction

Inhibins and activins are members of the transforming growth factor-β (TGF-β) superfamily, and are encoded by three separate genes known as inhibin α, inhibin/activin βA, and inhibin/activin βB (1). Inhibin, originally identified for its capacity to reduce synthesis and secretion of FSH, is a heterodimeric glycosylated protein the consists of two covalently linked subunits [αβA or αβB] known as inhibin A and inhibin B, respectively. Dimeric inhibin exists as different molecular weight forms ranging from 30/31 kDa to around 105 kDa, depending on the degree of glycosylation and posttranslational processing of each subunit. The FSH-suppressing activity of these forms decreases with increasing size. Free α subunit forms, pro-αC and αN, also exist in follicular fluid and serum, but they lack any known biological activity. Activin, originally identified for its capacity to increase synthesis and secretion of FSH, is a homo- or heterodimeric nonglycosylated protein that consists of two covalently linked β subunits [βAβA, βAβB, or βBβB] known as activin A, AB, or B, respectively. The activins can also exist in different molecular weight forms ranging from 24 kDa to 110 kDa, depending on the degree of posttranslational processing, with decreasing FSH stimulating activity with increasing molecular size. βC, βD, and βE genes have been identified, which suggests the existence of additional forms of activin. There is no evidence to date that these forms can dimerize with the α subunit to form inhibin, and their role in folliculogenesis is unknown, although the βC form is expressed in the ovary (2).

Both inhibin and activin are products of the follicular granulosa cells and corpus luteum [in primates]. Inhibin A and B act as gonadal feedback hormones that regulate the secretion of FSH. Activin, however, does not appear to serve as a classic peripheral hormone, but rather as a local regulator of FSH within the pituitary gland. As a result, it has been shown that both inhibin and activin have autocrine and paracrine actions within the ovarian follicle (1,3).

Estrogen, principally estradiol-17β [E2], also has an acknowledged pivotal role as an intrafollicular autocrine and paracrine regulator (4,5), in addition to its well-established feedback effects on gonadotropin secretion (4). There has been renewed interest in the local roles of E2 and its mechanism of action in ovarian function since the description of a second estradiol receptor [ERβ] (6), and mice with targeted deletions of the aromatase [ArKO] (7) and ERβ genes [ERKO] (8).

This chapter will summarize advances in knowledge of the local roles of inhibin, activin. and E2 in certain aspects of folliculogenesis.

A Functional Model of Folliculogenesis

Follicles in the ovary are either quiescent [primordial] or committed to growth [primary, secondary, tertiary/Graafian] or atresia. A functional scheme of folliculogenesis has been proposed (9) that divides committed follicles into categories according to their responsiveness to and dependence on gonadotropins, but retains the fundamental principal that no two follicles are functionally identical, although they may appear morphologically the same. The primordial follicle becomes committed to growth by a process not yet understood, but likely to involve local intraovarian regulation because it occurs spontaneously in the absence of pituitary luteinizing hormone (LH) and follicle stimulating hormone (FSH). Once committed to growth, follicles can grow independently of FSH and LH until the late preantral/early antral stage, although there is evidence that the presence of gonadotropins may facilitate this stage of development. Important early events in a committed follicle are the acquisition of responsiveness to FSH that is enhanced by local regulators, including activin, TGF-β and estradiol, and the formation of a functional, LH-responsive theca.

Dependence on gonadotropins, particularly FSH, is synonymous with the transition of a committed follicle from preantral to antral. At this time, when the proliferation of the somatic cells around the oocyte reaches a maximum, there is strong induction of aromatase activity and LH receptors in the granulosa layer. Widespread atresia is common in nondominant antral follicles, and local regulators (e.g., activin, IGF-1, and estradiol) can modulate the actions of LH and FSH. Finally, the dominant follicle is supported by the actions of peripheral LH and intrafollicular regulators until the levels of E2 rise sufficiently to trigger the gonadotropin surge and ovulation.

Sites of Production and Action

Inhibins and Activins

The inhibin–activin genes are all expressed in granulosa cells from a relatively early stage of folliculogenesis. Inhibin and activin are present in follicular fluid (1,3), although production of biologically active dimeric activin and inhibins early in folliculogenesis has not been fully described. There is evidence that small mouse preantral follicles (100–130 µm diameter) can synthesise dimeric activin A (10). We have demonstrated expression of the three inhibin–activin genes in preantral follicles of the postnatal rat that contain only 1–2 layers of granulosa cells (11). Little is known about the forms of inhibin and activin that are produced and the specific roles that they might play. There is evidence to suggest that inhibin B may be the predominant form in preantral, antral, and early antral follicles (12,13).

Activin receptors are members of the serine–threonine kinase family. Signal transduction involves activin binding to a type II receptor that recruits a type I receptor to form a complex that is phosphorylated and signals to the nucleus via a series of sMAD proteins (14). There are a number of isoforms of the type I and II receptors that can transmit the activin signal when complexed in the correct way. Activin receptors have been described on granulosa cells and oocytes from more advanced follicles (15), and type II and IIB receptors are found in rat ovarian extracts (16). Nothing is known about the expression of activin receptors on granulosa cells of early primary follicles or on theca cells. The field is complicated by the fact that folliculogenesis was observed in mice despite a deficiency in activin type II receptors (17), which infers that the type IIB receptor or some other form is involved.

Specific receptors for inhibin have not been described. Because inhibin antagonizes activin action, inhibin may act through the activin receptor complex (18) or an inhibin-specific binding component (19). Specific binding sites for inhibin have been described on ovine pituitary cells (20), a known target for inhibin action, and mouse ovarian tumor cells (21). Within the follicle, inhibin is known to act on theca (3) and granulosa cells (22), and on the oocyte (23), which implies that these are sites of inhibin binding/receptors.

Estradiol-17β

E2 is a product of the conversion of thecal androgen by granulosa cell aromatase activity, where LH drives thecal androgen production, and FSH and, subsequently, LH, drive aromatase activity (4). Both activities are subject to local regulation by E2 itself, inhibin, activin and insulinlike growth factor-1 (4). The actions of E2 are mediated by ERα (8) and ERβ which has several isoforms (6,24,25). We have used the postnatal ovarian rat model to define the relationship between ER subtype and folliculogenesis. By taking ovaries on Days 4, 8, and 12 after birth, it is possible to have ovarian tissue with known stages of folliculogenesis present that can be related to the responses obtained (26).

We examined the hypothesis that ERβ mRNA is the primary form of ER regulated in the follicle during development. This hypothesis is based on the fact that ERβ is the predominant form of ER in the ovary (6), and follicular growth appeared unperturbed up to the secondary and antral stages in mice with targeted disruption of the ERα gene (8). We also took the opportunity to compare the expression of the two isoforms, ERβ1 and ERβ2, in which the latter has a 54 nt or 18 amino acid insertion in the ligand binding domain (24), which lowers its affinity for E2 (25).

The postnatal rat ovary expressed both ERα and ERβ, but with different patterns and levels of expression (27). Total ovarian ERβ mRNA was more abundant than ER α mRNA. Both isoforms of ERβ mRNA were present, with the ERβ2 product consistently and statistically more predominant on Days 8 and 12. The expression of both forms increased during postnatal development up to Day 12. We were only able to detect ERβ amplicons in one of four RNA pools of Day 4 ovaries. The pattern of expression of ERα mRNA was different to that of ERβ mRNA, with no change in expression observed between Days 8 and 12 and the ERα amplicons detected in two of four pools of RNA prepared from Day 4 ovaries.

We concluded that expression of both ER first occurs early in folliculogenesis, most likely at the time committed primary follicles are formed, but not in primordial follicles. The increased expression of ERβ with advancing folliculogenesis could be due to increasing numbers of granulosa cells per ovary and/or an increase in receptor number per cell. The data is consistent with a role for ERβ in granulosa cell proliferation and differentiation, although the relative importance and specific roles of the ERα and ERβ isoforms remains unknown.

Actions During Folliculogenesis

Activin

FSH Receptors

It is obligatory for granulosa cells to acquire the capacity to respond to FSH for normal folliculogenesis to occur. This involves the expression of receptors for FSH [FSH-R] and maturation of the FSH receptor–signal transduction system, which are events that occur early in the life of a committed follicle. Detection of FSH-R mRNA by in situ hybridization and RT-PCR show that the FSH-R gene is expressed very early in folliculogenesis (28,29); however, the capacity of these cells to respond to FSH in terms of cyclic AMP (cAMP) production and steroidogenesis is very low until a later stage (30). We have examined the role of activin in expression of the FSH-R and its signal transduction system (11,31).

Early reports described FSH binding to postnatal rat ovarian membranes that increased between Days 4 and 8 (32,33). This increase was subsequently related to the expression of at least four alternately spliced forms of the FSH-R mRNA of which the 2.5 kb form on Northerns is believed to represent the mature form of the FSH-R (28,29,34). The full-length receptor mRNA is present at postnatal Day 1 in the rat ovary, although the truncated transcripts remain in greater abundance until Days 5–7. We (31) and others (34–36) showed that activin upregulated FSH binding to granulosa cells obtained from DES-treated 21-day-old rats, and that this was related to an increase in the steady-state levels of FSH-R mRNA, probably due to an increase in the transcription rate and stabilization of the mRNA. As a result, we examined by RT-PCR the expression of the different isoforms of FSH-R mRNA in postnatal rat ovaries at Days 4, 8, and 12 (Allen, Drummond and Findlay, unpublished observations). Three different isoforms were detected at Day 4 and four on Days 8 and 12, including the equivalent of the 2.5 kb form, and the relative expression of each increased with age and the stage of folliculogenesis. There was no evidence of a change in the ratio of each isoform with age.

We concluded that activin can upregulate the total expression of the FSH-R mRNA, but not the ratio of the alternatively spliced forms, and the binding of FSH to granulosa cells. It is not known if the initial expression of FSH-R mRNA is regulated by activin.

Responsive to FSH

Postnatal ovaries collected at Day 4 were steroidogenically responsive to cAMP agonists in the presence of a phosphodiesterase inhibitor, whereas responsiveness to FSH was limited until after Day 6–8 (30). We hypothesized that treatment with activin would enhance the actions of FSH on granulosa cells from postnatal rat ovaries (11). The addition of activin to dispersed ovarian cells from Day 4, 8, and 12 rats induced FSH-responsive progesterone production that was nondetectable in the absence of activin, and it enhanced both basal and FSH-stimulated inhibin production. These studies indicated that postnatal ovarian cells have a differential response to FSH in terms of progesterone and inhibin production, and that activin may play a facilitating role in the FSH signal transduction system. The mechanisms by which activin exerts these differential effects remains to be elucidated. The existence of the Type I and II receptors (15,16) and MAD expression in ovarian cells (37) suggests involvement of this pathway.

Inhibin

Dimeric inhibin upregulated the capacity of LH to stimulate thecal androgen synthesis (3) and the stimulatory action of FSH and LH on granulosa cell aromatase activity (22). This opens the possibility of a local positive feedback relationship in healthy [dominant] follicles in which dimeric inhibin enhances follicular production of E2. It is interesting that activin also facilitates FSH-induced estrogen production by granulosa cells, but it inhibits LH-induced androgen production by thecal cells (3). Further research is needed to resolve the relative importance of inhibin and activin in E2 production. The influence in this system of the activin-binding protein, follistatin, which inhibits the biological activity of activin, also needs resolution, especially because there is evidence of increased production of follistatin with advancing folliculogenesis (38).

Inhibin and activin added to cultures of immature oocytes assisted maturation and blastocyst formation with more transferable embryos (23). These actions could be mediated by a direct action on the oocyte, which is known to express activin receptor, (15) or indirectly via the cumulus cells.

The isolation of αN and pro-αC, which are posttranslational products of the inhibin α subunit precursor, from follicular fluid (1) prompted suggestions that these "free" peptides may play roles in folliculogenesis independent of the α subunit of dimeric inhibin. This hypothesis was tested by active and passive immunization against the peptides (39–42), not by direct administration because not enough is available. The major criticism of the immunization approach is its lack of specificity in that the antibodies will potentially recognize epitopes present on the high molecular weight forms of inhibin that contain these peptides, making it difficult to differentiate between actions of dimeric inhibins and the "free" α subunit forms. Nevertheless, the data suggest that αN or αN-containing inhibins do have an intraovarian role in fertility regulation that is independent of the endocrine effects of dimeric inhibins on pituitary secretion of FSH.

Active immunization against αN reduced oocyte recovery and the pregnancy rate of ewes (39), although, paradoxically, the number of apparent corpora lutea (CL) increased, probably as a result of increased circulating concentrations of FSH. Several of these CL-like structures had a cystic appearance similar to luteinized unruptured follicles. The 2-day-old CLs in immunized ewes differed from controls in that the luteal tissue remained thin, infolding was incomplete, and thecal–vascular invaginations were rare and failed to penetrate into the luteal tissue (40). Morphologically normal rupture stigma were seen at the apex of both control and αN-immunized ewes. The increase in both latent and active MMP-2 after the preovulatory LH surge was reduced in follicular fluid of immunized compared with control ewes. MMP-2 or gelatinase breaks down the components of basement membranes and is therefore an important component of the ovulatory cascade.

In a subsequent study, however, all antral follicles greater than 1 mm in the late follicular phase were atretic (41). We confirmed this observation in a more comprehensive experiment that also failed to show any significant effects of immunization on the circulating concentrations of FSH or any of the parameters of peripheral LH (42). It was concluded that αN or αN-containing peptides including inhibins are an important local component for maintaining the viability of antral follicles greater than 1 mm in the follicular phase of ewes. We believe that these effects are mediated primarily by modulation of gonadotropin action within the follicle. It also suggests that the effects of αN immunization on MMP-2 may have indirectly been due to atresia. It is apparent that what we call an "atretic follicle" may still be capable of undergoing luteinization even though its ovulating–tissue remodeling capacity is compromised—just like a luteinized unruptured follicle? It is interesting that we have observed similar effects of immunization against the inhibin αC peptide on atresia of antral follicles, despite an increase in FSH concentrations (42). Previous studies reported that this treatment increased ovulation rates and lambs born per ewe (43), and was associated with increased intrafollicular concentrations of activin and inhibin (44). More research is required to resolve these differences. A study on compound homozygous mutant mice (45) supports our conclusions. Mice lacking expression of both the inhibin α and GnRH genes [hpg mice] have small ovaries with relatively little follicular development beyond the primary stage; mice lacking the GnRH gene only have follicular development, which is normal through to the secondary stage.

We conclude that the α inhibin precursor or parts of the precursor protein may have paracrine or autocrine activity, quite distinct from inhibin's endocrine role, in the recruitment and selection of antral follicles from which the ovulatory follicle emerges.

Estradiol

Estrogen has an acknowledged pivotal role as an intrafollicular autocrine and paracrine modulator of the responses of follicular cells to the gonadotropins (4,5). E2 stimulates granulosa cell division and enhances their sensitivity to the actions of FSH and LH, including induction of the receptor systems for FSH, LH, and prolactin, cAMP production, and the steroidogenic pathways, particularly the induction of aromatase, the enzyme responsible for the production of E2 itself (4). Despite this abundance of evidence in support of a facilitatory role of E2 in follicular function, none of the models are completely free of estrogen or the capacity to synthesise estrogen. An obligatory role for E2 in folliculogenesis, therefore, has not been demonstrated.

Mice lacking a functional aromatase enzyme [ArKO] were generated by targeted disruption of exon 9 of the cyp19 gene (7). These animals should be free of endogenous estrogen. They were born at the expected Mendelian frequency from F1 parents, grew to adulthood, and displayed signs of hypoestrogenicity. The external genitalia and uterus were underdeveloped, and the skeleton had reduced bone mineral density. Serum E2 was below detection, whereas FSH, LH, and testosterone levels were markedly elevated compared with wild type (wt) animals. Aromatase activity was below detection in ovarian tissue and the females were infertile.

There was no significant difference in the mean ovarian weights of the ArKO, heterozygote [Het], or *wt* groups at 10–12 weeks or at 23 weeks of age (46). No CL were visible on the ovarian surface or in sections of ArKO ovaries, whereas ovaries of *wt* and Het animals apparently had normal CL. Although ArKO ovaries displayed follicles with abundant granulosa cells and evidence of antrum formation, development was arrested at or before the tertiary stage and the larger follicles in older animals were hemorrhagic. A particular feature of the ArKO ovary is the disorganized and hypertrophied interstitial region, with localized pockets of macrophagelike cells. Preliminary data based on RT-PCR of whole ovarian RNA suggests that the ArKO ovaries are capable of expressing inhibin α and βA, ERβ,17-20 lyase, but not ERα or inhibin βB. The levels of expression relative to age and the other genotypes are under investigation.

We conclude that estrogen is obligatory for folliculogenesis in mice beyond the early antral stage and consequently for fertility.

Acknowledgments. This work is supported by the National Health and Medical Research Council of Australia (RegKey 983212), the Victorian Breast Cancer Research Consortium, and the National Institutes of Health, USA. Our thanks to Faye Coates for help with preparation of the manuscript.

References

1. Findlay JK, Sai Xiao, Shukovski L, Michel U. Novel peptides in ovarian physiology: inhibin, activin, and follistatin. In: Adashi EY, Leung PCK, eds. Inhibin, activin and follistatin in the pituitary and ovary. New York: Springer-Verlag; 1997: 3–5.
2. Loveland KL, McFarlane JR, de Kretser DM. Expression of activin βC subunit mRNA in reproductive tissues. J Mol Endocrinol 1996;17:61–65.
3. Findlay JK. An update on the roles of inhibin, activin, and follistatin as local regulators of folliculogenesis. Biol Reprod 1993;48:15-23.
4. Hillier SG. Sex steroid metabolism and follicular development in the ovary. In: Clarke JR, ed. Oxford reviews of reproductive biology, Vol 7. Oxford: Clarendon Press; 1985: 168–222.
5. Hisaw FL. Development of the Graafian follicle and ovulation. Physiol Rev 1947;27:95–119.
6. Kuiper GGJM, Enmark E, Pelto-Huikko M, Nilsson S, Gustafsson J-A. Cloning of a novel estrogen receptor expressed in rat prostate and ovary. Proc Natl Acad Sci USA 1996;5925–30.
7. Fisher CR, Graves KH, Parlow AF, Simpson ER. Characterization of mice deficient in aromatase (ArKO) because of targeted disruption of the *cyp19* gene. Proc Natl Acad Sci USA 1998;95:6965–70.
8. Lubahn DB, Moyer JS, Golding TS, Couse JF, Korach KS, Smithies O. Alteration of reproductive function but not prenatal sexual development after insertional disruption of the mouse estrogen receptor gene. Proc Natl Acad Sci USA 1993;90: 11162–66.

9. Scaramuzzi RJ, Adams NR, Baird DT, Campbell BK, Downing JA, Findlay JK, et al. A model for follicle selection and the determination of ovulation rate in the ewe. Reprod Fertil Dev 1993;5:459–78.

10. Smitz J, Cortvrindt R, Hu Y, Vanderstichele H. Effects of recombinant activin A on in vitro culture of mouse preantral follicles. Mol Reprod Dev 1998;50:294–304.

11. Drummond AE, Dyson M, Mercer JE, Findlay JK. Differential responses of post-natal rat ovarian cells to FSH and activin. Mol Cell Endocrinol 1996;122:21–32.

12. Schwall RH, Mason AJ, Wilcox JN, Bassett SG, Zeleznik AJ. Localization of inhibin/activin subunit mRNAs within the primate ovary. Mol Endocrinol 1990;4:75–79.

13. Drummond AE, Dyson M, Robertson DM, Findlay JK. Regulation of inhibin-B production by cultured ovarian cells. Proceedings of the Twentieth-Eighth Annual Meeting of the Australian Society of Reproductive Biology 1997:31 (abstr.).

14. Mathews LS. Activin receptors and cellular signaling by the receptor serine kinase family. Endocrinol Rev 1994;15:310–25.

15. Cameron VA, Nishimura E, Mathews LS, Lewis KA, Sawchenko PE, Vale WW. Hybridization histochemical localization of activin receptor subtypes in rat brain, pituitary, ovary and testis. Endocrinology 1994;134:799–808.

16. Feng Z, Madigan MB, Chen CC. Expression of type II activin receptor genes in the male and female reproductive tissues of the rat. Endocrinology 1993;132:2593–600.

17. Matzuk MM, Kumar TR, Shou W, Coerver KA, Lau AL. Behringer RB, et al. Transgenic models to study the roles of inhibins and activins in reproduction, oncogenesis and development. Rec Prog Horm Res 1996;51:123–57.

18. Martens JWM, de Winter JP, Timmerman MA, McLuskey A, van Schaik RHN, Themmen APN, et al. Inhibin interferes with activin signaling at the level of the activin receptor complex in Chinese hamster ovary cells. Endocrinology 1997;138:2928–36.

19. Lebrun JJ, Vale WW. Activin and inhibin have antagonistic effects on ligand-dependent heteromerization of the Type I ad Type II activin receptors and human erythroid differentiation. Mol Cell Biol 1997;17:182–91.

20. Hertan R, Farnworth PG, Fitzsimmons KL, Robertson DM. Identification of high affinity binding sites for inhibin on ovine pituitary cells in culture. Endocrinology 1999;140:6–12.

21. Draper LB, Matzuk MM, Roberts VJ, Cox E, Weiss J, Mather JP, et al. Identification of an inhibin receptor in gonadal tumors from inhibin α-subunit knockout mice. J Biol Chem 1998;273:398–403.

22. Webb R, Campbell BK, Gong JG, Gutierrez CG, Armstrong DG. Growth factors: regulation of ovarian function. J Reprod Fert 1998;Abstr. Ser. 21, S5:6.

23. Stock AE, Woodruff TK, Smith LC. Effects of inhibin A and activin A during in vitro maturation of bovine oocytes in hormone- and serum-free medium. Biol Reprod 1997;56:1559–64.

24. Chu S, Fuller PJ. Identification of a splice variant of the estrogen receptor β gene. Mol Cell Endocrinol 1997;132:195–99.

25. Peterson DN, Tkalcevic GT, Koza-Taylor PH, Turi TG, Brown TA. Identification of estrogen receptor β_2, a functional variant of estrogen receptor β expressed in normal rat tissues. Endocrinology 1998;139:1082–92.

26. Carson RS, Smith J. Development and steroidogenic activity of preantral follicles in the neonatal rat ovary. J Endocrinol 1986;110:87–92.

27. Drummond AE, Baillie AJ, Findlay JK. Regulation of rat ovarian estrogen receptor α

and β expression of diethylstilboestrol. Proceedings of the Forthy-First Annual Meeting of the Endocrine Society of Australia 1998:109. Abstract 116.

28. Sokka T, Huhtaniemi IT. Ontogeny of gonadotrophin receptors and gonadotrophin-stimulated cyclic AMP production in the neonatal rat ovary. J Endocrinol 1990;127:297–303.

29. Rannikki AS, Zhang FP, Huhtaniemi IT. Ontogeny of follicle-stimulating hormone receptor gene expression in the rat testis and ovary. Mol Cell Endocrinol 1995;107:199–208.

30. Reddoch RB, Armstrong DT. Interactions of a phosphodiesterase inhibitor, 3-isobutyl-1-methyl xanthine, with prostaglandin E2, follicle-stimulating hormone, luteinizing hormone, and dibutyryl cyclic 3′ and 5′-adenosine monophosphate (cAMP) in cAMP and steroid production by neonatal rat ovaries in vitro. Endocrinology 1984;115:11–18.

31. Xiao S, Robertson DM, Findlay JK. Effects of activin and follicle-stimulating hormone (FSH)-suppressing protein/follistatin on FSH receptors and differentiation of cultured fat granulosa cells. Endocrinology 1992;131:1009–16.

32. White SS, Ojeda SR. Changes in ovarian luteinizing hormone and follicle-stimulating hormone receptor content and in gonadotropin-induced ornithine decarboxylase activity during prepubertal and pubertal development of the female rat. Endocrinology 1981;109:152–61.

33. Dunkel L, Tilly JL, Shikone T, Nishimori K, Hsueh AJ. Follicle-stimulating hormone receptor expression in the rat ovary: increases during prepubertal development and regulation by the opposing actions of transforming growth factors beta and alpha. Biol Reprod 1994;50:940–48.

34. Nakamura M, Minegishi T, Hasegawa H, Nakamura K, Igarashi S, Ito I, et al. Effect of an activin A on follicle-stimulating hormone (FSH) receptor messenger ribonucleic acid levels and FSH receptor expressions in cultured rat granulosa cells. Endocrinology 1993;133:538–44.

35. Tano M, Minegishi T, Nakamura K, Karino S, Ibuki Y, Miyamoto K. Transcriptional and post-transcriptional regulation of FSH receptor in rat granulosa cells by cyclic AMP and activin. J Endocrinol 1997;153:465–73.

36. Hasegawa Y, Miyamoto K, Abe Y, Nakamura T, Sugino H, Eto Y, et al. Induction of follicle stimulating hormone receptor by erythroid differentiation factor on rat granulosa cell. Biochem Biophys Res Commun 1988;156:668–74.

37. Draper LB, Woodruff TK. Smad Proteins are synthesized in the ovary. Proceedings of the Eightieth Annual Meeting Endocrine Society USA 1998:448(Poster No. P3 300).

38. Shintani Y, Dyson M, Drummond AE, Findlay JK. Regulation of follistatin production by rat granulosa cells in vitro. Endocrinology 1997;138:2544–51.

39. Russell DL, Findlay JK. The N-terminal peptide of inhibin α-subunit: what are its endocrine and paracrine roles? Trends Endocrinol Metab 1995;6:305–11.

40. Russell DL, Salamonsen LA, Findlay JK. Immunization against the N-terminal peptide of the inhibin α43-subunit (αN) disrupts tissue remodeling and the increase in matrix metalloproteinase-2 during ovulation. Endocrinology 1995;136:3657–64.

41. Dhar A, Salamonsen LA, Doughton BW, Brown RW, Findlay JK. Effect of immunization against the amino-terminal peptide (alpha N) of the alpha$_{43}$ subunit of inhibin on follicular atresia and expression of tissue inhibitor of matrix metalloproteinase (TIMP-1) in ovarian follicles of sheep. J Reprod Fert 1998;114:147–55.

42. Dhar A, Pruysers E, Doughton BW, Brown RW, Findlay JK. Effect of immunisation against the amino-terminal (αN) and carboxy terminal peptides (αC), of the alpha$_{43}$ subunit of inhibin on the pattern of gonadotrophins and follicular growth and atresia in the ewe. Proceedings of the Twenty-Ninth Annual Meeting of the Australian Society for Reproductive Biology 1998. Abstract 14.
43. Findlay JK, Doughton BW, Tsonis CG, Brown RW, Hungerford JW, Greenford PE, et al. Inhibin as a fecundity vaccine. Anim Reprod Sci 1993;33:325–43.
44. Tannetta DS, Feist SA, Bleach ECL, Groome NP, Evans LW, Knight PG. Effects of active immunization of sheep against an amino terminal peptide of the inhibin α_c subunit on intrafollicular levels of activin A, inhibin A and follistatin. J Endocrinol 1998;157:157–68.
45. Kumar TR, Wang Y, Matzuk MM. Gonadotrophins are essential modifier factors for gonadal tumor development in inhibin-deficient mice. Endocrinology 1996;137:4210–16.
46. Findlay JK, Britt K, Cox V, Dyson M, Jones M, Drummond AE, et al. Characterising the aromatase knockout (ArKO) mouse ovary. Proceedings of the Forty-First Annual Meeting Endocrine Society of Australia 1998. Abstract 72, p. 87.

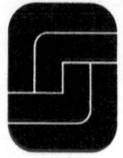

18

Prostaglandins and Ovulation: From Indomethacin to PGHS-2 Knockout

Jean Sirois, Jianmin Liu, Derek Boerboom, and Martine Antaya

The Prostaglandin Biosynthetic Pathway

The prostanoid family, which includes prostaglandins, prostacyclins, and thromboxanes, forms a group of potent mediators involved in numerous physiological processes, such as reproductive functions (ovulation, implantation, luteolysis,and parturition), immune and inflammatory responses, glomerular filtration, bone development, and hemostasis (1,2). They have also been implicated in various pathological conditions, including cardiovascular diseases, asthma, arthritis, gastric ulcers, bone resorption, and cancers (1,2). Prostanoid synthesis is initially dependent on the release of arachidonic acid from membrane phospholipids by phospholipase. Prostaglandin G/H synthase (PGHS, also known as COX) is the first rate-limiting enzyme in the biosynthetic pathway of all prostanoids from arachidonic acid (Fig. 18.1). Because of its key role in the generation of potent inflammatory signals, PGHS has been extensively studied biochemically. The enzyme is the target of a large group of nonsteroidal anti-inflammatory drugs (NSAIDs) and, on an economic basis, is one of the most important enzymes, considering the $5–10 billion received annually from the sale of NSAIDs (1). The enzyme, a membrane-bound glycoprotein, is a homodimer composed of two subunits of about 70,000 Mr (molecular weight) and one heme group (3). PGHS has two sequential enzymatic functions, a cyclooxygenase reaction responsible for the conversion of arachidonic acid to PGG_2, and a peroxidase reaction involved in the conversion of PGG_2 to PGH_2. PGH_2 is the common precursor for the synthesis of all prostanoids (Fig. 18.1).

The metabolism of PGH_2 into biologically active prostanoids is controlled by specific prostacyclin (PGI_2), prostaglandin (PGD_2, PGE_2, $PGF_2\alpha$) and thromboxane (TXA_2) synthases that are expressed in a cell-specific manner (1,3). Two isoforms of PGHS have been identified and are referred to as PGHS-1 and

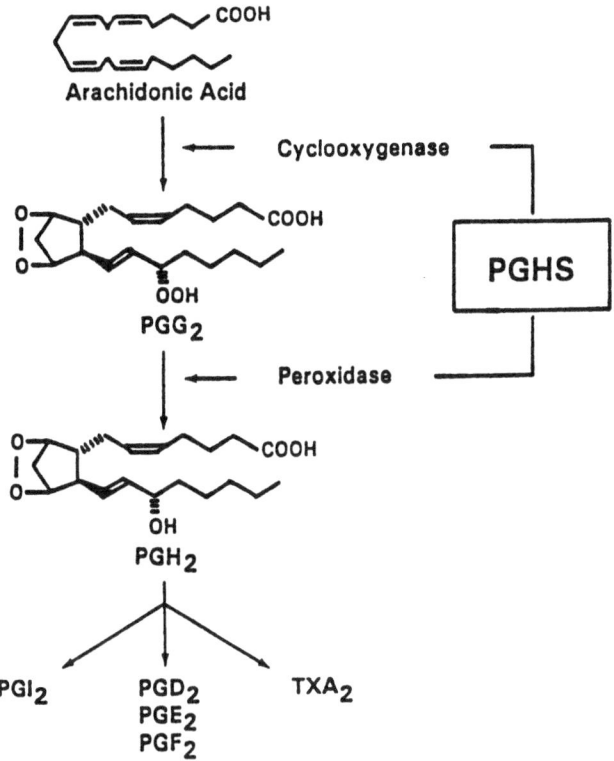

FIGURE 18.1. The prostaglandin biosynthetic pathway. PGHS: prostaglandin G/H synthase; PGI$_2$: prostacyclin; TXA$_2$: thromboxane.

PGHS-2. The first isoform (PHGS-1) was isolated 20 years ago from bovine and ovine seminal vesicles (4,5), whereas the second isoform (PGHS-2) was cloned from chicken and mouse fibroblasts and purified from rat granulosa cells in the early 1990s (6–8). The two isoforms share important similarities at the protein level: They are approximately the same size (600–604 amino acids; 70,000–72,000 Mr) and have conserved structural and functional domains, including a key tyrosine residue associated with the cyclooxygenase active site, two histidines involved in heme binding, and a serine residue located about 70 amino acids from the COOH-terminus that is responsible for inactivation by aspirin (6,7). PGHS-1 and –2, however, are clearly derived from distinct genes located on different chromosomes, and are encoded by mRNA of different sizes (about 2.8 vs. 4.0 kb for PGHS-1 and -2, respectively) (2). In addition, the two isoforms differ markedly in their expression (1, 2). PGHS-1 is present in a wide variety of tissues and is often referred to as *the constitutive form*. In contrast, PGHS-2 is generally undetectable is most tissues but can be induced by a variety of agonists and is referred to as *the inducible form.*

Prostaglandins and Ovulation

For more than 25 years, prostaglandins have been proposed as key mediators of the ovulatory process. This phenomenon has been the subject of excellent reviews (9–12). The story began in 1972 with the demonstration that inhibitors of prostaglandin synthesis blocked ovulation in rats and rabbits (13–15). Subsequent studies in other species, including mice, sheep, pigs, cattle, monkeys, and humans, confirmed the inhibitory effect of NSAIDs on ovulation in vivo (reviewed in Refs. 9 and 11). Indomethacin was also shown to block LH-induced ovulation in vitro in perfused rat and rabbit ovaries (16,17). It is interesting that the inhibitory action of NSAIDs appeared to be limited to the process of follicle wall rupture, and had little or no effect on other aspects of the response of the follicle to the preovulatory gonadotropin surge (luteinization and oocyte maturation). The role of prostaglandins during ovulation was further underscored by the demonstration that intrafollicular levels of PGE_2 and $PGF_{2\alpha}$ are dramatically increased in the hours preceding ovulation in several species (reviewed in Refs. 9–12).

Further evidence came from experiments in which the local (intrafollicular) or systemic administration of specific antisera to prostaglandins were shown to block ovulation in rabbits and mice (18,19); however, the dogma that prostaglandins are obligatory for the ovulatory process was challenged by conflicting studies showing that the antiovulatory action of indomethacin could not be overcome by the administration of specific prostaglandins (reviewed in Refs. 11,12). Other investigations also reported that ovulation could still occur at concentrations of indomethacin capable of inhibiting the normal preovulatory rise in ovarian prostaglandins (11,12). These studies, and others, raised doubts about the assumption that NSAIDs block ovulation solely by inhibiting prostaglandin synthesis, and suggested that redundant mechanisms involving alternative mediators could assure the fate of a normal ovulatory process. Furthermore, the specific functions of prostaglandins during ovulation have not been characterized. One putative mechanism of prostaglandin action is the activation of a proteolytic cascade leading to follicular rupture (10,20). Studies in rats showed that eicosanoid synthesis is required for the gonodotropin-dependent rise in ovarian interstitial collagenase mRNA prior to ovulation (21). Another potential mechanism of prostaglandin action is the promotion of a highly localized inflammatorylike reaction in preovulatory follicles (10). Future studies on the characterization and regulation of prostaglandin receptors during the ovulatory process should help unravel the precise site(s) of action of prostaglandins.

Induction of PGHS-2 in Rat Preovulatory Follicles

In 1987, the marked increase in follicular prostaglandin synthesis prior to ovulation in rats was first related to the induction of PGHS enzymes (22–24). Using two distinct models in vivo, Hedin et al. (22) clearly showed that the induction of immunoreactive PGHS was time-, tissue-, and gonadotropin dose-dependent in rats. Western blot analyses revealed that PGHS content was low in small antral and preovulatory follicles isolated prior to an ovulatory dose of hCG, but was selectively induced in preovulatory follicles after hCG treatment. The induction was transient (3–7 hours post-hCG), primarily restricted to the granulosa cell layer, and required high (ovulatory) dose of hCG. Curry et al. (25) reported that PGHS induction in granulosa cells was restricted to preovulatory follicles larger than 400 μm in rats, whereas PGHS immunoreactivity in theca cells was observed in preantral and antral follicles. The next important step involved the development of an in vitro system that mimicked induction of the enzyme in vivo (26). Using a model of incubated rat preovulatory follicles, Wong et al. (26) documented that a rapid increase in PGHS enzymes could be induced by LH, FSH, and forskolin in vitro, that the pattern of induction was unaltered by addition of exogenous prostaglandins and indomethacin to the media, but was blocked by inhibitors of transcription and translation. One puzzling outcome of this later study was the finding that the marked increase in PGHS protein was apparently related to a decrease in PGHS mRNA (2.8 kilobases). The fact that only one PGHS isoform was characterized at the time, and that only the PGHS-1 cDNA probe was available, would later provide the explanation for this discrepancy. The subsequent generation of two anti-PGHS polyclonal antibodies that recognized two molecular weight variants of PGHS (69,000 and 72,000 Mr) in the rat ovary provided the first evidence for the presence of distinct ovarian isoforms of the enzyme (27). The 72,000 Mr variant was the isoform induced by gonadotropins in granulosa cells prior to ovulation, whereas the 69,000 Mr variant was the form constitutively expressed in theca cells of small antral and preovulatory follicles, and in other tissues.

Sirois and Richards (8) then embarked on the purification and characterization of the PGHS isoform (72,000 Mr) responsible for increased follicular prostaglandin production prior to ovulation. Ovaries from hypophysectomized immature rats, primed with estradiol and FSH to stimulate preovulatory follicular development, were isolated 6 hours after an ovulatory dose of hCG. Solubilized cellular extracts were prepared from granulosa cells, the PGHS isoform was purified by anionic exchange chromatography and size fractionation, and the first 26 amino acid residues were characterized by amino-terminal microsequencing. These results provided a turning point in the field of eicosanoid research and ovulation because they first documented the purification of a novel PGHS isoform (PGHS-2) and revealed its implication in a normal physiological process (8). The PGHS isoform induced by gonadotropins in rat granulosa cells appeared to be distinct from the one characterized in the literature at the time, and was more similar to new PGHS-related cDNAs serendepidously cloned as early response gene products in mitogen-stimulated chicken and mouse fibroblasts (6,7). This novel finding allowed us to review the hormonal regulation of PGHS mRNA in the ovary, this time using a PGHS-2 specific cDNA probe (28). In three different in vivo and in vitro models, results clearly showed that high levels of gonadotropins caused a marked but transient induction of PGHS-2 transcripts (4.4 kb) in granulosa cells. PGHS-2 mRNA induction was rapid and preceded detection of PGHS-2 proteins by about 1 hour, thus resolving a previous discrepancy between protein and mRNA regulation.

Ovarian PGHS-1 and PGHS-2 in Other Mammalian Species

To determine whether the regulation of PGHS-2 in rat preovulatory follicles is a molecular process conserved in species with a different estrous cycle, the bovine follicle was used as a model for large monoovulatory species (29). Results from Northern and Western blots showed that hCG indeed caused a selective PGHS-2 induction in bovine granulosa cells prior to ovulation (29–31); however, a striking difference was observed in the time of PGHS-2 induction in rat (2–4 hours post-hCG) and bovine follicles (18 hours post-hCG). It is interesting that the interval from PGHS-2 induction to ovulation was remarkably similar in both species (about 10 hours; Fig. 18.2), suggesting that some of the molecular determinants involved in dictating the species-specific length of the ovulatory process (interval from LH/hCG to follicular rupture) may relate to differences in the control of PGHS-2 gene expression. To test the hypothesis that the time taken to induce PGHS-2 was responsible for the difference in ovulation interval seen between species, the mare was selected as another experimental model because the length of its ovulatory process (39–42 hours post-hCG) differs from that of the rat (12–14 hours post-hCG) and the cow (28–30 hours post-hCG). Results showed an induction of PGHS-2 in granulosa cells of equine follicles prior to ovulation (32,33). PGHS-2 was undetectable in equine preovulatory follicles isolated 0, 12, and 24 hours post-hCG, became apparent at 30 hours and reached maximal levels 39 hours after hCG treatment (32,33). The progressive delayed expression of PGHS-2 in species with longer ovulatory processes therefore supports its role as a determinant of the species-specific length of the ovulatory process (Fig. 18.2). Whereas the precise time course of PGHS-2 induction in vivo has not been determined in humans, Narko et al. (34) recently reported that PGHS-2 mRNA is present in granulosa cells obtained from women undergoing hormone treatment for in vitro fertilization. The potential role of PGHS-1 and other ovarian cells during the ovulatory process was suggested in a study

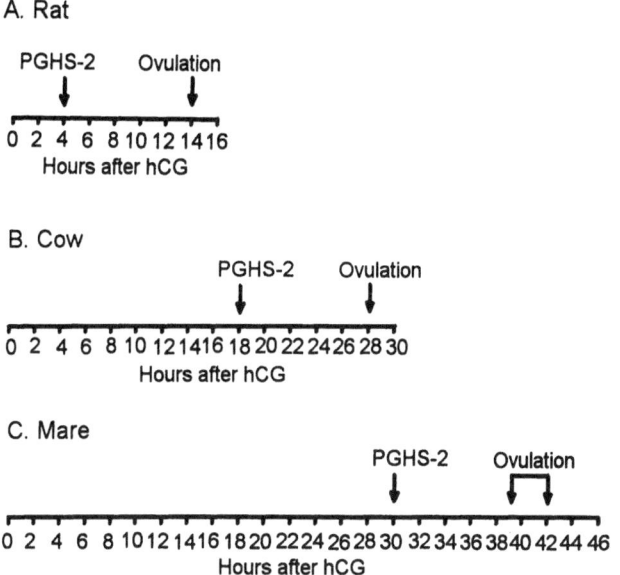

FIGURE 18.2. Relationship among PGHS-2 induction, time of ovulation, and length of the ovulatory process in rats (A), cows (B) and mares (C). *From* Sirois J, Doré M. The late induction of prostaglandin G/H synthase-2 in equine preovulatory follicles supports its putative role as a determinant of the ovulatory process. Endocrinology 1997;38:4427–34. © The Endocrine Society, with permission.

showing an increase in PGHS-1 mRNA in the thecal layer and germinal epithelium of ovine follicles just prior to ovulation (35).

The regulation of follicular PGHS-2 expression has also been studied in cattle during ovarian hyperstimulation (36). Follicular growth in heifers was stimulated with exogenous FSH, and ovulation was induced with hCG at the end of the superovulation treatment. Results revealed no PGHS-2 protein in any of the follicles isolated prior to hCG treatment or in small follicles (6– < 8 mm) obtained after hCG; however, up to 46% of medium (8– < 10 mm) and 91% of large (≥10 mm) follicles were PGHS-2 positive at 24 hours post-hCG. It is interesting that expression of PGHS-2 could be used to differentiate two subpopulations of superovulatory follicles with different steroidogenic capacities. PGHS-2 positive follicles were luteinized (high progesterone and low estradiol) and contained an expanded cumulus, whereas PGHS-2 negative follicles were not luteinized (low progesterone and high estradiol) and contained a compact cumulus. It is interesting that the incidence of PGHS-2 negative follicles larger than 8 mm at 24 hours post-hCG in this study (24%) was very similar to the incidence of anovulatory follicles detected by ultrasonography during superovulation. It can be hypothesized that the presence of PGHS-2 negative follicles larger than 8 mm represents an important drawback to the superovulatory response because these follicles remain anovulatory and because they are believed to provide an unfavorable local steroid environment. The ability to identify such follicles prospectively should help us understand the molecular basis for the development of large anovulatory follicles during ovarian hyperstimulation.

Molecular Regulation of PGHS-2 Gene Expression

LH, hCG, FSH, and other activators of the cAMP-dependent protein kinase pathway (PKA) were shown to induce PGHS-2 in granulosa cells of various species (22–33). PGHS-2 induction in ovarian cells, however, is not restricted to ligands activating the PKA pathway. GnRH, which is thought to act primarily but not exclusively through protein kinase-C (PKC), is a potent inducer of PGHS-2 in rat granulosa cells in vitro (37–39). Moreover, IL-1ß was also shown to induce PGHS-2 in human granulosa/luteal cells and in contact-dependent cocultures of rat granulosa and thecal-interstitial cells (34,40). The use of specific kinase inhibitors revealed that several cellular signaling pathways are involved in the LH/hCG induction of PGHS-2 in granulosa cells (38,39). Whereas PKA appears to play a primary role in PGHS-2 induction, PKC, and tyrosine kinases, but not calmodulin kinase-II, are also involved (38,39).

Further characterization of the molecular mechanisms responsible for PGHS-2 induction in granulosa cells were derived from studies on the isolation and regulation of the rat PGHS-2 promoter in vitro (41–43). The 5'-flanking region of the rat PGHS-2 gene was shown to contain several putative binding sites for known transcription factors, and deletion analyses of the promoter identified the first 200 bp upstream of the transcription start site to be essential for basal and forskolin inducible promoter activities. This DNA region contains several consensus cis-acting elements, including a C/EBP element, an E-box, and ATF/CRE. Results from electrophoretic mobility shift assays and site-directed mutagenesis studies showed that the E-box region binds USF proteins and is required for PGHS-2 promoter activity in granulosa cells (43). The cloning and characterization of the bovine and equine PGHS-2 promoters (Fig. 18.3) should help unravel the molecular basis for the differential control of PGHS-2 gene expression in species with a short versus a long ovulatory process.

PGHS-1 and PGHS-2 Knockouts

The different roles of PGHS-1 and PGHS-2 during the ovulatory process were further underscored in gene-targeting studies that produced PGHS-1– and PGHS-2–deficient mice (44–46). PGHS-1–deficient mice appeared to be fertile and

```
Rat  -201 AGGGAAGCTT CCTGGCTT-- CT-CTGGGCT CATTTGCGTG AGT-AA----
Bov  -200 CCCC...T.. ..GATT..-- ..AG.TT..G T.GC.AAAAA .AA-..GAAA
Equ  -212 .CC.C..... .TC..A..GC .G-A.TTT.. .......A.. .A.A..----
                                         C/EBP

Rat  -159 ---AG--CCT GCCCC-TA-- TGGGTATTAT GCAATTGGAA GCGGAGATGG
Bov  -153 GAA.T--... A.....-A.CC C....C..GC .....|.TTT AA.T...---
Equ  -167 ---..AT... .....A.C-- C....GG..C .....|.ACGC A.TC.A.A.T

Rat  -116 GGGAAAGCTG GGGGGGTGGG GGGGTGGGGA AAGCCGAGGC GGAAAGACAC
Bov  -109 --A.G..GG. .AAAA..TTT ..AAG....G ...GAA.... .......A..
Equ  -122 .A.TGG.GA. AAAA.T.T.A A...G.C..T ...GAA.... .....A.A..
              ATF/CRE        E-box
Rat   -66 AGTCACGAAG TCACGTGGAG TCCACTTTAC TAAGATTTAA AAGCAAGGTT
Bov   -61 .....T.CC. ..|.....-- G.T.T..C.. ----GCA... ...G.....C
Equ   -72 .....TTCCA ..|.....GC .T.-G...T. --.CGCA... ...G.....C

Rat   -16 CTCCGGGTTA GCGGCCAGTT GTCAAA--C-
Bov   -17 ...TCC.... ...TT..... ......GGA-
Equ   -25 ...TCC.... ...TT..... ......--.G
```

FIGURE 18.3. Comparison of the proximal region of the rat, bovine (Bov), and equine (Equ) PGHS-2 promoter. Identical nucleotides are indicated by a printed period. Arrowheads show the position of the transcription start site (+ 1) of the PGHS – 2 gene in each species.

ovulate normally because no difference was observed in litter size between null and wild type mice (45). Some evidence, however, suggests that normal parturition was impaired (45). In contrast, PGHS–2 deficient female, but not male, mice were infertile and exhibited failures in various reproductive processes, including ovulation, fertilization, implantation and decidualization (44,47). Administration of exogenous gonadotropins to PGHS-2 null mice induced follicular development but failed to produce a normal ovulatory response, suggesting that the ovary, and not the pituitary, was the primary site of the ovulatory defect (47). Although ovulation was severely comprised in PGHS-2 null mice, however, the blockage was never complete, prompting Russell and Richards (48) to suggest that occasional ovulations could result from PGHS-1 activity in the thecal cells. In future studies, PGHS-2 knockout mice will provide a powerful model to identify which prostanoid(s) is necessary to restore the ovulatory phenotype, and to characterize specific gene products regulated by the induction of prostaglandin synthesis.

References

1. Herschman HR. Review: prostaglandin synthase-2. Biochem Biophys Acta 1996;1299:125–40.
2. Williams CS, DuBois RN. Prostaglandin endoperoxide synthase: why two isoforms? Am J Physiol 1996;270:G393–400.

3. Smith WL, Marnett LJ. Prostaglandin endoperoxide synthase: structure and catalysis. Biochim Biophys Acta 1991;1083:1–17.
4. Hemler M, Lands WEM, Smith WL. Purification of the cyclooxygenase that forms prostaglandins. J Biol Chem 1976;251:5575–79.
5. Miyamoto T, Ogino N, Yamamoto S, Hayaishi O. Purification of prostaglandin endoperoxide synthetase from bovine vesicular gland microsomes. J Biol Chem 1976;251:2629–36.
6. Xie W, Chipman JG, Robertson DL, Erikson RL, Simmons DL. Expression of a mitogen-responsive gene encoding prostaglandin synthase is regulated by mRNA splicing. Proc Natl Acad Sci USA 1991;88:2692–96.
7. Kujubu DA, Fletcher BS, Varnum BC, Lim RW, Hershman HR. TIS10, a phorbol ester tumor promoter-inducible mRNA from Swiss 3T3 cells, encodes a novel prostaglandin synthase/cyclooxygenase homologue. J Biol Chem 1991;266:12866–72.
8. Sirois J, Richards JS. Purification and characterization of a novel, distinct isoform of prostaglandin endoperoxide synthase induced by hCG in granulosa cells of rat preovulatory follicles. J Biol Chem 1992;267:6382–88.
9. Armstrong DT. Prostaglandins and follicular functions. J Reprod Fert 1981;62:283–91.
10. Priddy AR, Killick SR. Eicosanoids and ovulation. Prostaglandins Leukotrienes and Essential Fatty Acids 1993;49:827–31.
11. Murdoch WJ, Hansen TR, McPherson. A review—role of eicosanoids in vertebrate ovulation. Prostaglandins 1993;46:85–115.
12. Espey LL, Lipner H. Ovulation. In: Knobil E, Neill JD, eds. Physiology of Reproduction, vol 1. New York: Raven Press; 1994:725–81.
13. Orczyk GP, Behrman HR. Ovulation blockade by aspirin and indomethacin: in vivo evidence for a role of prostaglandin in gonadotropin secretion. Prostaglandins 1972;1:3–21.
14. Armstrong DT, Grinwich DL. Blockade of spontaneous and LH-induced ovulation in rats by indomethacin, an inhibitor of prostaglandin synthesis. Prostaglandins 1972;1:21–28.
15. Grinwich DL, Kennedy TG, Amrstrong DT. Dissociation of ovulatory and steroidogenic actions of luteinizing hormone in rabbits with indomethacin, an inhibitor of prostaglandin synthesis. Prostaglandins 1972;1:89–96.
16. Brannstrom M, Koos RD, LeMaire WJ, Janson PO. Cyclic adenosine 3, 5'-monophosphate-induced ovulation in the perfused rat ovary and its mediation by prostaglandins. Biol Reprod 1987;37:1047–53.
17. Hamada Y, Bronson RA, Wright KH, Wallach EE. Ovulation in the perfused rabbit ovary: the influence of prostaglandins and prostaglandin inhibitors. Biol Reprod 1977;17:58–63.
18. Armstrong DT, Grinwich DL, Moon YS, Zamecnik J. Inhibition of ovulation in rabbits by intrafollicular injection of indomethacin and prostaglandin F antiserum. Life Sci 1974;14:129–40.
19. Lau IF, Saksena SK, Chang MC. Prostaglandins F and ovulation in mice. J Reprod Fert 1974;40:467–69.
20. Tsafriri A, Chun SY, Reich R. Follicular rupture and ovulation. In: Adashi EY, Leung PCK, eds. The Ovary. New York: Raven Press; 1993:227–44.
21. Reich R, Daphna-Iken D, Chun SY, Popliker M, Slager R, Adelmann-Grill MC, et al. Preovulatory changes in ovarian expression of collagenase and tissue metalloproteinase

inhibitor messenger ribonucleic acid: role of eicosanoids. Endocrinology 1991;129: 1869–75.

22. Hedin L, Gaddy-Kurten D, Kurten R, DeWitt DL, Smith WL, Richards JS. Prostaglandin endoperoxide synthase in rat ovarian follicles: content, cellular distribution, and evidence for hormonal induction preceding ovulation. Endocrinology 1987;121:722–31.

23. Huslig RL, Malik A, Clark MR. Human chorionic gonadotropin stimulation of immunoreactive prostaglandin synthase in the rat ovary. Mol Cell Endocrinol 1987;50:237–46.

24. Curry TE Jr, Malik A, Clark MR. Ovarian prostaglandin synthase: immunohistological localization in the rat. Am J Obstet Gynecol 1987;157:537–43.

25. Curry TE Jr, Bryant C, Haddix AC, Clark MR. Ovarian prostaglandin endoperoxide synthase: cellular localization during the rat estrous cycle. Biol Reprod 1990;42:307–16.

26. Wong WYL, DeWitt DL, Smith WL, Richards JS. Rapid induction of prostaglandin endoperoxide synthase in rat preovulatory follicles by luteinizing hormone and cAMP is blocked by inhibitors of transcription and translation. Mol Endocrinol 1989;3: 1714–23.

27. Wong WYL, Richards JS. Evidence for two antigenically distinct molecular weight variants of prostaglandin H synthase in the rat ovary. Mol Endocrinol 1991;5: 1269–79.

28. Sirois J, Simmons DL, Richards JS. Hormonal regulation of messenger ribonucleic acid encoding a novel isoform of prostaglandin endoperoxide synthase in rat preovulatory follicles: Induction in vivo and in vitro. J Biol Chem 1992;267:11586–92.

29. Sirois J. Induction of prostaglandin endoperoxide synthase 2 by human chorionic gonadotropin in bovine preovulatory follicles in vivo. Endocrinology 1994;135:841–48.

30. Liu J, Carrière P, Doré M, Sirois J. Prostaglandin G/H synthase is expressed in bovine preovulatory follicles after the endogenous surge of luteinizing hormone. Biol Reprod 1997;57:1524–31.

31. Tsai SJ, Wiltbank MC, Bodensteiner KJ. Distinct mechanisms regulate induction of messenger ribonucleic acid for prostaglandin (PG) G/H synthase-2, PGE (EP3) receptor, and PGF2α receptor in bovine preovulatory follicles. Endocrinology 1996;137:3348–55.

32. Sirois J, Doré M. The late induction of prostaglandin G/H synthase-2 in equine preovulatory follicles supports its putative role as a determinant of the ovulatory process. Endocrinology 1997;138:4427–34.

33. Boerboom D, Sirois J. Molecular characterization of equine prostaglandin G/H synthase-2 and regulation of its messenger ribonucleic acid in preovulatory follicles. Endocrinology 1998;139:1662–70.

34. Narko K, Ritvos O, Ristimaki A. Induction of cyclooxygenase-2 and prostaglandin $F_{2\alpha}$ receptor expression by interleukin-1β in cultured human granulosa cells. Endocrinology 1997;138:3638–44.

35. Murdoch WJ, Slaughter RG, Ji TH. In situ hydridization analysis of ovarian prostaglandin endoperoxide synthase mRNA throughout the periovulatory period in the ewe. Dom Anim Endocrinol 1991;8:455–57.

36. Liu J, Sirois J. Follicle size-dependent regulation of prostaglandin G/H synthase-2 during superovulation in cattle. Biol Reprod 1998;58:1527–32.

37. Wong WYL, Richards JS. Induction of prostaglandin H synthase in rat preovulatory follicles by gonadotropin-releasing hormone. Endocrinology 1992;130:3512–21.
38. Morris JK, Richards JS. Hormone induction of luteinization and prostaglandin endoperoxide synthase-2 involves multiple cellular signaling pathways. Endocrinology 1993;133:770–79.
39. Morris JK, Richards JS. Luteinizing hormone induces prostaglandin endoperoxide synthase-2 and luteinization in vitro by A-kinase and C-kinase pathways. Endocrinology 1995;136:1549–58.
40. Ando M, Kol S, Kokia E, Ruutiainen-Altman K, Sirois J, Rohan RM, et al. Rat ovarian prostaglandin endoperoxide synthase-1 and -2: periovulatory expression of granulosa cell-based interleukin-1-dependent enzymes. Endocrinology 1998;139: 2501–8.
41. Sirois J, Richards JS. Transcriptional regulation of the rat prostaglandin endoperoxide synthase 2 gene in granulosa cells: evidence for the role of a *cis*-acting C/EBPβ promoter element. J Biol Chem 1993;268:21931–38.
42. Sirois J, Levy L, Simmons DL, Richards JS. Characterization and hormonal regulation of the promoter of the rat prostaglandin endoperoxide synthase 2 gene in granulosa cells. J Biol Chem 1993;268:12199–206.
43. Morris JK, Richards JS. An E-box region within the prostaglandin endoperoxide synthase-2 (PGS-2) promoter is required for transcription in rat ovarian granulosa cells. J Biol Chem 1996;271:16633–43.
44. Dinchuk JE, Car BD, Focht KJ, Johnston JJ, Jaffee BD, Covington MB, et al. Renal abnormalities and an altered inflammatory response in mice lacking cyclooxygenase II. Nature 1995;378:406–9.
45. Langenbach R, Morham SG, Tiano HF, Loftin CD, Ghanayem BI, Chulada PC, et al. Prostaglandin synthase-1 gene disruption in mice reduces arachidonic acid-induced inflammation and indomethacin-induced gastric ulceration. Cell 1995;83:483–92.
46. Morham SG, Langenbach R, Loftin CD, Tiano HF, Vouloumanos N, Jennette JC, et al. Prostaglandin synthase 2 gene disruption causes severe renal pathology in the mouse. Cell 1995;83:473–82.
47. Lim H, Paria BC, Das SK, Dinchuc JE, Langenbach R, Trzaskos JM, et al. Multiple female reproductive failures in cyclooxygenase 2-deficient mice. Cell 1997;91:197–208.
48. Russell DL, Richards JS. Causes of infertility in mice with targeted deletion of the PGS-2 gene. Biol Reprod 1997;(suppl. 1)56:178.

Part V

Putative Periovulatory Intraovarian Messengers/Facilitators

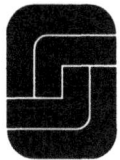

19

White Blood Cells: Active Participants in the Ovulatory Cascade

Mats Brännström and Eva Runesson

Introduction

There is now imposing evidence to suggest that the immune system is involved in physiological changes in the female genital organs. White blood cells, also commonly referred to as the leukocytes, are found in all these organs and may be involved in such disparate processes as cervical ripening (1), implantation/placentation (2), and oviductal function (3). In the ovary, white blood cells have been suggested to play important roles in most processes that involve changes in the structure or function of the follicle/corpus luteum. Thus, essential roles for these cells in the regulation of follicular development (4), atresia (5), corpus luteum function (6) and ovulation have been proposed. In this chapter, current concepts concerning the function of several subclasses of leukocytes in the process of ovulation will be covered.

The intraovarian events of the ovulatory cascade include all the local changes in and around the dominant follicle that occur from the onset of the LH-surge until follicular rupture with the subsequent expulsion of the oocyte from the interior of the follicle onto the surface of the ovary. The biochemical and structural changes involved in this cascade are reasonably uniform across all mammalian species thus far studied, although the time period of the ovulatory process varies from 12 to 15 hours in the widely used eCG/hCG-primed rat model (7) to about 35–38 hours in the human (8,9).

Current theory describing the intraovarian mechanisms involved in the ovulatory cascade (Fig. 19.1) is that of several LH-induced parallel biochemical mediator systems, working cooperatively to decrease the tensile strength of the follicle wall (10) and simultaneously to increase vascular permeability (11) as well as blood flow to the follicle vessels, particularly those positioned at the base of the follicle (12). The major structural change that occurs within the follicle wall, which gives rise to decreased tensility of this structure with

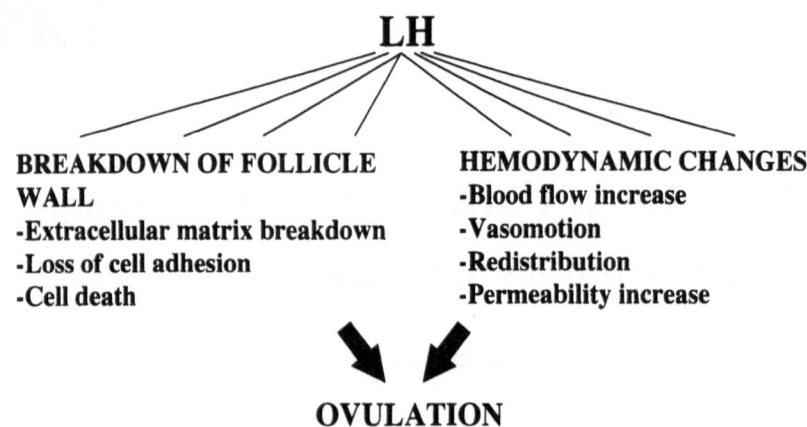

BREAKDOWN OF FOLLICLE WALL
-Extracellular matrix breakdown
-Loss of cell adhesion
-Cell death

HEMODYNAMIC CHANGES
-Blood flow increase
-Vasomotion
-Redistribution
-Permeability increase

OVULATION

FIGURE 19.1. Schematic diagram over LH induction of mediator systems and their major effects to cause ovulation.

time, is degradation of collagen fibers in the tunica albuginea, theca externa, and in the two basal membranes. The actions of serine proteases [e.g., plasminogen activator (PA) and plasmin (13), as well as metalloproteinases such as collagenase and gelatinase (14)] appear to be instrumental in this process. A transudation of increasing quantities of fluid from the blood into the antrum of the follicle may also be necessary to maintain and, during the last phase of the ovulatory process, slightly increase the follicular volume. This transport of fluid from the blood stream to the interior of the follicle would help to maintain stable positive intrafollicular pressure (15) and to counterbalance the marked loss of follicular fluid that occurs through the progressively degraded and perforated follicle wall (16). The major rupture of the exterior surface of the follicular wall will take place when the progressively decreasing tensile strength of the exterior follicle wall can no longer withstand the outward acting force of the positive intrafollicular pressure.

The circulating pool of leukocytes constitutes a readily available pool of cells specialized in tissue degradation/reorganization and in the induction of vascular changes through the release of enzymes and vasoactive substances. Thus, these cells are extremely suitable as effector cells in the ovulatory cascade.

General Characteristics of Leukocytes Found in the Ovary at Ovulation

Most blood cells, except lymphocytes, mature from a common hematopoietic stem cell. The different types of white blood cells were originally distinguished by their characteristic morphological features. Based on functional differences within these subgroups, we are today able to differentiate several types of cells within each subgroup, as exemplified by the Th1 and Th2 T-helper lymphocytes, which have different profiles of secreted cytokines. The characteristics of the distinct leukocyte subgroups, which have been linked to the ovulatory process, will be summarized.

Mast Cell

The mast cell, which is experimentally identified by large toluidine blue-stained secretory granules, is present in tissues adjacent to the microvasculature and at mucosal as well as epithelial surfaces. It is now generally accepted that at least two different subtypes of mast cells exist, the connective tissue mast cell (CTMC) and the mucosal mast cell (MMC). The two cell types differ in the quantity and composition of preformed secretory granules and in their response to external stimuli. The classic activation of the mast cell is immunological through binding of IgE, but nonimmunologic factors such as substance P, vasoactive intestinal polypeptide, and complement C5a may also act on the mast cell. Activation of mast cells results in degranulation of granules that contain several biologically active preformed mediators (i.e., histamine, serotonin, proteases), biosynthesis of newly formed eicosanoid mediators, and synthesis of a wide panel of cytokines. Several of these mediators have been proposed to be part of the biochemical ovulatory cascade as indicated in Table 19.1. Mast cells have estrogen receptors (17) and have been found in the ovaries of most species studied. They are typically located in the central medullary portion of the ovary (18), but, they also exist in the theca layer of the bovine follicle (19) and in the bursas surrounding the rat ovary (20).

Eosinophilic Granulocyte

The eosinophilic granulocytes constitute only a minor fraction of the circulating white blood cells, but they represent a large portion of tissue-bound cells in some organs, especially those lined by mucosa. For every eosinophilic granulocyte detected in blood, more than 100 exist in the tissues. The eosinophilic granules contain four major cationic proteins, all of which have cytotoxic effects on both invading parasites and on human cells. Eosinophils contain both progesterone- and estrogen-receptors (21) and are seen in great density in the ovary of the pig (22) as well as in the theca externa of the ovulating sheep follicle (23).

Neutrophilic Granulocyte

Neutrophils are the dominant immune cells that are recruited into sites of injury or acute inflammation during the initial phase of the inflammatory

TABLE 19.1. Mediators released by leukocytes following activation and that have been suggested to be involved in the ovulatory cascade.

	M.P	N.G	M.C.	E.G.
Histamine	-	-	×	-
Serotonin	-	-	×	-
Neutral proteases	-	-	×	-
Eosinophilic proteins	-	-	-	×
Plasminogen activators (PAs)	×	×	-	-
Elastase	×	×	-	-
Neutrophil serine protease	-	×	-	-
Collagenase	×	×	-	×
Gelatinase	×	×	-	-
Stromelysin	×	-	-	-
Leukotriene B4 (LTB4)	×	×	×	-
Hydroxytetraenoic acids (HETEs)	×	×	×	×
Prostaglandin E2 (PGE2)	×	×	×	×
Prostaglandin F2α (PGF2α)	×	×	×	-
Prostacyclin	×	×	-	-
Platelet activating factor (PAF)	×	×	×	×
Interleukin-1 (IL-1)	×	×	×	×
Interleukin-6 (IL-6)	×	×	×	×
Interleukin-8 (IL-8)	×	×	-	×
Granulocyte colony-stimulating factor (G-CSF)	×	×	-	-
Granulocyte-macrophage CSF (GM-CSF)	×	×	×	×
Macrophage CSF (M-CSF)	×	×	-	-
Macrophage migration inhibitory factor (MIF)	×	-	×	-
Tumor necrosis factor α (TNFα)	×	×	×	×
Reactive oxygen species (ROS)	×	×	-	×
Nitric oxide (NO)	×	×	×	×
Kallikrein	-	×	-	-
Angiotensin II	×	×	-	-

× = presence; - = absence
M.P. = macrophage; N.G. = neutrophilic granulocyte; M.C. = mast cell; E.G. = eosinophilic granulocyte.

process. Most mature neutrophils are pooled in the bone marrow and can be released into the blood stream, where they circulate only for some hours before entering the peripheral tissues at random or due to specific cytokine and chemokine signals. Mature neutrophils in the various tissues show differences in functional and structural parameters, possibly due to the local microenvironment of each specific tissue. Neutrophils are regarded as cells specialized in phagocytosis and tissue destruction, which are functions implemented by the release of several potent enzymes from the azurophilic and specific granules. This cell type, however, is also known to secrete an array of classical inflammatory mediators (e.g., eicosanoids and cytokines) (Table 19.1). Neutrophils have estrogen receptors (24) and are located in the ovarian medulla as well as in the theca layer of the preovulatory follicle in most species studied (23, 25–27).

Macrophage

Macrophages reside in every organ and tissue of the body, where they are of importance in the induction and regulation of immune responses, tissue remodeling, and in inflammatory processes. The precursor of the macrophage is the circulating monocyte, the majority of which circulate in the marginating pool and are thereby ready to penetrate into the tissue. Tissue infiltration may occur in a random fashion or be an active process driven by cytokine–chemokine influences. Once the monocyte enters the tissue, it differentiates into the functionally more active tissue macrophage, which survives in the tissue for up to several years, with its functional profile being determined by that particular tissue. Macrophages are the most active cells in inflammation and tissue remodeling, a process for which they are well equipped with several active substances (e.g., cytokines, eicosanoids, vasoactive amines, and tissue remodeling enzymes) (Table 19.1). Macrophages contain both estrogen and progesterone receptors (28) and are present within the ovary, where they commonly are concentrated to the medulla region (25,26,29).

Extravazation of Leukocytes in the Ovary

After the preovulatory LH surge, there are rapid and marked changes in the extensive capillary-venular networks spreading throughout the theca interna and theca externa. Even though there are several indications of changes in the structure of this endothelium (e.g., the appearance of fenestrations [30]), there are also changes in the properties that enable attachment and transmigration of leukocytes. Extravazation of leukocytes was suggested in early histological studies, where leukocytes were seen at several locations from the capillary lumen to the partly digested lamina propria and as far inside the follicle as the mural granulosa cell layer (30,31).

As in other tissues, the recruitment of leukocytes from the blood to the extravascular tissue of the preovulatory follicle is most likely to be regulated by complex mechanisms involving leukocyte–endothelial cell recognition. The specific design of this recognition determines the composition of the local inflammatory reaction by controlling the extent and time course of neutrophil, monocyte, eosinophil and/or lymphocyte extravazation. Expression of different types of adhesion molecules on endothelial cells and adhesion receptors on leukocytes regulates this process.

During the initial phase of the multistep adhesion cascade, there is a reversible binding between the leukocyte and the endothelial cell. This attachment is characterized by a rolling movement along the venular wall. In intravital microscopy observations of the microcirculatory changes in the rat follicle during the ovulatory phase, we could clearly observe this rolling phenomenon in venules (32). The margination of leukocytes was also observed in histological studies of the ewe ovary during the periovulatory period (23). The rolling greatly slows the transit of the leukocyte through the venule, allowing for exposure to activating and chemoattractant signals. The molecular basis of this loose and reversible attachment is the interaction between selectins on endothelium and white blood cells with their carbohydrate ligands on the opposing cell. In one study of ovarian expression of E-selectin and P-selectin in the ovary of the eCG-hCG–primed rat, a peak of the mRNA levels for these selectins was detected at 6 hours after hCG (33). Regulation of the expression in the ovary may be modulated by ovarian steroids because both progesterone and estradiol influence cytokine-induced expression of selectins on cultured endothelial cells (34).

During the next step of the extravasation process, there is a specific activation of the leukocytes, which will shed their selectin molecules at this point. The specific factors responsible for this process are endothelium-stroma-derived cytokines (particularly IL-1 and TNFα) and chemokines (see later) with leukocyte-activating properties. The activation process also involves increased expression of cell membrane-bound integrins (e.g., LFA-1 and Mac-1 on leukocytes and ICAM-1 and ICAM-2 on the endothelium). The expression of these adhesion molecules on the endothelium is also partly regulated by steroids (e.g., estradiol that increases TNFα-induced adhesion of neutrophils and monocytes to endothelial cells) (35). Thus, the very high follicular concentrations in and around the preovulatory follicle could by this mechanism promote the extravazation of the white blood cells to the follicular tissue. In one study, the cell- and time-specific expression of ICAM-1, which is of importance for extravazation of both monocytes and neutrophils, was investigated in the rat ovary during the periovulatory period (36). The ICAM-1 integrin was found mostly in the theca region of larger follicles, but with some expression in the stroma and none in the granulosa cell layer. In line with the concept of increased extravazation of leukocytes during the preovulatory phase, a 6 six-fold increase in both the ICAM-1 stained theca area and mRNA levels, with maximal levels at 12 and 6 hours, respectively, was seen (37).

This phase of firm binding between the leukocyte and endothelium, as described earlier, is followed by a change in leukocyte shape and migration through the basal membrane between the endothelial cells (transmigration).

Chemotaxis in the Preovulatory Follicle

Chemotactic substances are substances that have the ability to stimulate directed movement of specific leukocyte subtypes according to a concentration gradient of the substance in the extracellular matrix. Classical chemotactic substances are complement factor 5a, leukotriene B4 (LTB4) and platelet activating factor (PAF). The chemokines, which are members of the intecrine family, have been identified. Chemokines are a group of small (8–10 kDa) secreted cytokines with potent chemotactic and leukocyte-activating properties. They bind to glycosaminoglycans and heparin in the extracellular matrix as well as to endothelial cells. The chemokines are divided into the α-subfamily, which are largely specific for neutrophils, and the β-subfamily, which primarily act upon monocytes and T-cells. Most of the chemokines exert their effects via binding to G protein-coupled cell surface receptors on the respective leukocyte subtypes, resulting in plasma membrane and cytoskeleton changes. The leukocyte will then move along the chemokine gradient with typically broad lamellopodia at the leading edge of the cell and a short tail at the rear.

It has been clear for a long time that follicular fluid of most mammalian species contains chemotactic activity. In human follicular fluid chemotactic activity toward neutrophils was identified, where the levels of this bioactivity were related to the maturity of the follicle (38). In this study a correlation existed between the capacity of an oocyte to give rise to a successful pregnancy at IVF and high levels of chemotactic activity in the follicle. The presence of this chemotactic activity has since been confirmed by the same group using a sparse-pore membrane, which only takes into account true chemotaxis, excluding cell movement due to chemokinesis (39). In a study of chemotactic activity in the bovine follicle, it was found that follicular fluid from mature follicles and conditioned medium of follicular tissue, granulosa cells, and early luteal tissue possess significant leukocyte attractant activity (40). Similar results have been obtained with follicular fluid from the mare (41). In the ewe, the follicle secretes a chemotactic collagen-degradation product, with increased secretion after the LH surge (42). Intrafollicular injection of a neutralizing antibody resulted in a reduction of the progesterone levels in blood during the luteal phase, but a normal ovulation rate, which suggests that this specific blockage may inhibit the luteinization component of the ovulatory process (43).

Several chemokines have been identified in human ovarian tissue. Interleukin-8 (IL-8), which is also named neutrophil activating peptide (NAP)-1, is a chemotactic cytokine released by a variety of cells, including endothelial cells, fibroblasts, epithelial cells, and some leukocyte subtypes. It is a chemoattractant for neutrophils and, to a lesser degree, is active on eosinophils and T-lymphocytes. In addition to its chemotactic properties, it also activates neutrophils to undergo respiratory burst and mediator synthesis/release. Local mRNA expression of this chemokine was identified in granulosa–lutein cells from IVF-patients, in follicular wall biopsies taken during late follicular phase (44) and in ovarian stromal cells (45). The local expression in both the theca and granulosa cell compartment of the human antral follicle has since been confirmed by in situ hybridization (5). A considerable local production of IL-8 was indicated by the 14- to 30-fold higher concentrations found in follicular fluid of IVF patients as compared with peripheral blood (44,45). A gonadotropin-dependent induction of IL-8 expression was verified by the 10-fold elevated levels in follicular fluids of IVF patients after hCG administration as compared with before (45) and in follicular fluid of naturally cycling women after the LH surge as compared to midfollicular phase (46). In the latter study, we could also demonstrate a gonadotropin-induced increase in the secretion of IL-8 from cultured granulosa cells obtained from human preovulatory follicles of the natural cycle. The gonadotropin effect may be mediated by the proinflammatory cytokines IL-1 and TNFα, which both have the capacity to increase IL-8 production in granulosa–lutein cells in culture (44) and the expression of IL-8 mRNA in ovarian stromal cells (45).

In the rabbit ovary, maximal levels of IL-8 were found at 4 hours after hCG, which is a time about 2–5 hours before maximal ovarian levels of myeloperoxidase and neutrophil elastase, markers of neutrophil presence and activation, were attained (47). It is interesting that exogenous administration of human recombinant IL-8 to rats, which is a species where IL-8 has not yet been identified, induced an increase in the follicle size that was comparable to that after injection of hCG (48). A functional role of this chemokine in the ovulatory cascade was demonstrated in the rabbit because anti-IL-8 antiserum given 30 minutes prior to hCG decreased the ovulation rate by about one third (47).

Growth regulated oncogene α (GROα) is another α-chemokine, which binds to the same receptors as IL-8 and has chemotactic activity towards neutrophils, basophils and T-lymphocytes. The levels of this chemokine is low in peripheral blood with no variations in the serum levels during the menstrual cycle or during controlled hyperstimulation (49). In this study we found that the levels were considerably higher in follicular fluid, that purified granulosa lutein cells secrete GROα, and that the human preovulatory follicle show intense GROα immunostaining in the theca layer and moderate staining in the granulosa layer. Thus, the presence and distribution pattern of this chemokine in the human follicle are similar to IL-8.

The macrophage-specific chemokines belong to the β-chemokine family. Monocyte chemotactic protein-1 (MCP-1) is found in high levels in human follicular fluid (50,51) and secreted by a variety of cell types, including cultured human granulosa cells and ovarian stromal cells, where secretion is stimulated by luteinizing hormone (LH) (50). Expression of the MCP-1 gene is upregulated in both of these cell types by LH and the proinflammatory cytokines IL-1 and TNFα (51). Some degree of selectivity seems to exist concerning the panel of β-chemokines induced by LH in the human follicle. For instance, the chemokine RANTES, with monocytes, eosinophils, and T-lymphocytes as its primary target cells, is not detectable in the human preovulatory follicle (49).

Granulocyte-macrophage colony-stimulating factor (GM-CSF) is a glycosylated cytokine with the capacity to recruit, regulate, and activate macrophages and granulocytes in peripheral tissues. The perfused rat ovary secretes large quantities of GM-CSF bioactivity, with an increase from ovaries obtained just prior to follicular rupture in comparison with preovulatory ovaries (52). The mRNA for this cytokine is not present in the preovulatory mouse follicle, but it appears in the theca layer of the follicle after the initiation of the ovulatory process and is then present in the corpus luteum (53). In the human, we found higher concentrations in follicular fluids from hyperstimulated women as compared with naturally cycling women and both the receptor and ligand were present in human granulosa-lutein cells (54).

Macrophage-colony stimulating factor (M-CSF) is primarily involved in controlling proliferation and differentiation of the monocyte–macrophage lineage, but it does also play a role in the recruitment of these cells into peripheral tissues. This cytokine and its receptor (c-fms) is found in high concentrations in the human ovary (55). Mice lacking functional M-CSF exhibit decreased ovulation rate (56), and we have found that an increase in the follicular fluid levels in the human occurs after the spontaneous LH surge (unpublished observation). Taken together, these results indicate that this cytokine plays a functional role in ovulation, possibly by facilitating recruitment and activation of macrophages.

Leukocyte Increase in the Follicle at Ovulation

A great number of reports have indicated a general increase in leukocyte content in and around the ovulating follicle. With the use of monoclonal antibodies and other specific markers for leukocyte subtypes, there is now evidence for a selectivity in the increase of specific leukocyte subtypes at ovulation.

A high density of mast cells has been confirmed to exist in the ovarian medulla, cortex, and bursas of the rat ovary and to increase during proestrus (20). Moreover, a preovulatory increase in histamine content observed in the rabbit follicle (57) and human ovary (58) is indirect evidence for increased number of mast cells in these regions during the ovulatory cascade.

The numbers of neutrophils in the theca layer of the ovulating follicle appear to increase after the preovulatory LH surge. We found that an eight-fold increase in the number of neutrophils, identified with a specific monoclonal antibody, occurred from the preovulatory stage in the rat to a time 10 hours later (25). The neutrophils were typically located in the inner region of the theca layer. There was also an increase, although somewhat less pronounced, in the density of these cells in the central medulla part of the ovary. In the human ovary, we detected an increase of the number of these cells in the tunica albuginea and theca layer of the ovulatory follicle (26). Studies using conventional histological techniques in the sheep (23) and in the rabbit (27) likewise established the significant increase of these cells in the follicle wall during the ovulatory process. Indirect evidence for an increase of this cell type in the rat ovary at ovulation is the five-fold periovulatory increase in the follicular concentration of myeloperoxidase (59). This neutrophilic marker enzyme, as well as neutrophil elastase, which reflects neutrophil activity, showed an increase of similar magnitude, in the rabbit ovary 6–9 hours after hCG administration (47).

A large population of macrophages is present adjacent to capillaries in the stroma of the human ovary (60,61). The numbers of these cells increase in the tunica albuginea and the thecal layer of the human follicle wall just prior to ovulation (26,61). They are also present in human follicular fluid (62,63). We detected a five-fold increase in number of these cells in the rat in the theca layer during the ovulatory process, but with no changes in the medulla of the ovary during the same time period (25).

Eosinophils are fairly scarce in the ovary of the human and rat, but they are the most prominent blood cell type present in the theca layer of the preovulatory pig follicle, where a significant increase in the density in the follicle is observed at ovulation (22). Likewise, in the ewe the largest increase is observed just after the time of follicular rupture (23).

Leukocyte Participation in Ovulation

There now exist both in vitro and in vivo data to suggest that leukocytes are active participants in the ovulatory cascade.

The in vitro perfused ovary model adapted for the rabbit, rat and mouse ovary (64) has been used extensively to study the influences of various substances on the ovulatory process. In these studies, the ovary is perfused with a synthetic medium devoid of blood cells and plasma products. A general finding in these experiments has been that although LH–hCG given in vitro induce ovulations, the ovulation rate in vitro is considerably lower than that obtained in vivo. Because the leukocytes mostly extravazate to the ovarian tissue after the LH surge, they may be one of several important in vivo factors lacking during ovulation taking place in vitro. To test this hypothesis, we performed experiments in rat ovaries, where a crude extract of peripheral blood leukocytes obtained from male rats was added to the perfusion system to attain the same number of total white blood cells per volume as in the circulation. The leukocyte addition increased the LH-induced ovulation rate almost three-fold, but was unable to induce ovulations in the absence of LH (65). In this study it was also demonstrated that the leukocytes extravazate and accumulate close to the lamina propria. A study (66) using cytostatic drugs to depress the bone marrow in rats showed a statistically insignificant 30% reduction in ovulation rate when the peripheral leukocyte counts were depressed to 25% of normal levels. The rather small sample size ($n = 5$) may account for the lack of statistical significance in this particular study. A similar decrease in ovulation rate (27%) was seen in our experiments where we depleted neutrophils from the peripheral blood of eCG–hCG-primed rats by administration of a neutrophil-specific cytotoxic monoclonal antibody (67). In this study, the neutrophil numbers were reduced by 70% in peripheral blood. There was also a significantly lower density of neutrophils in the theca-lutein area of the newly ruptured follicles.

There are several lines of evidence to suggest that macrophages are important in ovulation. The CSF-1 deficient op/op mouse, which has very few macrophages in peripheral organs, has a disrupted estrous cycle and decreased ovulation rate (56). The ovulation rate of these animal is partly restored by administration of exogenous CSF-1 (4). Intrabursal injection in the rat of liposome-encapsulated dichloromethylene diphosphate 3 days before hCG injection, which will allow in vivo elimination of macrophages from the ovarian tissue, reduces ovulation rate about 40% on the treated side, compared with the control side in the eCG–hCG-primed rat model (68), which indicates a functional role of macrophages in late follicular development or ovulation.

Leukocyte-Derived Mediators with Effects on Ovulation

Several biological mediators have been demonstrated to be associated with the changes in the follicle at ovulation. Some of these mediators are also released from white blood cells upon activation (Table 19.1). The experimental evidence for a role of these leukocyte-linked mediators in the ovulatory cascade are summarized later.

Histamine and Serotonin

Histamine and serotonin are biogenic amines released by activated mast cells. Serotonin is not present in human mast cells, but it is abundant in mast cells of the rat and mouse. It was revealed that serotonin enhances estradiol production of preovulatory follicles in vitro (69) and induces ovulations in the perfused rat ovary model, albeit at a decreased rate (70).

Histamine, which acts through three classes of receptors (H1–H3), is present in about 10-fold higher quantities in CTMCs as compared with MMCs. Histamine promotes ovulation in the in vitro perfused rat ovary (71), and the effect is mediated through both H1 and H2 receptors (72). The mechanism of action of histamine in ovulation is not fully clear, although effects on several ovulation-associated mediators have been observed. Histamine may work by influencing smooth muscle cells in the ovary because it has been demonstrated that spontaneous contractions in the rabbit ovary are inhibited by an H1 antagonist (73) and that the contractile response of human follicle strips increases upon histamine stimulation (74). In experiments with bovine follicle strips, histamine induces a dose-dependent contraction pattern, which is inhibited by an H1 receptor antagonist (75). Other significant mechanisms in ovulation may be a histamine-induced increase in follicular progesterone (76), a steroid that is fundamental for ovulation (77) and vasodilatation of the ovarian artery (78).

Neutral Proteases

Mast cell granules contain neutral proteases, which are also named *mast cell proteases*. In vitro data obtained from other tissues have demonstrated that tryptase enzymes are active in the breakdown of connective tissue, which is a major component of the follicle wall, by degradation of fibronectin (79) and activation of prostromelysin and procollagenase (80). Mast cell chymase may be effective in ovulation by converting precursor IL-1β to active IL-1β (81), degrading basement membrane (82), and converting angiotensin I to angiotensin II (83).

Eosinophilic Proteins

Eosinophilic cationic protein and major basic protein may promote ovulation by causing disintegration of cellular membranes, plasminogen activation, and degradation of type I collagen (84), present in the theca externa and tunica albuginea. It is also noteworthy that eosinophil peroxidase activates mast cells in vitro (85).

Serine Proteases

PA is a serine protease with broad substrate specificity, that is secreted from macrophages and neutrophils upon activation. A role in ovulation has been proposed via plasmin activation, which in turn activates several latent prometalloproteinases into active forms. Plasmin degrades follicle wall tissue in vitro (13), whereas intrabursal injection of PA-neutralizing antibody in the rat (86) or null mutations of the PA genes in the mouse (87) result in decreased ovulation rate.

Elastase is another serine protease secreted from macrophages and neutrophils. It may be important in the degradation of collagen in the follicle wall by its capacity to cleave the telopeptide nonhelical regions containing collagen cross-links and by its capacity to activate metalloproteinases (88). Neutrophil-serine protease could also contribute to the degradation of the follicle wall because it has been shown to degrade extracellular matrix of other tissues (89).

Metalloproteinases

There are three major types of metalloproteinases (i.e., collagenase, stromelysin, and gelatinase), which are secreted predominantly from macrophages and neutrophils (Table 19.1). Collagenolytic activity increases in the ovary prior to follicular rupture (90,91) and inhibitors of metalloproteinases and collagenase inhibits ovulation in the rat ovary (92).

Eicosanoids

Most subtypes of leukocytes contain cyclooxygenase and 5-lipoxygenase enzymes that have the capacity to initiate arachidonic acid metabolism to biologically active prostaglandin and leukotriene derivatives. The cysteinyl leukotrienes (LTC4, LTD4, LTE4) are produced selectively by eosinophils, basophils, and mast cells. Macrophages and neutrophils produce predominantly LTB4. Intraovarian levels of leukotrienes and hydroxytetraenoic acids (HETEs) increase following hCG administration during the preovulatory phase (7,93), whereas a lipoxygenase inhibitor decreases ovulations in the rat ovary in vitro, which is an effect that is reversed by exogenous administration of LTB4 (94). The leukotriene-induced effects that may facilitate ovulation include vasodilatation, increased permeability, and an increase in collagenolytic activity.

Prostaglandin E2, F2α and prostacyclin are secreted by most leukocytes upon activation (Table 19.1) and are produced in increasing amounts by the ovulating follicle upon LH stimulation (95). Prostaglandins are integral parts of the ovulatory cascades (96–98) and the effects may be related to stimulation of vasodilatation, permeability, PA, and collagenolysis.

Platelet-Activating Factor (PAF)

PAF is produced by most types of leukocytes, but it is mainly cell-associated other than a readily releasable pool of PAF existing in mast cells (99). This substance has been shown to be critically involved in ovulation, as demonstrated by inhibition of ovulation by intrabursal injection of a PAF antagonist (100). Known actions of PAF that can potentially promote ovulation include the activation and chemotaxis of neutrophils and macrophages, release of granule mediators from eosinophils, release of platelet-derived vasoactive mediators, and contraction of smooth muscle cells.

Interleukin-1

Interleukin-1 is a proinflammatory, multifunctional cytokine, secreted in particularly high quantities by activated macrophages as well as by neutrophils, mast cells, and eosinophils. Interleukin-1 induces ovulations and amplifies the LH-induced ovulatory response in ex vivo–perfused rat ovaries (101), whereas

IL-1 receptor antagonist attenuates LH-supported ovulation in vitro (102) and in vivo (103). The effects of IL-1 may be related to promotion of prostaglandin synthesis (104), induction of gelatinase activity (105), modulation of PA activity (106), and stimulation of nitric oxide (NO) production (107).

Other Cytokines

Tumor necrosis factor α is fairly analogous to IL-1 in function and produced by most types of white blood cells. This cytokine increases the ovulation rate after LH stimulation in the in vitro perfused rat ovary (108). This effect may be related to stimulation of follicular prostaglandin (104) and progesterone (109) production. It is also possible that TNFα acts in an autocrine pattern upon tissue, bound leukocytes in the ovary by causing further degranulation and release of collagenolytic enzymes (110) and generation of reactive oxygen species (ROS; 111).

Interleukin-6 is produced in large amounts from ovarian tissue at the time of ovulation (52), and a role ovulation in the human ovary has been suggested (112). IL-6, unexpectedly, does not inhibit LH-induced ovulation in the rat ovary (113). Several other cytokines (Table 19.1) are produced by leukocytes upon activation, and their role in ovulation may be related to recruitment and activation of ovarian leukocytes as described earlier.

Reactive Oxygen Species (ROS)

ROS are formed within neutrophils, macrophages, and eosinophils through activation of an NADPH oxidase enzyme. They are mostly used for microbicidal purposes, but they may also be harmful to the tissue of the host. These free radicals may be important in inducing tissue degradation at sites of inflammation by increasing the susceptibility of proteins to degradation by proteolytic agents (114). It was shown in a study in the rabbit that inclusion of free radical scavening enzymes in the medium during ovarian in vitro perfusion reduced the ovulation rate (115).

Nitric Oxide (NO)

NO is released in large quantities by activated macrophages and neutrophils, but studies have suggested that NO is also produced in mast cells and eosinophils. Inhibitors of NO synthesis decrease ovulation rate when administered to rat ovaries (107). The effects by NO to promote ovulation may be related to cytotoxic action (116) and blood flow regulation (107).

Kallikrein

Kallikreins are tissue-bound enzymes that convert liver-derived plasma kininogens into kinins (e.g., bradykinin). Neutrophil granules contain kal-

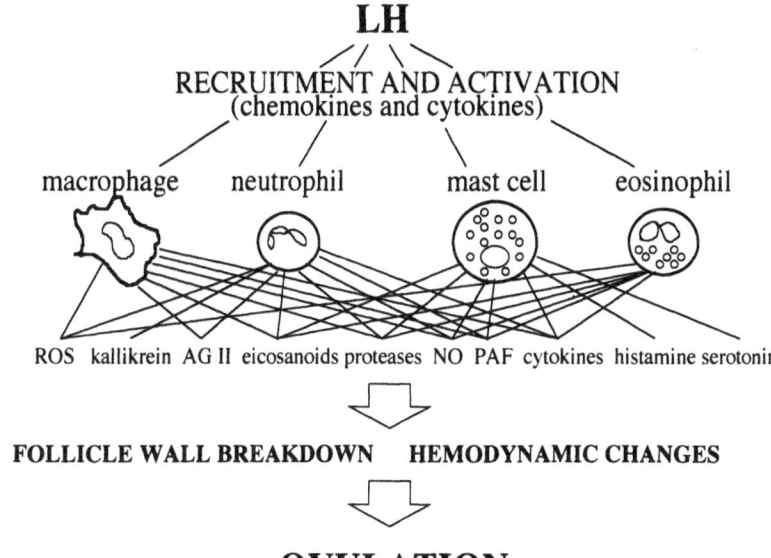

FIGURE 19.2. Summary of LH-induced effects on ovarian leukocytes and their release of ovulatory mediators. ROS = reactive oxygen species; AG II = angiotensin II; NO = nitric oxide; PAF = platelet activating factor.

likrein. The activity of kallikrein enzymes in ovarian tissue increase just prior to ovulation (117). Bradykinin amplifies the LH-induced ovulatory response in the ex vivo-perfused rat ovary (118) and induces ovulations in the rabbit ovary (119).

Angiotensin II

The vasoactive mediator angiotensin II is produced in leukocytes by de novo synthesis or by conversion of angiotensin I. Angiotensin II receptor antagonists inhibit ovulation in the rat (120), and angiotensin II induces follicular rupture and oocyte maturation in the rabbit ovary (121). The mechanisms involved in the ovulation promoting affect by this mediator are not clear.

Summary

During the ovulatory process LH sets biochemical changes in motion in the follicle that lead to recruitment and activation of several types of white blood cells. The activated cells invade the theca layer, where, by secretion of a variety of biological mediators, they act to degrade the exterior follicle wall and induce hemodynamic changes (Fig. 19.2), which ultimately leads to ovulation.

References

1. Bokström H, Brännström M, Alexandersson M, Norström A. Leukocyte subpopulations in the human uterine cervical stroma at early and term pregnancy. Hum Reprod 1997;12:586–90.
2. Robertson SA, Allanson M, Mau VJ. Molecular regulators of uterine leukocyte recruitment during early pregnancy in the mouse. Trophoblast Res 1998;11:101–19.
3. Givan AL, White HD, Stern JE, Colby E, Gosselin EJ, Guyre PM, et al. Flow cytometric analysis of leukocytes in the human female reproductive tract: comparison of fallopian tube, uterus, cervix, and vagina. Am J Reprod Immunol 1997;38:350–59.
4. Araki M, Fukumatsu Y, Katabuchi H, Schultz LD, Takahashi K, Okamura H. Follicular development and ovulation in macrophage colony-stimulating factor-deficient mice homozygous for the osteopetrosis (op) mutation. Biol Reprod 1996;54:478–84.
5. Chang RJ, Gougeon A, Erickson GF. Evidence for a neutrophil-interleukin-8 system in human folliculogenesis. Am J Obstet Gynecol 1998;178:650–57.
6. Brännström M, Friden BE. Immune regulation of corpus luteum. Semin Reprod Endocrinol 1998;15:363–70.
7. Espey LL, Tanaka N, Okamura H. Increase in ovarian leukotrienes during hormonally induced ovulation in the rat. Am J Physiol 1989;256:E753–59.
8. Edwards RG, Steptoe PC, Fowler RE, Baillier J. Observations on preovulatory human ovarian follicles and their aspirates. Br J Obstet Gynecol 1980;87:769–79.
9. Andersen AG, Als-Nielsen B, Hornes PJ, Franch-Andersen L. Time interval between human chorionic gonadotropin (hCG) injection to follicular rupture. Hum Reprod 1995;10:3202–5.
10. Espey LL. Ultrastructure of the apex of the rabbit Graafian follicle during the ovulatory process. Am J Physiol 1967;212:1397–401.
11. Hess KA, Chen L, Larsen WJ. The ovarian blood follicle barrier is both charge- and size-selective in mice. Biol Reprod 1998;58:705–11.
12. Brännström M, Zackrisson U, Hagström HG, Josefsson B, Hellberg P, Granberg S, et al. Preovulatory changes of blood flow in different regions of the human follicle. Fertil Steril 1998;69:435–42.
13. Beers WH. Follicular plasminogen activator and the effect of plasmin on ovarian follicle wall. Cell 1975;6:379–86.
14. Reich R, Daphna-Iken D, Chun SY, Popliker M, Slager R, Adelmann-Grill BC, et al. Preovulatory changes in ovarian expression of collagenases and tissue metalloproteinase inhibitor messenger RNA: role of eicosanoids. Endocrinology 1991;129:1869–75.
15. Espey LL, Lipner H. Measurerment of intrafollicular pressure in the rabbit ovary. Am J Physiol 1963;205:1067–72.
16. Löfman CO, Brännström M, Holmes PV, Janson PO. Ovulation in the isolated perfused rat ovary as documented by intravital microscopy. Steroids 1989;54:481–90.
17. Pang X, Cotreau-Bibbo MM, Sant GR, Theoharides TC. Bladder mast cell expression of high affinity oestrogen receptors in patients with interstitial cystitis. Br J Urol 1995;75:154–61.
18. Jones RE, Duvall D, Guillette LJ. Rat ovarian mast cells: distribution and cyclic changes. Anat Rec 1980;197:489–90.
19. Nakamura Y, Smith M, Krishna A, Terranova PF. Increased number of mast cells in the dominant follicle of the cow: relationships among luteal, stromal, and hilar regions. Biol Reprod 1987;37:546–49.

20. Gaytan F, Aceitero J, Bellido C, Sanchez-Criadon JE, Aquilar E. Estrous cycle-related changes in mast cell numbers in several ovarian compartments in the rat. Biol Reprod 1991;45:27–33.

21. Bonini S, Lambiase A, Schiavone M, Centofanti M, Palma LA, Bonini S. Estrogen and progesterone receptors in vernal keratoconjunctivitis. Ophthalmology 1995;102:1374–79.

22. Standaert FS, Zamor CS, Chew BP. Quantitative and qualitative changes in blood leukocytes in the porcine ovary. Am J Reprod Immunol 1991;215:163–68.

23. Cavender JL, Murdoch WJ. Morphological studies of the microcirculatory system of periovulatory ovine follicles. Biol Reprod 1988;39:989–97.

24. Ito I, Hayashi T, Yamada K, Kuzuya M, Naito M, Iguchi A. Physiological concentration of estradiol inhibits polymorphonuclear leukocyte chemotaxis via a receptor mediated system. Life Sci 1995;56:2247–53.

25. Brännström M, Mayrhofer G, Robertson S. Localization of leukocyte subsets in the rat ovary during the periovulatory period. Biol Reprod 1993;48:277–86.

26. Brännström M, Pascoe V, Norman RJ, McClure N. Localization of leukocyte subsets in the human follicle wall and in the corpus luteum throughout the menstrual cycle. Fertil Steril 1994;61:488–95.

27. Gerdes U, Gåfvels M, Bergh A, Cajander S. Localized increases in ovarian vascular permeability and leukocyte accumulation after induced ovulation in rabbits. J Reprod Fertil 1992;5:539–50.

28. McLaren J, Prentice A, Charnock-Jones DS, Millican SA, Muller SA, Sharkey AM, et al. Vascular endothelial growth factor is produced by peritoneal fluid macrophages in endometriosis and is regulated by ovarian steroids. J Clin Invest 1996;98:482–89.

29. Hume DA, Halpin D, Charlton H, Gordo S. The mononuclear phagocyte system of the mouse defined by immunohistochemical localization of antigen F4/80: macrophages of endocrine organs. Proc Natl Acad Sci USA 1988;81:4174–77.

30. Bjersing L, Cajander S. Ovulation and the mechanism of follicle rupture. I. Light microscopic changes in rabbit ovarian follicles prior to induced ovulation. Cell Tiss Res 1974;149:287–300.

31. Parr EL. Histological examination of the rat follicle prior to ovulation. Biol Reprod 1974;11:483–503.

32. Brännström M, Löfman CO, Mikuni M, Janson PO, Zackrisson U. Morphological and vascular changes during ovulation in the rat (Abstr.). Biol Reprod 1997;56(suppl. 1):117.

33. Bonello N, Lomas J, Norman RJ. Periovulatory expression of ICAM–1, VCAM-1, E-selectin and P-selectin mRNA in the rat ovary. Proceedings of the Sixteenth Annual Meeting of Fertility Society of Australia 1997:118–19.

34. Aziz KE, Wakefield D. Modulation of endothelia cell expresion of ICAM-1, E-selectin, and VCAM-1 by beta-estradiol, progesterone and dexamethasone. Cell Immunol 1996;167:79–85.

35. Cid MC, Kleinman HK, Grant DS, Schapner HW, Fauci AS, Hoffman GS. Estradiol enhances leukocyte binding to tumor necrosis factor (TNF)-stimulated endothelial cells via an increase in TNF-induced adhesion molecules E-selectin, intercellular adhesion molecule type 1, and vascular cell adhesion molecule. J Clin Invest 1994;93:17–25.

36. Bonello N, Norma RJ. Localization and quantification of rat ovarian intercellular adhesion molecule type 1 (ICAM-1) across the periovulatory period (Abstr.). Biol Reprod 1997;56(suppl. 1):118.

37. Bonello N, Norman RJ. Expression of leukocyte-endothelial adhesion molecules in the rat ovary across the periovulatory period (Abstr.). Proceeding of the Twenty-Eighth Annual Conference of Australian Society for Reproductive Biology 1997:74.
38. Herriot DM, Warnes GM, Kerin JF. Pregnancy-related chemotactic activity of human follicular fluid. Fertil Steril 1986;45:196–201.
39. Harkin DG, Bignold LP, Herriot-Warnes DM, Kirby CA. Chemotaxis of polymorpho-nuclear leukocytes towards human preovulatory follicle fluid and serum using a sparse-pore polycarbonate filtration membrane. J Reprod Immunol 1994;27:151–55.
40. Sirotkin AW, Luck MR. Potential leukocyte attractants in the bovine periovulatory ovary. Reprod Nutr Dev 1995;35:675–83.
41. Watson ED, Sertich PL, Zanecosky HG. Detection of chemotactic factors in preovula-tory follicular fluid from mares. Am J Vet Res 1991;52:1412–15.
42. Murdoch WJ, McCormick RJ. Production of low molecular weight chemoattractants for leukocytes by periovulatory ovine follicles. Biol Reprod 1989;40:86–90.
43. Murdoch WJ, McCormick RJ. Mechanisms and physiological implications of leuco-cyte chemoattractants into periovulatory ovine follicles. J Reprod Fert 1993;97:375–80.
44. Runesson E, Boström E-K, Janson PO, Brännström M. The human preovulatory follicle is a source of the chemotactic cytokine interleukin-8. Molec Hum Reprod 1996;2:245–50.
45. Arici A, Oral E, Bukulmez O, Buradagunta S, Engin O, Olive DL. Interleukin-8 expression and modulation in human preovulatory cycles and ovarian cells. Endocri-nology 1996;137:3762–69.
46. Runesson E, Hellberg P, Brännström M. The chemokine interleukin-8 in follicle from normal menstrual cycles—one possible mediator of the inflammatory events causing ovulation (Abstr.). Proceedings of the Keystone Symposia on Molecular and Cellular Biology, 1998:23.
47. Ujioka T, Matsukawa A, Tanaka N, Matsuura K, Yoshinaga M, Okamura H. Interleukin-8 as an essential factor in the human chorionic gonadotropin-induced rabbit ovulatory process: interleukin-8 induces neutrophil accumulation and activation in ovulation. Biol Reprod 1998;58:526–30.
48. Goto J, Kanayama N, Asahina T, Okada Y, Kobayashi T, Terao T. Induction of follicular growth by exogenous interleukin-8. Human Reprod 1997;12:2729–34.
49. Karström-Encrantz L, Runesson E, Boström E-K, Brännström M. Selective presence of the chemokine growth-regulated oncogene alpha (GRO alpha) in the human follicle and secretion from cultured granulosa-lutei cells at ovulation. Mol Human Reprod 1998;4:1077–83.
50. Brännström M, Boström E-K, Encrantz L, Runesson E. Chemotactic cytokines in the human follicle at ovulation (Abstr.). Biol Reprod 1996;54(suppl. 1):68.
51. Arici A, Oral E, Bukulmez O, Buradagunta S, Bahtiyar O, Jones EE. Monocyte chemo-tactic protein-1 expression in human preovulatory follicles and ovarian cells. J Reprod Immunol 1997;32:201–9.
52. Brännström M, Norman RJ, Seamark RF, Robertson SA. Rat ovary produces cytokines during ovulation. Biol Reprod 1994;50:88–94.
53. Jasper MJ, Norman RJ, Robertson SA. Tissue compartment specific mRNA expres-sion of the GM-CSF cell signalling system in the mouse ovary (Abstr.). Proceeding of the Twenty-Eighth Annual Conference of Australian Society for Reproductive Biology 1997:82.

54. Jasper MJ, Brännström M, Olofsson JI, Petrucco OM, Mason H, Robertson SA, et al. Granulocyte-macrophage colony stimulating factor: presence in human follicular fluid, protein secretion and mRNA expression by ovarian cells. Mol Hum Reprod 1996;2: 55–62.
55. Witt BR, Pollard JW. Colony stimulating factor-1 in human follicular fluid. Fertil Steril 1997;68:259–64.
56. Cohen PE, Zhu L, Pollard JW. Absence of colony stimulating factor-1 in osteopetrotic (csfm op/csf mop) mice disrupts estrous cycles and ovulation. Biol Reprod 1997;56:110–18.
57. Morikawa H, Okamura H, Okazaki T, Nishimura T. Changes of histamine in rabbit ovary during ovulation. Acta Obstet Gynecol Jap 1976;28:504–8.
58. Morikawa H, Okamura H, Takenaka A, Morimoto K, Nishimura T. Histamine concentration and its effects on ovarian contractility in humans. Int J Fertil 1981;26:283–86.
59. Abisogun AO, Daphna-Iken D, Reich R, Kranzfelder D, Tsafriri A. Modulatory role of eicosanoids in vascular changes during the preovulatory period in the rat. Biol Reprod 1988;38:756–62.
60. Katabuchi H, Fukumata Y, Okamura H. Immunohistochemical and morphological observations of macrophages in the human ovary. In: Hirshfield AN, ed. Growth factors and the ovary. New York: Plenum Press; 1989:409–13.
61. Takaya R, Fukuaya T, Sasano H, Suzuki T, Tamura M, Yajima A. Macrophages in normal cycling human ovaries; immunohistochemical localization and characterization. Hum Reprod 1997;12:1508–12.
62. Loukides JA, Loy RA, Edwards R, Honig J, Visintin I, Polan ML. Human follicular fluids contain tissue macrophages. J Clin Endocrinol Metab 1990;71:1363–67.
63. Wang LJ, Brännström M, Pascoe V, Norman RJ. Cellular composition of primary cultures of human granulosa-lutein cells and the effect of cytokines on cell proliferation. Reprod Fertil Dev 1995;7:21–26.
64. Brännström M. In vitro perfused ovary. In: Chapin J, Heidel JJ, eds. Methods in reproductive toxicology. New York: Academic Press; 1993:160–69.
65. Hellberg P, Thomsen P, Janson PO, Brännström M. Leukocyte supplementation increases the luteinizing hormone-induced ovulation rate in the in vitro-perfused rat ovary. Biol Reprod 1991;44:791–97.
66. Chun S-Y, Daphna-Iken D, Calman D, Tsafriri A. Severe leukocyte depletion does not affect follicular rupture in the rat. Biol Reprod 1993;48:905–9.
67. Brännström M, Bonello N, Norman RJ, Robertson SR. Reduction of ovulation rate in the rat by administration of a neutrophil-depleting monoclonal antibody. J Reprod Immunol 1995;29:265–70.
68. Van der Hoek K, Woodhouse CM, Van Rooijen N, Maddocks S, Norman RJ. The effect of intrabursal injection of liposome encapsulated diphosphonate on ovulation in the mouse (Abstr.). Proceedings of the Twenty-Eighth Annual Conference of Australian Society for Reproductive Biology 1997:73.
69. Terranova PF, Uilenbroek J, Saville L, Horst D, Nakamura Y. Serotonin enhances oestradiol production by hamster preovulatory follicles in vitro: effect on experimentally induced atresia. J Endocrinol 1990;125:433–38.
70. Schmidt G, Kannisto P, Owman C, Sjöberg NO. Is serotonin involved in the ovulatory process of the rat ovary perfused in vitro? Acta Physiol Scand 1988;132:251–56.
71. Schmidt G, Owman C, Sjöberg NO. Histamine induces ovulation in the isolated perfused rat ovary. J Reprod Fertil 1986;78:159–66.
72. Schmidt G, Owman C, Sjöberg NO. Cellular localization of ovarian histamine, its

cyclic variations and histaminergic effects on ovulation in the rat ovary perfused in vitro. J Reprod Fertil 1988;82:409–17.

73. Wallach EE, Wright KH, Hamada Y. Investigation of mammalian ovulation with an in vitro perfused rabbit ovary preparation. Am J Obstet Gynecol 1978;132:728–38.

74. Morikawa H, Okamura H, Takenaka A, Morimoto K, Nishimura T. Histamine concentration and its effects on ovarian contractility in humans. Int J Fertil 1981;26:283–86.

75. Schmidt G, Kannisto P, Owman C, Walles B. Characterization of histamine receptors mediating contraction and relaxation of the bovine ovarian follicle wall. Int J Fertil 1987;87:399–406.

76. Schmidt G, Ahren K, Brännström M, Kannisto P, Owman C, Sjöberg NO. Histamine stimulates progesterone synthesis and cyclic AMP accumulation in isolated preovulatory follicles. Neuroendocrinology 1987;46:69–74.

77. Brännström M, Janson PO. Progesterone is a mediator in the ovulatory process of the in vitro perfused rat ovary. Biol Reprod 1989;40:1170–78.

78. Schmidt G, Kannisto P, Owman C. Histaminergic effects on the isolated rat ovarian artery during the estrous cycle. Biol Reprod 1990;42:762–68.

79. DuBuske L, Austen KF, Czop J, Stevens RL. Granule associated serine neutral proteases of the mouse bone marrow-derived mast cell that degrade fibronectin: their increase after sodium butyrate treatment of the cells. J Immunol 1984; 133:1535–41.

80. Gruber BL, Schwartz LB, Ramamurthy NS, Irani AM, Marchese MJ. Activation of latent rheumatoid synovial collagenase by human mast cell tryptase. J Immunol 1988;140: 3936–42.

81. Mizutani H, Schechter N, Lazarus GS, Black RA, Kupper TS. Rapid and specific conversion of precursor interleukin 1β (IL-1β) to an active IL-1 species by human mast cell chymase. J Exp Med 1991;174:821–25.

82. Briggaman RA, Schecter NM, Fraki J, Lazarus GS. Degradation of the epidermal-dermal junction by a proteolytic enzyme from human skin and polymorphonuclear leukocytes. J Exp Med 1984;160:1027–42.

83. Reilly CF, Tewksbury DA, Schecter NM, Travis J. Rapid conversion of angiotensin I to angiotensin II by neutrophil and mast cell proteinases. J Biol Chem 1982;257:8619–22.

84. Hibbs MS, Mainardi CL, Kang AH. Type-specific collagen degradation by eosinophils. Biochem J 1982;207:621–24.

85. Henderson WR, Chi EY, Klebanoff SJ. Eosinophil peroxidase-induced mast cell secretion. J Exp Med 1980;152:265–79.

86. Tsafriri A, Bicsak TA, Cajander SB, Ny T, Hsueh AJ. Suppression of ovulation rate by antibodies to tissue-type plasminogen activator and alpha 2-antiplasmin. Endocrinology 1989;124:415–21.

87. Leonardsson G, Peng XR, Liu K, Nordström L, Carmeliet P, Mulligan R, et al. Ovulatory efficiency is reduced in mice that lack plasminogen activator gene function: functional redundancy among physiological plasminogen activators. Proc Natl Acad Sci USA 1995;92:12446–50.

88. Okada Y, Nakanishi I. Activation of matrix metalloproteinase 3 (stromelysin) and matrix metalloproteinase 2 (gelatinase) by human neutrophil elastase and cathepsin G. FEBS Lett 1989;249:353–58.

89. Palmgren MS, de Shuzo RD, Carter RM, Zimmy ML, Shan SV. Mechanisms of neutrophil damage to human alveolar extracellular matrix: the role of serine and metalloproteases. J Allergy Clin Immunol 1992;89:905–15.

90. Curry TE, Mann JS, Huang M, Keeble SC. Gelatinase and proteoglycanase activity during the preovulatory period in the rat. Biol Reprod 1992;46:256–64.
91. Reich R, Tsafriri A, Mechanic GC. The involvement of collagenolysis in ovulation in the rat. Endocrinology 1988;116:522–27.
92. Brännström M, Woessner JF, Koos RD, Sear CHJ, LeMaire WJ. Inhibitors of mammalian tissue collagenase and metalloproteinases suppress ovulation in the perfused rat ovary. Endocrinology 1988;122:1715–21.
93. Espey LL, Tanaka N, Adams RF, Okamura H. Ovarian hydroxyeicosatetraenoic acid compared with prostanoids and steroids during ovulation in the rat. Am J Physiol 1991;290:E163–69.
94. Mikuni M, Yoshida M, Hellberg P, Peterson CA, Edwin SE, Brännström M, et al. The lipoxygenase inhibitor, nordihydroguaiaretic acid, inhibits ovulation and reduces leukotriene and prostaglandin levels in the rat ovary. Biol Reprod 1998; 58:1211–16.
95. Larson L, Olofsson J, Hellberg P, Brännström M, Selstam G, Hedin L. Regulation of prostaglandin biosynthesis by luteinizing hormone and bradykinin in rat preovulatory follicles in vitro. Prostaglandins 1991;41:111–21.
96. Tsafriri A, Koch Y, Lindner HR. Ovulation rate and serum LH levels in rats treated with indomethacin or prostaglandin E2. Prostaglandins 1973;3:461–67.
97. Brännström M, Larson L, Basta B, Hedin L. Regulation of prostaglandin endoperoxide synthase by cAMP in the in vitro perfused rat ovary. Biol Reprod 1989;41:513–21.
98. Hellberg P, Brännström M. A prostacyclin analogue, Iloprost, augments LH-induced follicular rupture in the perfused rat ovary. Prostaglandins 1990;40:361–71.
99. Mencia-Huerta JM, Lewis RA, Razin E, Austen KF. Antigen-initiated release of platelet-activating factor (PAF-acether) from mouse bone marrow-derived mast cells sensitized with monoclonal IgE. J Immunol 1983;131:2958–64.
100. Abisogun AO, Braquet P, Tsafriri A. The involvement of platelet activating factor in ovulation. Science 1989;243:381–83.
101. Brännström M, Wang L, Norman R. Ovulatory effect of interleukin-1β on the perfused rat ovary. Endocrinology 1993;132:399–04.
102. Peterson CM, Hales HA, Hatasaka HA, Mitchell MD, Rittenhouse L, Jones KP. Interleukin-1β modulates prostaglandin production and the natural interleukin-1 receptor antagonist inhibits ovulation in the optimally stimulated rat ovarian perfusion system. Endocrinology 1993;133:2301–6.
103. Simon C, Tsafriri A, Chun S-Y, Piquette GN, Dang W, Polan ML. Interleukin-1 receptor antagonist suppresses hCG-induced ovulation in the rat. Biol Reprod 1994;51:662–67.
104. Brännström M, Wang L, Norman RJ. Effects of cytokines on prostaglandin production and steroidogenesis of incubated preovulatory follicles of the rat. Biol Reprod 1993;48:165–71.
105. Hurwitz A, Dushnik M, Solomon H, Ben-Chetrit A, Finci-Yeheskel Z, Milwidsky A, et al. Cytokine-mediated regulation of ovarian function: interleukin-1 stimulates the accumulation of 92 kD gelatinase. Endocrinology 1993;132:2709–14.
106. Bonello N, Norman RJ, Brännström M. Interleukin-1β inhibits luteinizing hormone-induced plasminogen activator activity in rat preovulatory follicles in vitro. Endocrine 1995;3:49–54.
107. Bonello N, McKie K, Andrew L, Ross N, Braybon E, Jasper M, et al. Inhibition of nitric oxide: effects on interleukin-1β - enhanced ovulation rate, steroid hormones, and

ovarian leukocyte distribution at ovulation in the rat. Biol Reprod 1996;54:436–45.

108. Brännström M, Bonello N, Wang LJ, Norman RJ. Effects on tumor necrosis factor α (TNFα) on ovulation in the rat ovary. Reprod Fertil Dev 1995;7:67–73.

109. Zolti M, Meirom R, Shemesh M, Wollach D, Mashiach S, Shore L, et al. Granulosa cells as a source and target organ for tumor necrosis factor-α. FEBS Lett 1990;261:253–55.

110. Klebanoff SJ, Vadas MA, Harlan JM, Sparks LH, Gamble JR, Agostim JM, et al. Stimulation of neutrophils by tumor necrosis factor. J Immunol 1986;136:3311–19.

111. Ferrante A, Hauptmann BM, Seckinger P, Dayer JM. Inhibition of tumor necrosis factor α (TNFα)-induced neutrophil respiratory burst by a TNFα inhibitor. Immunology 1991;72:440–42.

112. Machelon V, Emilie D, Lefevre A, Nome F, Durand-Gasselini I, Testart J. Interleukin-6 biosynthesis in the human preovulatory follicle: some of its potential roles at ovulation. J Clin Endocrinol Metab 1992;130:1750–52.

113. Van der Hoek KH, Woodhouse CM, Brännström M, Norman RJ. Effects of interleukin (IL)-6 on luteinizing hormone- and IL-1β-induced ovulation and steroidogenesis in the rat ovary. Biol Reprod 1998;58:1266–71.

114. Capodici C, Berg RA. Neutrophil collagenase activation: the role of oxidants and cathepsin G. Agents Actions 1991;34:8–10.

115. Miyazaki T, Sueko K, Dharmarajan AM, Atlas SJ, Bulkley GB, Wallach EE. Effect of inhibition of oxygen free radical on ovulation and progesteron production by the in-vitro perfused rabbit ovary. J Reprod Fert 1991;91:207–12.

116. Ellman C, Corbett J, Misko T, McDaniel M, Beckerrman K. Nitric oxide mediates interleukin-1 induced cellular cytotoxicity in the rat ovary. J Clin Endocrinol Metab 1993;71:3053–56.

117. Espey LL, Miller DH, Margolius HS. Ovarian increase in kinin-generating capacity in PMSG/hCG-primed immature rats. Am J Physiol 1986;251:E362–65.

118. Brännström M, Hellberg P. Bradykinin potentiates LH-induced follicular rupture in the rat ovary perfused in vitro. Human Reprod 1989;4:475–81.

119. Yosimura Y, Espey LL, Hosoi Y, Adashi T, Atlas SG, Ghodgaonkar RB, et al. The effects of bradykinin on the ovulatory process on the in vitro perfused rat ovary. Endocrinology 1988;122:2540–46.

120. Mikuni M, Brännström M, Hellberg P, Peterson CA, Pall M, Edwin S, et al. Saralasin-induced inhibition of ovulation in the rat ovary is not replicated by the angiotensin II type-2 (AT2) receptor antagonist PD123319. Am J Obstet Gynecol 1998:179:35–40.

121. Yoshimura Y, Karube M, Koyama N, Shoikawa S, Nanno T, Nakamura Y. Angiotensin II directly induces follicle rupture and oocyte maturation in the rabbit. FEBS Lett 1992;307:305–8.

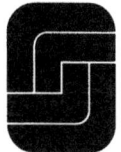

20

Ovarian Nitric Oxide: A Modulator of Ovulation and Oocyte Maturation

Lisa M. Olson, Albina Jablonka-Shariff, and Angeline N. Beltsos

Introduction

Nitric oxide (NO) is a highly diffusable and lipophilic gas that has been identified as a major secretory product of mammalian cells (1–3). It is synthesized from
arginine by nitric oxide synthase (NOS), yielding NO and citrulline (1–3). Three
isoforms of NOS have been identified, each of which is encoded by a separate
gene (4,5). Two constituitive isoforms, first identified in the endothelium and
brain, require calcium and calmodulin for activity and respond to stimuli by
producing small quantities of NO for short periods (1,2,5,6). A third inducible
NOS (iNOS) is transcriptionally regulated by a number of cytokines and hormones, and results in a sustained synthesis of NO over long periods (1,2,4).

NO is synthesized by rat and human ovarian cells and has been implicated
as an important signaling molecule during the periovulatory period (7–15).
Ovarian NOS activity is increased by human chorionic gonadotropin (hCG)
(16), and inhibition of NOS with pharmacological agents lowers the number
of ovulated oocytes both in perfused ovaries (14,15) and in vivo (9,11,12). In
addition, the rodent ovary expresses endothelial NOS (eNOS) and iNOS, both
of which are regulated by gonadotropins (13,17–19). eNOS has been localized to granulosa cells, thecal cells, stroma (13,18), and the surface of the
oocyte in developing follicles (13). In contrast, iNOS staining was observed
only in somatic cells of the follicle (13,20).

The cell–specific expression of ovarian eNOS and iNOS suggest that unique
functions may exist for eNOS-derived NO versus iNOS-derived NO in the
developing follicle. To determine if isoform-selective functions for NO exist
during ovulation and oocyte maturation, we studied mice in which the genes
for either eNOS or iNOS have been disrupted (eNOS-KO and iNOS-KO, respectively). We superovulated wildtype (WT), eNOS-KO and iNOS-KO im-

mature female mice and examined the number and quality of the oocytes released, as well as the histology of the ovaries following ovulation.

Materials and Methods

Hormones, Chemicals, and Antibodies

Pregnant mare's serum gonadotropin (PMSG) was obtained from Calbiochem (La Jolla, CA) and hCG (Profasi) was purchased from Serono (Randolph, MA). Hyaluronidase (Type 3), mineral oil, pronase, and bovine serum albumin (BSA; fraction V) were purchased from Sigma Chemical Company (St. Louis, MO). Normal rabbit serum was obtained from Vector Laboratories (Burlingame, CA), and propidium iodide from Boehringer Mannheim (Indianapolis, IN). The eNOS polyclonal rabbit antiserum was a gift from Monsanto/G. D. Searle Company (St. Louis, MO), and was prepared using a peptide fragment corresponding to amino acids 1173–1192 of bovine eNOS (21).

Superovulation of Animals and Tissue Collection

Immature WT (129 Sv/Ev) mice were originally obtained from Taconic Laboratories (Germantown, NY). Homozygote iNOS-KO breeding pairs were obtained from Drs. John Mudgett and Carl Nathan, Merck Research Laboratories (Rathway, NJ) and Columbia University (New York), respectively. Homozygote eNOS-KO breeding pairs were obtained from Drs. Paul Huang and Mark Fishman, Harvard Medical School (Boston, MA). Mice were housed in a 25°C room with a 12-hour light, 12-hour dark cycle. They received chow and tap water ad libitum. At 27 days of age, they were given a single i.p. injection of 5 IU of PMSG, followed 52 hours later by an i.p. injection of 5 IU of hCG. Mice were weighed and sacrificed 16 hours later using CO_2 asphyxiation, followed by cervical dislocation. For each mouse, both ovaries with the attached oviducts were removed into prewarmed (37°C) Dulbecco's PBS. Ovaries were dissected free from the oviduct, weighed, and fixed in Bouin's solution. Ovarian weight is expressed as a ratio of ovarian weight to body weight. After 20 hours of fixation, the tissue was dehydrated in a graded ethanol series, embedded in paraffin wax, and stored until sectioned for histological examination. The animal protocol used was approved by the Washington University Medical School institutional committee on laboratory animal care and was conducted in accordance with the NIH guidelines for the care and use of laboratory animals.

Histological Examination of Ovaries

We examined the ovaries of WT and eNOS-KO mice ($n = 3$ mice/genotype), 16 hours following hCG administration. Serial sections of ovaries (6 μm thick) were stained with hematoxylin and eosin. For each ovary (approximately 250 sections per WT ovary and 200 sections per eNOS-KO ovary) every fifth section was examined and the total number of corpora lutea (CL), unruptured luteinized Graafian follicles with a remnant oocyte (LGF), and atretic Graafian follicles (AGF) was quantified. The total number of all three structures was designated as 100% and the relative percentages of CL, LGF, and AGF per ovary were calculated.

Immunofluorescent Staining of Ovulated Oocytes

Ovulated oocytes obtained from WT mice ($n = 80$) were mounted on poly-L-lysine-coated slides and fixed with Carnoy's solution (ethanol–chloroform–glacial acetic acid, 6:3:1, respectively). The presence of eNOS in ovulated oocytes was visualized using immunofluorescence techniques as previously described (13,22,23). All slides were incubated with eNOS polyclonal antiserum at a 1:100 dilution and were counterstained with propidium iodide to visualize oocyte chromosomes, respectively. Control staining ($n = 20$ oocytes) consisted of replacing the primary antiserum with normal rabbit serum. Ovulated oocytes from eNOS-KO females ($n = 30$) served as an additional control. Incident light fluorescence was monitored with a Nikon light microscope equipped with a mercury lamp (Boyce Scientific, St. Louis, MO). In addition, the cytoplasm of ovulated oocytes was analyzed with a laser scanning confocal microscope (Carl Zeiss, Thornwood, NY).

Ovulation Efficiency and Oocyte Classification

Oocyte–cumulus complexes were recovered from the enlarged ampulla of each oviduct. Cumulus cells were removed using hyaluronidase (0.25 mg/ml) and by gentle mouth-pipetting the oocytes through a glass micropipette. The denuded oocytes were washed three times with DPBS supplemented with BSA (5 mg/ml). After washing, oocytes from each mouse were pooled and placed in a final droplet of 200 μL DPBS with BSA and covered with mineral oil. The total number of oocytes for each mouse were counted. The average number of oocytes ovulated per eNOS-KO or iNOS-KO mouse were divided by the average number of ovulated oocytes per WT mouse. Thus, the data for the KO mice is expressed as a percentage of the WT result. To check their viability, oocytes were treated with 3 mg/mL pronase at 37°C for 5 minutes to remove the zona pellucida, washed with DPBS, and stained with 0.5% eosin stain. The viability of all oocytes was 99.1 ± 0.6%. To determine the influence of genotype on oocyte maturation, ovulated oocytes were examined with an inverted microscope at 200–400 magnification with phase contrast optics and classified as achieving one of the following stages of meiosis: (1) metaphase I (MI) stage included oocytes with no germinal vesicle or extruded polar body; (2) metaphase II (MII) stage included oocytes with one extruded polar body; or (3) atypical stage included all oocytes with abnormalities such as cytoplasmic fragmentation, loss of spherical shape, enlarged polar body, more than one polar body and/or cytoplasmic extrusions (23). The percentage of oocytes in each stage of meiosis was calculated by dividing the number of oocytes at each stage by the total number of ovulated oocytes for each mouse.

Statistical Analysis

All data are presented as the mean ± SEM. Significant effects of genotype on the number of ovulated oocytes, the percentage of CL, LGF, and AGF in ovaries, and the percentage of oocytes at MI, MII, or atypical stages of maturation were determined by ANOVA followed with the Fishers least significant difference posthoc test of means (24). A p-value < 0.05 was considered significant. Data were analyzed using Systat software (Systat, Inc., Evanston, IL).

Results

Ovarian function of immature eNOS-KO and iNOS-KO mice was assessed by determining the ovary's response to superovulation with exogenous gonadotropins. Ovaries obtained from eNOS-KO mice were significantly smaller than were ovaries obtained from WT mice (Table 20.1). Although eNOS-KO females did ovulate in response to hCG, the number of ovulated oocytes reduced to 37.5% compared with that observed with WT females (Table 20.1). In contrast, disruption of the iNOS gene resulted in a less severe phenotype following superovulation. We observed no significant influence of iNOS deficiency on ovarian weight, but did see a modest reduction in the number of ovulated oocytes (Table 20.1). As the eNOS-KO mice showed a more severe ovulation defect than the iNOS-KO mice, we continued our studies only with the eNOS-KO mice.

TABLE 20.1. The effect of genotype on ovarian weight and the number of ovulated oocytes.

Genotype	Ovarian weight (percent of WT)	Number of ovulated oocytes (percent of WT)
eNOS-KO	51 ± 4*	37.5 ± 4.5*
	($n = 15$)	($n = 22$)
iNOS-KO	91 ± 7	69.9 ± 9.1†
	($n = 22$)	($n = 26$)

Data were calculated as a percentage of the ratio of ovarian weight to body weight or the number of ovulated oocytes observed with WT mice ($n = 14$–16) and are expressed as the mean ± SEM.
*Significantly different from WT mice, $p < 0.001$, †$p < 0.05$

Histological Examination of WT and eNOS-KO Ovaries

As eNOS-KO females showed a significant reduction in the number of ovulated oocytes, we wondered whether eNOS was important for follicular rupture or whether fewer follicles had developed in eNOS-KO ovaries. To address this question, we carefully examined the ovaries of WT and eNOS-KO females. We observed that ovaries from eNOS-KO females contained fewer CL than WT ovaries; however, the number of CL in each genotype was very consistent with the number of oocytes ovulated. Thus, eNOS-KO females ovulated fewer oocytes and therefore contained fewer CL. During this analysis, however, we consistently observed fully luteinized Graafian follicles with trapped oocytes as well as Graafian follicles that were undergoing atresia in eNOS-KO mice (Figs. 20.1 and 20.2). Indeed, after counting these structures in the ovaries, eNOS-KO females showed a significant increase in the number of luteinized unruptured Graafian follicles as well as atretic Graafian follicles compared with WT females (Fig. 20.3).

Expression of eNOS in Mouse Oocytes

Utilizing an eNOS-specific polyclonal antibody, we observed strong positive immunofluoresent staining for eNOS in the cytoplasm of oocytes obtained from WT mice (Fig. 20.4A). No staining was observed when normal rabbit serum was used in lieu of the primary antibody or with ovulated oocytes collected from eNOS-KO mice (Fig. 20.4B).

Abnormal Oocyte Meiotic Maturation in eNOS-KO Mice

During the course of quantifying the influence of genotype on ovulation, we noted that ovulated oocytes from eNOS-KO mice often looked abnormal. For this reason, and the fact that oocytes express eNOS, freshly isolated unstained ovulated oocytes obtained from WT and eNOS-KO mice were carefully examined and classified (Table 20.2). The majority of oocytes obtained from WT mice were at MII, which is the appropriate stage of meiosis for ovulated oocytes. Approximately 28% of WT oocytes remained at MI, which indicates a failure of these oocytes to progress through meiosis in a timely fashion. A very small percentage of WT oocytes showed any abnormalities. In contrast, oocytes obtained from eNOS-KO mice showed severe deficiencies in their ability to progress normally through meiosis ($p < 0.002$). Only 14% of all oocytes were at the normal MII stage of meiosis with roughly 47% remaining in MI and 40% showing signs of atypical development (Table 20.2).

Discussion

NO is synthesized by ovarian cells of several species and, when inhibited during the periovulatory period results in fewer ovulations (7–11,13–15).

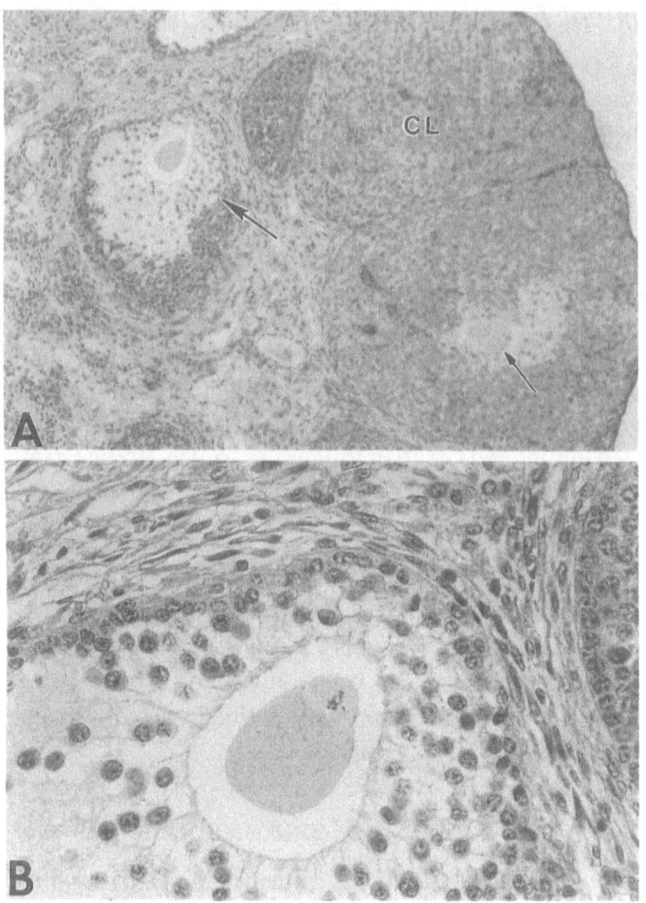

FIGURE 20.1. A representative paraffin section of an ovary obtained from an eNOS-KO mouse 16 hours following hCG administration. (A) Fragment of an ovary showing an atretic Graafian follicle (long arrow), a luteinized Graafian follicle with a remnant oocyte (short arrow), and a CL, 100×. (B) Higher magnification of the atretic Graafian follicle from (A) showing the oocyte with the first polar body, 400×.

These data provide compelling evidence that NO plays a critical role in the ovulatory process; however, the situation becomes complicated as the rodent ovary expresses both eNOS and iNOS in a cell-specific manner and both isoforms are regulated by the hormones that drive the ovulatory cycle (13,17–19). To study the potential unique functions for eNOS-derived NO versus iNOS-derived NO in the ovary, we studied the response of ovaries obtained from eNOS-KO and iNOS-KO mice to a superovulation protocol. Following the administration of exogenous gonadotropins to these mice, we observed a

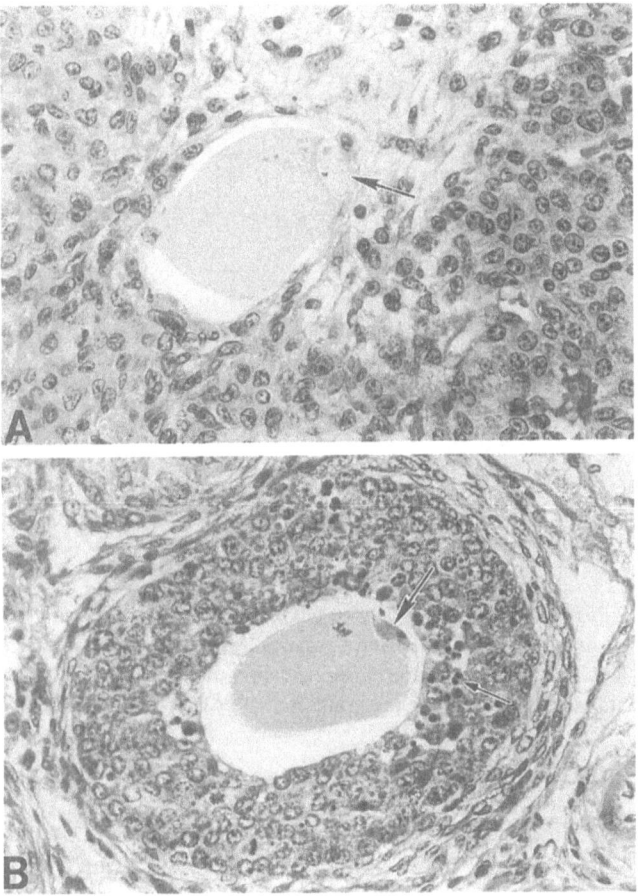

FIGURE 20.2. A representative paraffin section of an ovary obtained from an eNOS-KO mouse 16 hours following hCG administration, 400×. (A) Luteinized unruptured Graafian follicle with a trapped ocyte (arrow). (B) Atretic secondary follicle with many pyknotic nuclei in granulosa cells (arrow) and containing an oocyte with an abnormal polar bodylike structure (long arrow).

significant reduction in ovarian weight and the number of ovulated oocytes from ovaries obtained from eNOS-KO mice compared with ovaries from WT mice. There was no effect of disrupting the iNOS gene on ovarian weight, and we observed only a modest reduction in the number of ovulated oocytes from ovaries obtained from iNOS-KO mice relative to WT controls. These data suggest that eNOS-derived NO plays a more critical role in the ovulatory process than does iNOS-derived NO.

Because eNOS-KO mice showed a more severe phenotype, we examined ovaries obtained from eNOS-KO mice, 16 hours following hCG administra-

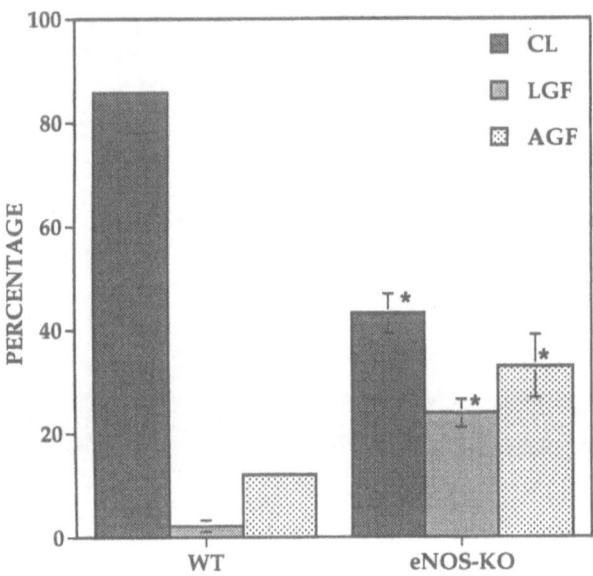

FIGURE 20.3. Distribution of corpora lutea (CL), luteinized unruptured grafian follicles with remnant oocyte (LGF), and atretic graafian follicles (AGF) in ovaries from WT and eNOS-KO mice after ovulation. * Significantly different from WT mice, $p < 0.05$; absence of standard error bars on the graph indicates that the SEM < 1%.

tion, and compared them with WT ovaries. The reduction in ovulated oocytes observed with eNOS-KO mice could be explained by a requirement for eNOS-derived NO for the rupture process, perhaps via its modulation of adequate blood flow. Indeed, we found significantly greater numbers of luteinized unruptured Graafian follicles in ovaries obtained from eNOS-KO mice compared with ovaries obtained from WT mice, which suggests that at least part of the reduction in ovulated oocytes was due to an inability of these follicles to rupture and release the oocytes.

We had previously shown that eNOS is expressed in both theca and granulosa cells, as well as in the oocyte in preantral and antral follicles (23). We also therefore considered that eNOS-derived NO may play a critical role in follicular development and that the reduction in ovulated oocytes could be a result of fewer Graafian follicles developing in response to the gonadotropin stimulation. We observed significantly greater numbers of atretic Graafian follicles in ovaries from eNOS-KO mice relative to WT ovaries. NO has been shown to inhibit follicular atresia and act as a "follicle survival factor"; thus, it is entirely possible that fewer ovulations in eNOS-KO mice are a result of greater atresia occurring in Graafian follicles and a rupture defect as a result of a lack of eNOS-derived NO.

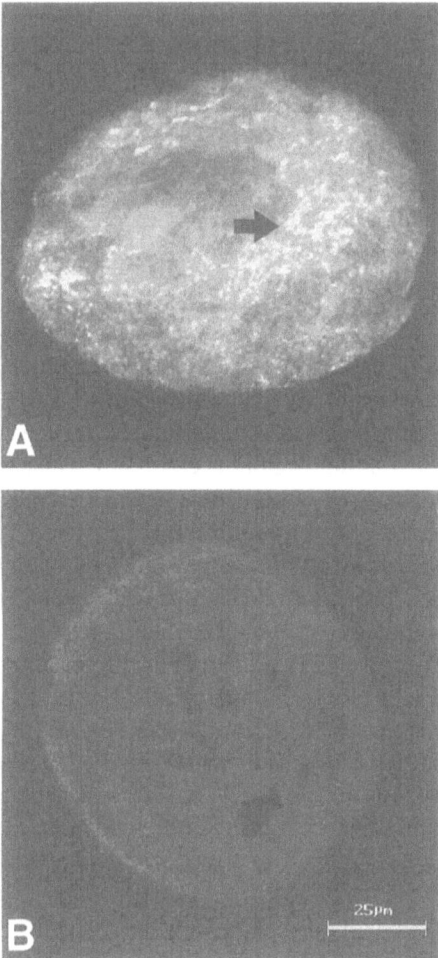

FIGURE 20.4. Immunofluorescent localization of eNOS in ovulated oocytes using laser-scanning confocal fluorescence microscopy. (A) WT oocyte showing strong positive cytoplasmic staining for eNOS (arrow). (B) No staining was observed in an oocyte collected from an eNOS-KO mouse.

In addition to the lowered ovulation rate, we have also documented that oocytes obtained from eNOS-KO mice show a distinctly abnormal pattern of oocyte maturation. In response to the LH surge, resident ovarian oocytes resume meiosis, undergo germinal vesicle breakdown (GVBD), and release their first polar body, before arresting for a second time at MII (25). Compared with oocytes from WT mice, a greater percentage of eNOS-KO oocytes remained at MI and fewer oocytes were at MII, which indicates a failure of these

TABLE 20.2. The effect of eNOS deficiency on oocyte meiotic maturation in mice.

| Genotype | Percentage of oocytes at each stage of meiosis | | |
	MI	MII	Atypical
WT	27.7 ± 0.7	68.1 ± 0.6	4.2 ± 1.2
eNOS-KO	46.5 ± 0.3*	14.4 ± 1.1*	39.3 ± 0.8*

Data are expressed as the mean ± SEM (n = 10 mice/genotype).
*Significantly different from WT mice, $p < 0.002$

oocytes to progress through meiosis. In addition, a much greater percentage of ovulated oocytes showed atypical morphology.

The resumption of meiosis is very dependent on the interaction between the oocyte and its surrounding cumulus cells (26). Thus, the abnormalities in meiotic maturation observed suggests that eNOS-derived NO functions as an important signaling molecule either for the oocyte itself and/or for communications between the oocyte and its surrounding cumulus cells. One mechanism through which NO may participate in oocyte maturation is via its regulation of the synthesis of cyclic nucleotides. Nitric oxide is a known regulator of guanylate cyclase and stimulates the production of cyclic GMP (cGMP) in target cells (1). Cyclic nucleotides synthesized by cumulus cells have long been recognized as important modulators of oocyte maturation (27,28). Indeed, cGMP has been shown to stimulate the resumption of meiosis in both rat and hamster oocytes (28). Thus, it is clearly possible that oocyte NO functions to regulate the level of cGMP synthesized by the cumulus cell mass during later stages of meiotic maturation that results in abnormal oocyte maturation.

In addition, the distinct morphological defects observed with NOS inhibition suggest that oocyte NOS may also be critical for structural events during meiosis. Important structural alterations that occur during meiosis include microtubule reorganizations that influence meiotic spindle assembly and chromosome segregation (29,30). The unusual cytoplasmic extensions observed may be due to an inability of the metaphase spindle to translocate to the cell surface properly.

In conclusion, eNOS-KO mice show a significant reduction in the number of ovulated oocytes in response to gonadotropin stimulation compared with WT mice. Examination of ovaries obtained from eNOS-KO mice suggest that eNOS-derived NO may be critical for both follicular development as well as adequate follicular rupture. Because ovulated oocytes express eNOS and a lack of eNOS-derived NO results in abnormal meiotic maturation, we suggest that eNOS-derived NO is a key modulator of ovulation and oocyte maturation.

Acknowledgments. The authors thank Drs. Paul Huang and Mark Fishman and Drs. John Mudgett and Carl Nathan for providing the original eNOS-KO and iNOS-KO breeding pairs, respectively. We are grateful to Dr. Tom Misko for his gift of polyclonal eNOS antibody and to Dr. David G. Beebe for his assistance with the confocal microscope.

References

1. Nathan C. Nitric oxide as a secretory product of mammalian cells. FASEB J 1992;6:3051–64.
2. Moncada S, Palmer RM, Higgs EA. Nitric oxide: physiology, pathophysiology, and pharmacology. Pharmacol Rev 1991;43:109–42.
3. Ignarro LJ. Biosynthesis and metabolism of endothelium-derived nitric oxide. Annu Rev Pharmacol Toxicol 1990;30:35–60.
4. Xie Q-W, Cho HJ, Calaycay J, et al. Cloning and characterization of inducible nitric oxide synthase from mouse macrophages. Science 1992;256:225–28.
5. Lamas S, Marsden PA, Li GK, Tempst P, Michel T. Endothelial nitric oxide synthase: molecular cloning and characterization of a distinct constitutive enzyme isoform. Proc Natl Acad Sci USA 1992;89:6348–52.
6. Bredt DS, Hwang PM, Glatt CE, Lowenstein C, Reed RR, Snyder SH. Cloned and expressed nitric oxide synthase structurally resembles cytochrome P-450 reductase. Nature 1991;351:714–18.
7. Ben-Shlomo I, Kokia E, Jackson MJ, Adashi EY, Payne DW. Interleukin-1β stimulates nitrite production in the rat ovary: evidence for heterologous cell-cell interaction and for insulin-mediated regulation of the inducible isoform of nitric oxide synthase. Biol Reprod 1994;51:310–18.
8. Ellman C, Corbett JA, Misko TP, McDaniel M, Beckerman KP. Nitric oxide mediates interleukin-1β induced cellular cytotoxicity. A potential role for nitric oxide in the ovulatory process. J Clin Invest 1993;92:3053–56.
9. Shukovski L, Tsafriri T. The involvement of nitric oxide in the ovulatory process in the rat. Endocrinology 1995;135:2287–90.
10. Chun S-Y, Eisenhauer KM, Kubo M, Hsueh AJW. Interleukin-1$_b$ suppresses apoptosis in rat ovarian follicles by increasing nitric oxide production. Endocrinology 1995;136:3120–27.
11. Powers RW, Chen L, Russell PT, Larsen WJ. Gonadotropin-stimulated regulation of blood-follicle barrier is mediated by nitric oxide. Am J Physiol 1995;269:E290–98.
12. Olson LM, Jablonka-Shariff A, Salvemini D, Masferrer J. Inhibitors of nitric oxide synthase (NOS) lower ovulation rate: interaction between nitric oxide and prostaglandin synthesis (Abstr.). Eleventh Ovarian Workshop 1996;43.
13. Jablonka-Shariff A, Olson LM. Hormonal regulation of nitric oxide synthases and their cell-specific expression during follicular development in the rat ovary. Endocrinology 1997;138:460–68.
14. Bonello N, McKie K, Jasper M, et al. Inhibition of nitric oxide: effects of interleukin-β-enhanced ovulation rate, steroid hormones, and ovarian leukocyte distribution at ovulation in the rat. Biol Reprod 1996;54:436–45.
15. Yamauchi J, Miyazaki T, Iwasaki S, et al. Effects of nitric oxide on ovulation and ovarian steroidogenesis and prostaglandin production in the rabbit. Endocrinology 1997;138:3630–37.
16. Nakamura Y, Ono M, Nakata M, et al. Nitric oxide synthase (NOS) activity in the ovary

during ovulation in immature rats injected with pregnant mare serum gonadotropin (PMSG)-human chorionic gonadotropin (HCG) (Abstr.). Biol Reprod 1996;54:68.

17. Van Voorhis BJ, Moore K, Strijbos PJLM, et al. Expression and localization of inducible and endothelial nitric oxide synthase in the rat ovary. J Clin Invest 1995;96:2719–26.

18. Zackrisson U, Mikuni M, Wallin A, Delbro D, Hedin L, Brannstrom M. Cell-specific localization of nitric oxide synthases (NOS) in the rat ovary during follicular development, ovulation and luteal formation. Hum Reprod 1996;11:2667–73.

19. Powers RW, Chambers C, Larsen WJ. Diabetes-mediated decreases in ovarian superoxide dismutase activity are related to blood-follicle barrier and ovulation defects. Endocrinology 1996;137:3101–10.

20. Tao M, Kodama H, Kagabu S, et al. Possible contribution of follicular interleukin-1β to nitric oxide generation in human pre-ovulatory follicles. Hum Reprod 1997;12:2220–25.

21. Corbett JA, Wang JL, Misko TP, Shao W, Hickey WG, McDaniel ML. Nitric oxide mediates IL-1β -induced islet dysfunction and destruction: prevention by dexamethasone. Autoimmunity 1993;15:145–53.

22. Olson LM, Jones-Burton CM, Jablonka-Shariff A. Nitric oxide decreases estradiol synthesis of rat luteinized ovarian cells: possible role for nitric oxide in functional luteal regression. Endocrinology 1996;137:3531–39.

23. Jablonka-Shariff A, Olson LM. The role of nitric oxide in oocyte meiotic maturation and ovulation: meiotic abnormalites of endothelial nitric oxide synthase knock-out mouse oocytes. Endocrinology 1998;139:2944–54.

24. Steel RGD, Torrie JH. Principles and procedures of statistics: a biometrical approach. Second ed. New York: McGraw-Hill; 1980:137–67.

25. Wassarman PM, Albertini DF. The mammalian ovum. In: Knobil E, Neill JD, eds. The physiology of reproduction. New York: Raven Press; 1994:79–115.

26. Eppig JJ. Intercommunication between mammalian oocytes and companion somatic cells. BioEssays 1991;13:569–74.

27. Sato E, Koide SS. Biochemical transmitters regulating the arrest and resumption of meiosis in oocytes. Int Rev Cytol 1987;106:1–33.

28. Tornell J, Billing H, Hillensjo T. Regulation of oocyte maturation by changes in ovarian levels of cyclic nucleotides. Hum Reprod 1991;6:411–22.

29. Messinger SM, Albertini DF. Centrosome and mircrotubule dynamics during meiotic progression in the mouse oocyte. J Cell Sci 1991;100:289–98.

30. Albertini DF. Cytoplasmic reorganization during the resumption of meiosis in cultured preovulatory rat oocytes. Dev Biol 1987;120:121–31.

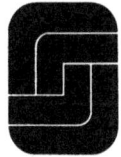

21

Oxidants and Antioxidants in Follicle/Oocyte Function

HAROLD R. BEHRMAN, SANDRA L. PRESTON, PINAR H. KODAMAN,
MASASHI TAKAMI, MICHAEL J. ROSSI, AND ERVIN E. JONES

The reactive oxygen "tone" in cells and tissues is in a dynamic balance that is set by the rate of production and degradation of these short-lived compounds. Much of what is known about reactive oxygen in biology concerns damaging or pathological processes, including aging, cancer, radiation damage, various diseases, and toxicity of xenobiotics. In this chapter, a different perspective will be brought to bear, where potentially important functional roles of reactive oxygen species are discussed with respect to the follicle. A notable characteristic of follicular development is the intrinsic plasticity of this process that involves a host of developmental and regressive states. It may not seem unnatural, therefore, that reactive oxygen species serve as important mediators in follicle remodeling, signaling, steroidogenesis, and germ-cell function. Although this field of investigation is just emerging, an overview of information on the general nature and actions of reactive oxygen species, and the possible role of antioxidant vitamins, most notably ascorbic acid, on follicular/oocyte function will be presented.

Nature of Reactive Oxygen Species

Free radicals have been described as molecular entities that contain at least one unpaired electron in an atomic or molecular orbital (1). The enhanced reactivity of free radicals over more stable molecules results from the fact that more energy is required, for example, to maintain two separate species that each have an unpaired electron than to allow them to come together and share electrons. The reactivity of a free radical is inversely related to its stability.

Oxygen radicals are intermediate, short-lived species produced by the reduction of oxygen (addition of electrons), ultimately forming water. The addition of a single electron to oxygen leads to the formation of the superoxide *anion radical*, gaining another electron produces hydrogen peroxide, and trivalent reduction generates the hydroxyl radical. Some enzymes catalyze either single (NADPH oxidase) or double (glucose oxidase) electron additions to oxygen that form superoxide or hydrogen peroxide, respectively. The hydroxyl radical can be generated from hydrogen peroxide in the presence of ferrous or cuprous ions and is one of the most reactive radicals known. The hydroxyl radical reacts so quickly with neighboring molecules that it rarely strays from its site of production (1). Other agents that play a role in free radical chemistry are not free radicals themselves; rather, they become such in the appropriate environment. These reactive oxygen species include hydrogen peroxide, singlet oxygen, hypochlorous ion, and lipid hydroperoxides. Transition elements, notably iron and copper, can propagate reactions via redox cycling because of their multivalent capacity (1).

Defense Against Reactive Oxygen Species

Oxygen radicals and reactive oxygen species are ubiquitous in aerobic organisms, and the reproductive system must be protected from their potentially damaging effects. One avenue of defense against reactive oxygen species is to provide a low oxygen environment (e.g., that seen with developing germ cells within the avascular environment of the follicle) and a barrier of protective nurse cells that surrounds the oocyte. Other avenues of protection include scavenging by antioxidants, inhibition of radical production, enzyme-catalyzed degradation, and repair of damaged cell products.

A major line of defense is enzymatic detoxification of superoxide anion, hydrogen peroxide, and lipid hydroperoxides that are catalyzed by superoxide dismutase, catalase, and glutathione peroxidase, respectively (2–4). Both mitochondria and cytosol contain unique enzymes that catalyze the dismutation of superoxide into hydrogen peroxide and oxygen. Cytosolic superoxide dismutase is a copper–zinc metalloenzyme (also found in the extracellular fluid); the mitochondrial form is a manganese metalloenzyme (2). It is interesting that mice that lack copper–zinc superoxide dismutase are subfertile and their ovaries display only primary and small preantral follicles along with increased stroma, but few corpora lutea, which indicates poor follicular development or increased atresia (5). Hydrogen peroxide is detoxified by two major enzymes: catalase and glutathione peroxidase. Catalase is found primarily within peroxisomes of most cells; this iron metalloenzyme catalyzes the conversion of hydrogen peroxide into water and oxygen (3). Glutathione peroxidase, in contrast to catalase, is a selenium-containing enzyme and catalyzes the degradation of lipid peroxides as well as hydrogen peroxide (3).

A major source of protection against the damaging effects of oxygen radicals is provided by antioxidant vitamins, with vitamin E serving such a role in the lipid-rich environment of membranes and vitamin C in aqueous compartments; carotenoids also play a role. Membranes are major sites of damage by radicals, and the protective role of vitamin E is of paramount importance in terminating peroxidative chain reactions of unsaturated lipids. Vitamin C recycles oxidized vitamin E back to the reduced state, and the resulting vitamin C radical can be regenerated by transhydrogenases or replaced from extracellular sources.

The final cellular approach to counter deleterious effects of free radicals involves repair processes invoked to remove damaged cellular components. The replacement of peroxidized fatty acids in membrane phospholipids by activation of phospholipase A2 and acyltransferases is one example. Another is the activation of poly(ADP-ribose) polymerase, which serves a vital role in the repair of damaged DNA (6). There appears to be less information on the role of proteases in removal or repair of proteins subjected to oxidative damage, but such phenomena would be expected.

Reactive Oxygen Blocks the Action of FSH in Granulosa Cells

A common feature of follicular atresia is the loss of action of FSH. We showed that rat granulosa cells are extremely sensitive to hydrogen peroxide with abrogation of the action of gonadotropic hormones (7). The reaction of the cells to hydrogen peroxide is very rapid in onset and occurs at the level of DNA, the cell membrane, and other sites. The effects of peroxide are characterized by an abrupt depletion of ATP and abrogation of the actions of both follicle stimulating hormone (FSH) and luteinizing hormone (LH) on cyclic AMP and progesterone synthesis. The depletion of ATP produced by hydrogen peroxide in granulosa cells can be prevented by 3-aminobenzamide (an inhibitor of DNA repair). FSH-stimulated cyclic AMP and progesterone production are severely inhibited by hydrogen peroxide, and these effects are independent of cellular ATP levels. These effects of hydrogen peroxide are also not due to an inhibition of binding of FSH to granulosa cells or to a change in the biological activity of FSH. Because hydrogen peroxide also inhibits cholera toxin- but not forskolin-stimulated cyclic AMP production, it appears that peroxide may abrogate the interaction of the occupied FSH receptor with adenylyl cyclase via coupling to G-proteins. The inhibition of steroidogenesis by hydrogen peroxide is only partially due to inhibition of cyclic AMP production as steroidogenesis stimulated by 8-bromocyclic AMP is also inhibited by peroxide.

Regulation of Ascorbic Acid Transport in Granulosa Cells

Ascorbic acid serves a vital role as the preeminent, water soluble antioxidant (8,9). Infertility is a benchmark of ascorbic acid deficiency in the guinea pig, and such animals display marked ovarian atrophy along with widespread follicular atresia and premature resumption of meiosis (10,11). It is interesting that ascorbic acid and other antioxidants inhibit follicular apoptosis in cultured rat follicles (12). Although most vertebrates other than primates, guinea pigs, and fruit-eating bats do not have a dietary requirement for this vitamin, ascorbic acid is synthesized only in the liver of these mammals (13–15). Peripheral tissues of all mammals are therefore dependent upon delivery and cellular uptake of ascorbic acid to meet localized requirements of this essential oxidant scavenger. The need for membrane transporters is further emphasized by the fact that ascorbic acid is present almost totally as the negatively charged anion at physiological pH (16) and is therefore excluded from cells.

We showed that the uptake of ascorbic acid in granulosa cells is driven by Na^+- and energy-dependent transporters. These transporters are positively regulated by FSH, IGF-1, and GnRH, and by second messengers such as cyclic AMP and diacylglycerol. The upregulation of ascorbic acid transport appears to be induced by a common tyrosine specific protein kinase-dependent pathway for FSH, IGF-1, and GnRH (17).

FSH responsiveness is vital for the prevention of follicular atresia and for selection of the dominant follicle (18), and this effect may be mediated by IGF-1 (19,20). Incubation of rat granulosa cells with FSH produces a marked increase in ascorbic acid uptake, which demonstrates that the ability of granulosa cells to accumulate ascorbic acid is a regulated and potentially vital determinant in preventing follicular atresia (11,12). IGF-1 was similarly shown to increase ascorbic acid uptake, and this response was additive to the action of FSH. This is in accordance with previously reported synergistic effects of IGF-1 and FSH on differentiation of granulosa cells (21–25). Although the stimulatory effect of FSH is apparent within 4 hours of treatment, IGF-1 requires 48 hours to show a significant increase in ascorbic acid uptake, and responses to both hormones are independent of an effect on cell proliferation.

It was previously shown that the binding of FSH to specific cell surface receptors coupled to adenylyl cyclase leads to cyclic AMP production and the activation of the cyclic AMP-dependent protein kinase A pathway in granulosa cells (26,27). FSH has also been reported to increase intracellular Ca^{++}, which activates the protein kinase C pathway (28). Thus, to determine if ascorbic acid uptake is influenced by these pathways, granulosa cells were incubated for 24 hours with 8-bromocyclic AMP. A significant increase in ascorbic acid uptake indicates that the induction of ascorbic acid transport is mediated by the cyclic AMP pathway. Phorbol ester similarly caused a significant increase in ascorbic acid uptake, indicating a role of the protein kinase C pathway. When the maximum effective dose was used for both phorbol ester and 8-bromocyclic AMP, as determined from a dose–response curve constructed for both agents, a further synergistic increase in ascorbic acid uptake occurs, which indicates independent regulation by both agents, as well as that ascorbic acid transport may be regulated by both kinase pathways.

Evidence has shown that the actions of IGF-1 and FSH are mediated by tyrosine-specific protein kinases in granulosa cells (25,29). For example, the highly specific tyrosine kinase inhibitor AG-18 blocks FSH-induced transcription of steroidogenic enzymes in granulosa cells, which indicates the importance of this kinase pathway in the cellular responses to FSH (29). We similarly found that a tyrosine kinase pathway mediates induction of ascorbic acid transport by FSH, IGF-1, and GnRH, as AG-18 abolished the actions of these diverse ligands.

Granulosa cells accumulate ascorbic acid in a time- and cell-dependent manner. Uptake is substrate-dependent and a saturable process with a K_m of 50.8 µM and a V_{max} of 3.3 pmol/10^6 cells/minute. As such, the granulosa cell ascorbic acid transport system shows similar characteristics to transporters that we and others have shown in other cells (30–32). The K_m of ascorbic acid uptake in granulosa cells is well within the range for blood levels of ascorbic acid, which are about 50–100 µM (16). Furthermore, the same K_m was obtained after treatment with different inducers and was similar to the K_m of ascorbic acid transport that we found in rat luteal cells (32). This implies that the same transporter for ascorbic acid is probably present in both granulosa and luteal cells; however, the transporters appear to be less numerous in the granulosa cells (V_{max} = 3.3 pmol/10^6 cells/minute) than it is in luteal cells (V_{max} = 14 pmol/10^6 cells/minute) (32).

Ascorbic acid uptake in granulosa cells is energy-dependent as dinitrophenol, which is an inhibitor of mitochondrial proton transport that significantly inhibited ascorbic acid uptake. Ouabain, an inhibitor of Na^+/K^+ ATPase, and incubation of granulosa cells in a low Na^+ milieu also significantly inhibited ascorbic acid uptake, which suggests that the transport of ascorbic acid by granulosa cells involves an active transport process that depends on the sodium gradient established by the Na^+/K^+ ATPase system.

Thus, ascorbic acid uptake in rat granulosa cells is hormonally regulated. Our findings along with previously reported information on the regulation of apoptosis in granulosa cells (11,12,33), suggest that ascorbic acid plays a vital role in the selection of the dominant follicle and in the prevention of atresia or apoptosis. The evidence that many second messengers are involved in regulation of the cellular accumulation of this essential antioxidant further emphasizes the vital role of ascorbic acid in the developing follicle.

Role of Ascorbic Acid in the Follicle/Oocyte

The ascorbic acid content of certain tissues (e.g., the corpus luteum) is rapidly depleted by LH. This response can be used as sensitive and specific bioassay for LH (34). In addition, prostaglandin $F_{2\alpha}$ severely depletes ascorbic acid in the corpus luteum within a few minutes (32,35), and this response is inversely associated with the production of reactive oxygen species (35,36). High levels of LH, however, occur only before ovulation, which ultimately induces follicular rupture and signals the oocyte within the follicle to resume meiosis. Although ascorbic acid depletion in the entire ovary with attendant corpora lutea of previous cycles is known to occur at this time (37–39), no studies have directly addressed the ascorbic acid status of the preovulatory follicle in response to LH. Our preliminary findings show that LH depletes ascorbic acid in the preovulatory follicle within 2 hours, and agents that deplete ascorbic acid in the follicle [e.g., gonadotropin and menadione (a redox-cycling agent that generates oxygen radicals)] induce the resumption of meiosis (40). Although incubation of the oocytes- or oocyte-cumulus complexes with ascorbic acid does not prevent the spontaneous resumption of meiosis, we found that the direct microinjection of ascorbic acid into the oocyte delays the onset of oocyte maturation.

The depletion of ascorbic acid in preovulatory ovaries confirms earlier reports in both the rat and guinea pig (37–39). To our knowledge, however, this is the first report of the depletion of ascorbic acid in the preovulatory follicle by go-nadotropin both in vivo and during incubation. We have previously observed that the mere isolation of tissue and the preparation of primary cells for culture results in a total depletion of ascorbic acid (17,32). An identical response is seen with isolation of oocytes and oocyte–cumulus complexes, which may contribute to the induction of spontaneous oocyte maturation; however, the isolation and incubation of intact preovulatory follicles, in which maturation of oocytes is well known not to occur (41–43), results in only the partial depletion of ascorbic acid. Thus, in contrast to isolated oocytes or cumulus-enclosed oocytes, intact incubated follicles contain a reserve of ascorbic acid, which may provide a con-tinuous supply of this antioxidant to the oocyte or other cells and may thereby prevent the onset of oocyte maturation.

The mechanism of ascorbic acid depletion in the follicle by LH is not known. In the corpus luteum, this response is associated with stimulation of ascorbic acid secretion and steroidogenesis because treatment with aminoglutethimide, a po-tent steroidogenesis inhibitor, partially blocked ascorbic acid depletion by LH (32). A similar mechanism of action of LH for ascorbic acid depletion may occur in the follicle, or possibly via other oxidant-generating mechanisms. The time course for the onset of oocyte maturation by incubation of preovulatory follicles with LH is about 3–4 hours (43,44), and this event is later than the time-course we found for depletion of ascorbic acid by LH, which occurs within 2 hours. Deple-tion of ascorbic acid in follicles incubated with menadione is probably the result of oxidant production (e.g., superoxide) that is generated by this well-estab-lished redox-cycling agent (45–48). Ascorbic acid is a known scavenger of super-oxide (49) as well as other oxidant radicals, including alkoxy, alkyl peroxy, glutathione, and tocopherol radicals (8,9), that may also be produced by the formation of the archetypal oxygen radical, superoxide.

The mechanism by which depletion of ascorbic acid may initiate the onset of meiosis is unknown. One possibility is that antioxidants directly inhibit meiosis or act indirectly to maintain intraoocyte levels of cyclic AMP, which is well known to inhibit oocyte maturation (50–52). On the other hand, because ascorbic acid depletion occurs in response to the generation of oxygen radicals, radicals such as superoxide may serve to mediate the resumption of meiosis, and ascorbic acid depletion may be merely a side-effect of such a response. Neither possibility can be excluded at the present time. It is interesting that findings show that superoxide increases mitosis (53,54), and that the resumption of meiosis may occur by similar mechanisms.

Further support for a role of antioxidants in oocyte maturation was provided by other studies in which we found that the spontaneous resumption of meiosis in cumulus-enclosed oocytes was inhibited by a wide variety of phenolic antioxidants, all of which are lipophillic and are therefore expected to penetrate cells readily (55). The most potent of the antioxidants were nordihydroguaiaretic acid (NDGA) and 2,3-tert-butyl-4-hydroxyanisole (BHA). The inhibition of oocyte maturation by NDGA and BHA was long lasting, at least in oocyte–cumulus complexes, but it was not permanent. In addition, their inhibitory activity could also be reversed by washing. Phenolic antioxidants also inhibit oocyte maturation in denuded oocytes and this response is similar to that seen in oocyte–cumulus complexes. BHA, however, is significantly more potent in denuded oocytes than NDGA, in contrast to that found in oocyte–cumulus complexes.

In summary, ascorbic acid is depleted by LH in the preovulatory follicle, and this response is associated with the resumption of meiosis because other agents that deplete ascorbic acid also induce oocyte maturation. Moreover, cell permeant phenolic antioxidants are potent inhibitors of the spontaneous resumption of meiosis; however, the present results do not rule out the possibility that ascorbic acid depletion may be an effect of oxidant production and that the generation of such oxidants (e.g., superoxide) may be important mediators for the induction of oocyte maturation.

References

1. Halliwell B, Gutteridge JMC. Free radicals in biology and medicine. Oxford: Oxford University Press; 1989.
2. Fridovich I. The biology of oxygen radicals: general concepts. In: Halliwell B, ed. Oxygen radicals and tissue injury. Bethesda: FASEB; 1988:1–8.
3. Chance B, Sies H, Boveris A. Hydroperoxide metabolism in mammalian organs. Physiol Rev 1979;59:527–605.
4. Fridovich I. Biological effects of the superoxide radical. Arch Biochem Biophys 1986;247:1–11.
5. Matzuk MM, Dionne L, Guo Q, Kumar TR, Lebovitz RM. Ovarian function in superoxide dismutase 1 and 2 knockout mice. Endocrinology 1998;139:4008–11.

6. Schraufstetter IU, Hyslop PA, Hinshaw DB, Spragg RG, Sklar LA, Cochrane CG. Hydrogen peroxide-induced injury of cells and its prevention by inhibitors of poly(ADP-ribose) polymerase. Proc Natl Acad Sci USA 1986;83:4908–12.

7. Margolin Y, Aten RF, Behrman HR. Antigonadotropic and antisteroidogenic actions of peroxide in rat granulose cells. Endocrinology 1990;127:245–50.

8. Buettner GR. The pecking order of free radicals and antioxidants: lipid peroxidation, α-tocopherol, and ascorbate. Arch Biochem Biophys 1993;300:535–43.

9. Rose RC, Bode AM. Biology of free radical scavengers: an evaluation of ascorbate. FASEB J 1993;7:1135–42.

10. Bessesen DH. Changes in organ weights of the guinea pig during experimental scurvy. Am J Physiol 1923;63:245–56.

11. Kramer MM, Harman MT, Brill AK. Disturbances of reproduction and ovarian changes in the guinea-pig in relation to vitamin C deficiency. Am J Physiol 1933;106:611–22.

12. Tilly JL, Tilly KI. Inhibitors of oxidative stress mimic the ability of follicle-stimulating hormone to suppress apoptosis in cultured rat ovarian follicles. Endocrinology 1995;136:242–52.

13. Sauberlich HE. Pharmacology of vitamin C. Annu Rev Nutr 1994;14:371–91.

14. Frei B. Reactive oxygen species and antioxidant vitamins: mechanisms of action. Am J Med 1994;97:3A–5S.

15. Meister A. Glutathione-ascorbid acid antioxidant system in animals. J Biol Chem 1994;269:9397–400.

16. Levine M, Morita K. Ascorbic acid in endocrine systems. Vitamin Horm 1985; 42:1–64.

17. Behrman HR, Preston SL, Aten RF, Rinaudo P, Zreik TG. Hormone induction of ascorbic acid transport in immature granulosa cells. Endocrinology 1996;137:4316–21.

18. Gougeon A. Regulation of ovarian follicular development in primates: facts and hypotheses. Endocrine Rev 1996;17:121–55.

19. Chun S-Y, Billig H, Tilly JL, Furuta I, Tsafriri A, Hsueh AJW. Gonadotropin suppression of apoptosis in cultured preovulatory follicles: mediatory role of endogenous inulin-like growth factor I. Endocrinology 1994;135:1845–53.

20. Chus S-Y, Eisenhauer KM, Minami S, Billig H, Perlas E, Hseuh AJW. Hormonal regulation of apoptosis in early antral follicles: follicle-stimulating hormone as a major survival factor. Endocrinology 1996;137:1447–56.

21. Adashi EY, Resnick CE, Brodie AMH, Svoboda ME, Van Wyk JJ. Somatomedin-C-mediated potentiation of follicle-stimulating hormone-induced aromatase activity of cultured granulosa cells. Endocrinology 1985;117:2313–20.

22. Adashi EY, Resnick CE, Brodie AMH, Svoboda ME, Van Wyk JJ. Somatomedin-C enhances induction of luteinizing hormone receptors by follicle-stimulating hormone in cultured rat granulose cells. Endocrinology 1985;116:2369–75.

23. Adashi EY, Resnick CE, Svoboda ME, Van Wyk JJ. Somatomedin-C synergizes with follicle-stimulating hormone in the aquistion of progestin biosynthetic capacity by cultured rat granulose cells. Endocrinology 1985;116:2135–42.

24. Giudice LC. Insulin-like growth factors and ovarian follicular development. Endocrine Rev 1992;13:641–69.

25. Costrici N, Elberg G, Lunenfeld B, et al. A cytosolic protein tyrosine kinase activity is induced by follicle stimulating hormone and insulin like growth factor-I in human granulosa cells. Endocrinology 1995;136:4705–8.

26. Hunzicker-Dunn M, Birnbaumer L. Adenylyl cyclase activities in ovarian tissues. III. Regulation of responsiveness to LH, FSH, and PGE1 in the prepubertal, cycling, pregnany, and pseudopregnant rat. Endocrinology 1976;99:198–210.

27. Ratoosh SL, Richards JS. Regulation of the content and phosphorylation of R(II) by adenosine 3',5'-monophosphate, follicle-stimulating hormone, and estradiol in cultured granulosa cells. Endocrinology 1985;117:917–27.

28. Grasso P, Reichert LE Jr. Follicle-stimulating hormone receptor-mediated uptake of $^{45}Ca^{2+}$ by cultured rat Sertoli cells does not require activation of cholera toxin- or pertussis toxin-sensitive guanine nucleotide binding proteins or adenylate cyclase. Endocrinology 1990;127:949–56.

29. Orly J, Rei Z, Greenberg NM, Richards JS. Tyrosine kinase inhibitor AG18 arrests follicle-stimulating hormone-induced granulosa cell differentiation: use of reverse transcriptase-polymerase chain reaction assay for multiple messenger ribonucleic acids. Endocrinology 1994;134:2336–46.

30. Rose RC. Transport of ascorbic acid and other water-soluble vitamins. Biochim Biophys Acta 1988;947:335–66.

31. Moger WH. Uptake and release of ascorbic acid by rat Leydig cells in vitro. J Androl 1987;8:398–402.

32. Musicki B, Kodaman PH, Aten RF, Behrman HR. Endocrine regulation of ascorbic acid transport and secretion in luteal cells. Biol Reprod 1996;54:399–406.

33. Tilly JL, Tilly KI, Kenton ML, Johnson AL. Expression of members of the Bcl-2 gene family in the immature rat ovary: equine chorionic gonadotropin-mediated inhibition of granulosa cell apoptosis is associated with decreased Bax and constitutive Bcl-2 and Bcl-x$_{long}$ messenger ribonucleic acid levels. Endocrinology 1995;136: 232–41.

34. Parlow AF. Influence of difference in the persistence of luteinizing hormones in blood on their potency in the ovarian ascorbic acid depletion bioassay. Endocrinology 1972;91:1109–12.

35. Aten RF, Duarte KM, Behrman HR. Regulation of ovarian antioxidant vitamins, reduced glutathione, and lipid peroxidation by luteinizing hormone and prostaglandin F$_{2\alpha}$. Biol Reprod 1992;46:401–7.

36. Riley JCM, Behrman HR. In vivo generation of hydrogen peroxide in the rat corpus luteum during luteolysis. Endocrinology 1991;128:1749–53.

37. Mills JM, Schwartz NB. Ovarian ascorbic acid as an endogenous and exogenous assay for cyclic proestrous LH release. Endocrinology 1961;69:844–50.

38. Astrade JJ, Caligaris L. Ovarian ascorbic acid concentration and its modifications during sexual and reproductive activity in the rat. Acta Physiol 1966;16:1–5.

39. Paeschke KD. Untersuchung des ascorbinsaure-stoffwechsels zure bestimmung des ovulationstermins. Arch Gynaek 1967;204:274–77.

40. Guarnaccia MM, Preston SL, Toyloy V, Behrman HR. Depletion of ascorbic acid by LH in the preovulatory follicle may mediate the resumption of meiosis. Biol Reprol 1997;56(suppl. 1):178.

41. Pincus G, Enzmann EV. The comparative behavior of mammalian eggs in vivo and in vitro. I. The activation of ovarian eggs. J Exp Med 1935;62:665–75.

42. Hillensjo T. Oocyte maturation and glycolysis in isolated preovulatory follicles of PMS-injected immature rats. Acta Endocrinol (Copenh) 1976;82:809–30.

43. Pellicer A, Parmer TG, Stoane JM, Behrman HR. Desensitization to FSH in cumulus cells is coincident with hormone-induction of oocyte maturation in the rat follicle. Mol Cell Endocrinol 1989;64:179–88.

44. Tsafriri A, Lindner HR, Zor U, Lamprecht SA. In vitro induction of meiotic division in follicle-enclosed rat oocytes by LH, cyclic AMP and prostaglandin E2. J Reprod Fertil 1972;31:39–50.
45. Thor H, Smith MT, Hartzell P, Bellomo G, Jewell SA, Orrenius S. The metabolism of menadione (2-methyl-1,4-naphthoquinone) by isolated hepatocytes. J Biol Chem 1982;257:12419–25.
46. Frei B, Winterhalter KH, Richter C. Menadione- (2-methyl-1,4-napthoquinone-) dependent enzymatic redox cycling and calcium release by mitochondria. Biochemistry 1986;25:4438–43.
47. Bellomo G, Mirabelli F, Vairetti M, Iosi F, Malorni W. Cytoskeleton as a target in menadione-induced oxidative stress in cultured mammalian cells: I. Biochemical and immunocytochemical features. J Cell Physiol 1990;143:118–28.
48. Schweinzer E, Goldenberg H. Monodehydroascorbate reductase activity in the surface membrane of leukemic cells. Eur J Biochem 1993;143:1057–62.
49. Nishikimi M. Oxidation of ascorbic acid with superoxide anion generated by the xanthine-xanthine oxdase system. Biochem Biophys Res Commun 1975;63:463–68.
50. Magnusson C, Hillensjo T. Inhibition of maturation and metabolism in rat oocytes by cyclic AMP. J Exp Zool 1977;201:139–47.
51. Eppig JJ. The participation of cyclic adenosine monophosphate (cAMP) in the regulation of meiotic maturation of oocytes in the laboratory mouse. In: Greve T, Hyttel P, Weir B, eds. Cell biology of mammalian egg manipulation. The Journals of Reproduction and Fertility, volume supplement 38; Cambridge; 1989:3–8.
52. Buccione R, Schroeder AC, Eppig JJ. Interactions between somatic cells and germ cells throughout mammalian oogenesis. Biol Reprod 1990;43:543–47.
53. Sen CK, Packer L. Antioxidant and redox regulation of gene transcription. FASEB J 1996;10:709–20.
54. Irani K, Xia Y, Zweier JL, et al. Mitogenic signaling mediated by oxidants in ras-transformed fibroblasts. Science 1997;275:1649–52.
55. Takami M, Preston SL, Jones EE, Behrman HR. Antioxidants reversibly inhibit the spontaneous resumption of meiosis. Biol Reprod 1998;58(suppl. 1):142.

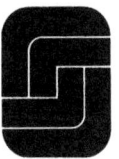

22

Periovulatory Changes in Ovarian Metalloproteinases and Tissue Inhibitors of Metalloproteinases (TIMPS) Following Indomethacin Treatment

THOMAS E. CURRY, JR., CAROLYN M. KOMAR, PATRICK D. BURNS, AND WARREN B. NOTHNICK

Introduction

The periovulatory luteinizing hormone (LH) surge sets in motion a series of biochemical and biophysical changes culminating in follicular rupture and release of the oocyte. Among these biochemical events is a stimulation of prostaglandin production in conjunction with a stimulation of proteolytic enzyme activity (reviewed in Refs. 1,2). The LH-stimulated increase in prostaglandins (PGs) has been suggested to be of pivotal importance in the ovulatory process (1,2). Such a postulate is supported by reports that $PGF_{2\alpha}$ (3,4) and prostacyclin (5) are able to induce follicular rupture in the absence of gonadotropins. Further evidence for the role of PGs in ovulation is the observation that blockade of PG production by various PG synthase inhibitors (e.g., indomethacin) results in an inhibition of ovulation in the rat, rabbit, sheep, pig, primate, and human (reviewed in Refs. 1,2). The mechanism(s) by which PGs may regulate follicular rupture, however, is unknown. It is hypothesized that local PG production may impact ovarian blood flow, smooth muscle contractility, oxygen-free radical formation, and action, as well as proteolysis associated with apical connective tissue degradation and oocyte extrusion (1,2).

Periovulatory follicular proteolysis is postulated to occur via the coordinated action of a series of different proteolytic enzyme systems, including the metalloproteinases (MMPs) and the plasminogen activators. The metalloproteinases are a multigene family of zinc-dependent proteinases that act on the extracellular connective tissue matrix throughout the body. Metalloproteinases are synthesized and secreted as latent enzymes that must be activated in the extracellular space. The four major subclasses of MMPs include the collagenases, gelatinases, stromelysins, and membrane type MMPs (6). Following the preovulatory LH surge (or exogenous hCG to mimic the LH surge), there is a stimulation of MMP mRNA expression and activity (reviewed in Refs. 1,6,7). Concomitant with the increase in enzyme activity, there is an 80% thinning of the apex of the preovulatory follicle (1), a fragmentation of the follicular collagen fibrils (8), and a decrease in the content of follicular collagen (9). Administration of putative chemical inhibitors of MMPs blocks ovulation both in vitro (10) and in vivo (11). In toto, these findings demonstrate the central role of MMPs in the dynamic process of follicular rupture.

The activity of the matrix metalloproteinases in the extracellular space is regulated by MMP inhibitors found in both the serum and produced locally within tissues. The TIMPs are a family that differ in their mode of action toward the MMPs (reviewed in Refs. 6,12). Four distinct TIMPs have been identified based on their biological action (TIMP-1, TIMP-2, TIMP-3, and TIMP-4). TIMP-1 is a 28 kDa secreted glycoprotein capable of binding to all active forms of MMPs as well as the latent form of the 92 kDa gelatinase. TIMP-2 is also secreted, has been shown to be differentially regulated from TIMP-1, and has been shown to have different affinities for the various MMPs. For example, TIMP-2 has a high affinity for the latent and active forms of 72 kDa gelatinase. TIMP-3 is a 21 kDa protein that is bound to the extracellular matrix after secretion and, unlike TIMP-1 or TIMP-2, has been suggested to act as an additional regulatory stop point for MMP action (6,12). TIMP-4 has been cloned, but there is limited information regarding this inhibitor's substrate specificity or mode of action, although preliminary studies suggest that it has traits similar to those of TIMP-2 (13,14).

The current study examined the potential interaction between prostaglandin production and the matrix MMP system during the periovulatory period. Inhibition of the LH-stimulated increase in either PG synthesis or the MMP system compromises oocyte release, which suggests that these pathways are of pivotal importance for follicular rupture. The significance of these experiments is to determine the interplay between these two LH-stimulated cascades that has not been fully characterized. The present experiments examined the mRNA expression of collagenase, the gelatinases, and the TIMPs in ovaries from animals treated with indomethacin to inhibit prostaglandin synthesis during the ovulatory period.

Materials and Methods

Animal Treatment

Immature female Sprague–Dawley rats (Harlan Sprague-Dawley, Indianapolis, IN) were injected with 20 IU of pregnant mare's serum gonadotropin (PMSG) to induce follicular development on Days 23–24 of age. Animals were injected with 10 IU of hCG 48 hours latter, followed 30 minutes later by indomethacin (1 mg/200 µl, i.p.) or vehicle (i.e., control). Rats were killed at the time of hCG administration (i.e., 0 hours) or 4, 8, or 12 hours later. Ovaries were removed, cleaned, and processed for either measurement of $PGF_{2\alpha}$ to confirm inhibition of PG synthesis by indomethacin treatment or Northern analysis of metalloproteinase and TIMP mRNA expression. All animal procedures for these experiments were approved by the University of Kentucky Institutional Animal Care and Use Committee.

$PGF_{2\alpha}$ Radioimmunoassay

Whole ovaries were homogenized in 0.5 ml of homogenization buffer (saline containing 10^{-6} M indomethacin), acidified with formic acid, and extracted with ethyl acetate. Extracts were reconstituted in 1 ml of 0.01 M phosphate buffered saline + 0.1% gelatin, diluted 1:20 and assayed for $PGF_{2\alpha}$ by RIA as described previously for the ewe (15) and validated in the present study for rat ovarian tissue. Intra- and interassay coefficients of variation for the three pools across two assays were 8.8 and 15.5%, respectively. All samples were run in duplicate and the sensitivity of the assay was 10 pg/tube.

Progesterone and Estradiol Radioimmunoassay

Serum steroid content was determined by radioimmunoassay using Coat-A-Count tubes (Diagnostic Products Corp., Los Angeles, CA) as routinely performed in our laboratory (16). Progesterone and estradiol assay sensitivities were 30 pg/ml and 8 pg/ml, respectively. Intraassay and interassay coefficients of variation were 4.7% and 9.0% for progesterone and 5.4% and 8.4% for estradiol, respectively.

Northern Blot Analysis: Detection of mRNA for MMPs and TIMPs

Total ovarian RNA was isolated from the control and indomethacin-treated rats by the method of Chomczynski and Sacchi (17) using an acid guanidinium thiocyanate-phenol-chloroform extraction procedure as described previously (18). Total RNA samples (20 µg/lane) underwent electrophoresis through a 1% agarose gel containing formaldehyde and were transferred to a Nytran membrane (Schleicher and Schuell, Keene, NH). Complementary DNA probes for murine 72 kDa (MMP-2) and 92 kDa gelatinase (MMP-9) as well as murine TIMP-1, TIMP-2, TIMP-3, and TIMP-4 (supplied by Dr. D. Edwards) and rat 18S ribosomal RNA were prepared for random primer labeling to a specific activity of $1.0–2.5 \times 10^8$ cpm/µg using [α-^{32}P] dCTP (New England Nuclear, Boston, MA). Membranes were hybridized with the radiolabeled cDNAs for 18 hours at 45°C and subsequently washed. The reaction product was visualized by autoradiography on Kodak X-AR film (Eastman Kodak, Rochester, NY). Resulting blots were analyzed with a LKB Ultroscan XL laser (LKB instruments, Rockville, MD). To assess equality of sample loading and capillary transfer to the membrane, the blots were quantitated against the 18S ribosomal band to normalize the mRNA expression of the MMPs and TIMPs. Relative mRNA content for each enzyme or inhibitor was then expressed as arbitrary units that were calculated by setting the control 0-hour transcript level equal to 1.0 and expressing all other transcript levels as a fold change from that value.

Ribonuclease Protection Assay

Levels of mRNA for rat collagenase-3 were quantitated by an RNase protection assay according to Ambion's RPAII kit instructions (Ambion, Inc., Austin, TX). The cDNA probes for rat collagenase-3 (MMP-13, supplied by Dr. L. Matrisian) and the ribosomal protein L32 (supplied by Dr. Park-Sarge) were linearized and ^{32}P-labeled antisense probes were transcribed using a Maxiscript kit (Ambion, Inc.). Protected fragments were visualized by electrophoresis through a 5% acrylamide–8 M urea gel. Relative levels of mRNA for collagenase-3 were calculated by normalizing the intensity of the protected collagenase fragment to that of the L32 internal control using a phosphoimager (Molecular Dynamics, Sunnyvale, CA).

Experimental Design

Each experiment was designed to test the effects of indomethacin treatment on ovarian $PGF_{2\alpha}$ content, serum steroid concentrations, and mRNA levels for the MMPs and TIMPs. To normalize the variability between different experimental replicates, data are expressed as the mean fold change ± SEM compared with the control (i.e., 0-hour time point). Each experimental replicate represents tissue generated from a separate group of rats collected at the previously identified different time points. Differences in ovarian $PGF_{2\alpha}$ content, serum steroid concentrations, and mRNA levels between treatments were tested with a one way analysis of variance (ANOVA). Student-Neuman-Keuls procedure was used for posthoc group comparisons. A value of $p < 0.05$ was considered significant.

Results

Effect of Indomethacin on Ovarian Weight, $PGF_{2\alpha}$ Content, and Steroidogenesis

The effect of indomethacin treatment on ovarian weight, ovarian $PGF_{2\alpha}$ content, and serum steroid levels is shown in Table 22.1. Administration of hCG resulted in an increase in ovarian weight that was unaffected by indometha-

TABLE 22.1. Effect of indomethacin (Indo) administration on ovarian weight, ovarian PGF$_{2\alpha}$ content, and serum estradiol and progesterone levels.

Treatment	Ovarian weight (mg)	Estradiol (pg/ml)	Progesterone (ng/ml)	PGF$_{2\alpha}$ (pg/mg tissue)
0 hour Vehicle	31 ± 4	318 ± 51	12.2 ± 1.1	130 ± 12
0 hour Indo	33 ± 2	357 ± 38	11.5 ± 2.5	110 ± 11
4 hour Vehicle	34 ± 3	618 ± 43	31.0 ± 2.2	130 ± 14
4 hour Indo	35 ± 2	581 ± 75	31.9 ± 1.9	85 ± 9
8 hour Vehicle	45 ± 3	405 ± 52	67.6 ± 5.5	1820 ± 92
8 hour Indo	41 ± 3	381 ± 41	63.3 ± 5.9	80 ± 12*
12 hour Vehicle	58 ± 4	237 ± 53	50.9 ± 3.0	1530 ± 68
12 hour Indo	48 ± 3	219 ± 54	35.5 ± 4.8	75 ± 11*

*Significantly different from vehicle treated rats, mean + SEM, $n = 3$.

cin treatment. The concentrations of PGF$_{2\alpha}$ were elevated by hCG treatment within 8 hours (14-fold increase compared with 0 hours vehicle). Treatment with indomethacin 30 minutes after hCG, however, blocked the gonadotro-pin-induced increase and maintained PGF$_{2\alpha}$ levels at or below the 0-hour level (Table 22.1).

Levels of estradiol and progesterone were initially increased following hCG administration before declining at the 12-hours time point (Table 22.1). Treatment with indomethacin had no effect on hCG-stimulated levels of es-tradiol or progesterone.

Effect of Indomethacin on Ovarian Metalloproteinase mRNA Expression

For collagenase-3, hCG induced a 4.4-fold increase in mRNA expression at 12 hours after hCG administration, which was inhibited by administration of indomethacin (Figure 22.1, $n = 5$). Although levels of the 72 kDa gelatinase mRNA increased 3.6-fold by 12 hours after hCG treatment, indomethacin had no effect on mRNA expression of this metalloproteinase (Figure 22.2, $n = 4$). Unlike collagenase-3 and the 72kDa gelatinase, levels of the 92 kDa gelatinase mRNA were unchanged by hCG stimulation or indomethacin treatment ($n = 3$, data not shown).

Effect of Indomethacin on Ovarian TIMP mRNA Expression

For the TIMPs, hCG induced a 4.2-fold increase in TIMP-1 mRNA levels within 8 hours after hCG injection (Figure 22.3, $n = 3$). TIMP-2 mRNA expres-

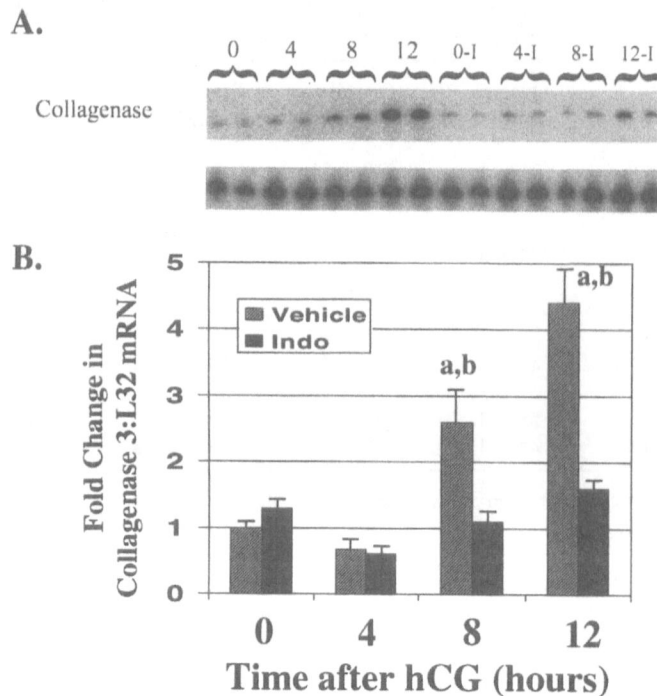

FIGURE 22.1. Ribonuclease protection analysis of collagenase-3 mRNA in ovarian tissue from animals treated with or without indomethacin. (A) A single protected fragment of approximately 273 base pairs was detected in ovarian tissue from vehicle- and indomethacin-treated animals. The depicted blot is a representation of five separate experiments where 0 = collection at 0 hours after hCG, 0-I = 0 hour indomethacin group. (B) Changes in ovarian collagenase-3 mRNA following indomethacin (Indo) treatment during the periovulatory period. The mRNA levels for collagenase-3 were normalized to the ribosomal L32 transcript expression. Data are expressed as the fold change in collagenase-3 mRNA/L32 mRNA expression (mean ± SEM, $n = 5$) compared with the 0-hour vehicle value. (a) Significantly different from 0-hour vehicle ($p < 0.05$). (b) Significantly different from indomethacin value at the same collection time (i.e., 8 or 12 hours).

sion was unchanged (data not shown, $n = 3$), whereas TIMP-3 mRNA levels decreased to 60% of the 0-hour vehicle levels at 8 hours after hCG treatment (Figure 22.4, $n = 4$). Administration of indomethacin had no effect on the levels of mRNA expression for any of the various TIMPs. TIMP-4 mRNA was undetectable by Northern analysis using up to 45 μg of total RNA or 2–3 μg of polyadenylated mRNA.

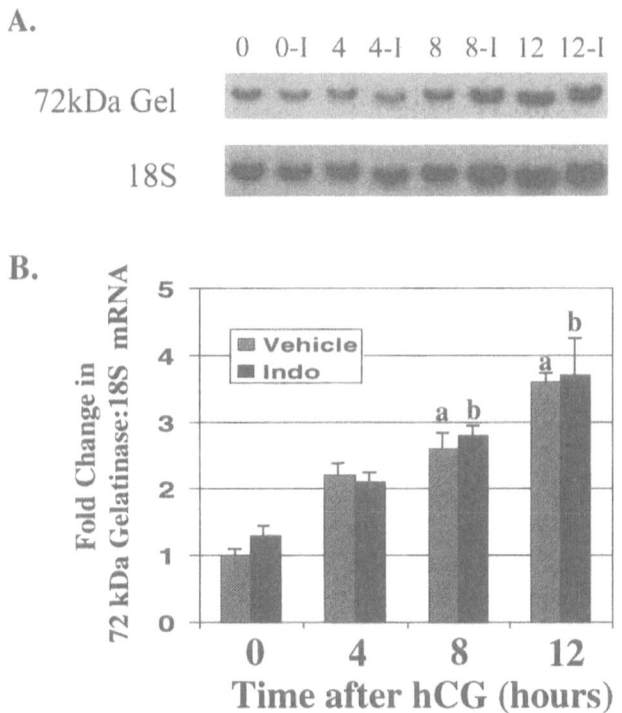

FIGURE 22.2. Northern analysis of the 72 kDa gelatinase mRNA in ovarian tissue from animals treated with or without indomethacin. (A) Northern analysis was performed using 20 μg of total RNA per lane as described in Materials and Methods. A single transcript of approximately 3100 base pairs, which is consistent with the size of the 72 kDa gelatinase, was detected in ovarian tissue from vehicle- and indomethacin-treated animals. The depicted blot is a representation of three separate experiments. 0 = 0 hour vehicle, 0-I = 0 hour indomethacin group. (B) Changes in ovarian 72 kDa gelatinase mRNA following indomethacin treatment (Indo) during the periovulatory period. The mRNA levels for the 72 kDa gelatinase were normalized to the 18S transcript expression. Data are expressed as the fold change in 72 kDa gelatinase mRNA/18S mRNA expression compared with the 0 hour vehicle value (mean ± SEM, $n = 3$). (a) Significantly different from 0 hour vehicle ($p < 0.05$). (b) Significantly different from 0 hour Indomethacin group ($p < 0.05$).

Discussion

It is well documented that the endogenous LH surge (or exogenous hCG administration) induces the expression and activity of the MMP system during the ovulatory process. This chapter demonstrates that hCG stimulates an increase in collagenase-3, 72 kDa gelatinase and TIMP-1 mRNA expression

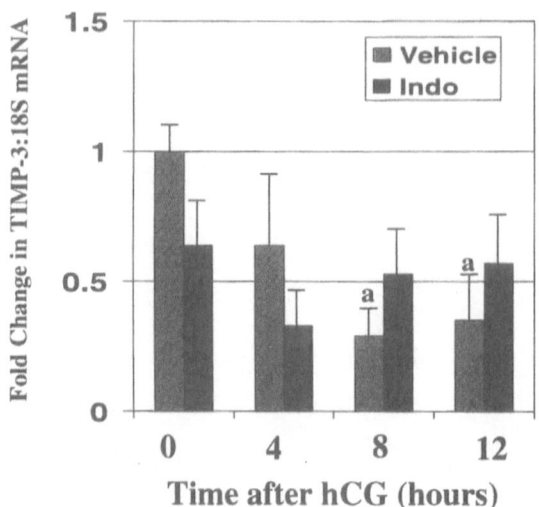

FIGURE 22.3. Changes in TIMP-1 mRNA expression following indomethacin treatment during the periovulatory period. The mRNA levels for TIMP-1 were normalized to the 18S transcript expression. Data are expressed as the fold change in TIMP-1 mRNA/ 18S mRNA expression compared with the 0 hour vehicle value (mean ± SEM, $n = 4$). (a) Significantly different from 0 hour vehicle ($p < 0.05$). (b) Significantly different from 0 hour Indo group ($p < 0.05$).

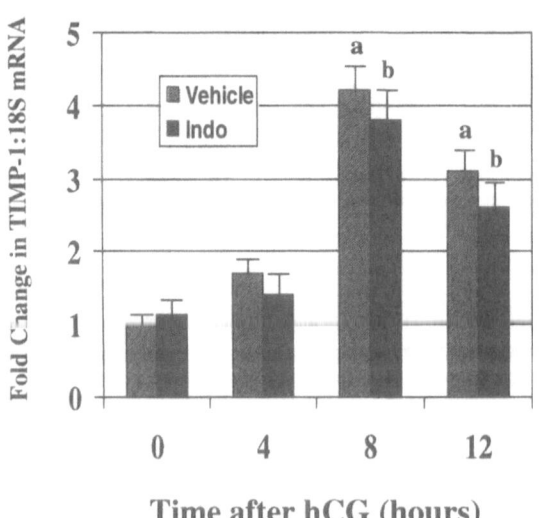

FIGURE 22.4. Changes in TIMP-3 mRNA expression following indomethacin treatment during the periovulatory period. The mRNA levels for TIMP-3 were normalized to the 18S transcript expression. Data are expressed as the fold change in TIMP-3 mRNA/ 18S mRNA expression compared with the 0 hour vehicle value (mean ± SEM, $n = 4$). (a) Significantly different from 0 hour vehicle ($p < 0.05$).

while decreasing the expression of TIMP-3 mRNA. Relatively little is known, however, about the regulation of ovarian MMPs or TIMPs. This chapter explored the possible impact of prostaglandins on MMP and TIMP mRNA expression because prostaglandins have been postulated as key mediators of follicular rupture (1,2). Our findings demonstrate that only collagenase-3 mRNA levels were diminished by indomethacin administration. Inhibition of the periovulatory increase in PGs had no effect on the hCG-stimulated increase in the 72 kDa gelatinase or TIMP-1. Our findings are in concordance with previous reports (19) that inhibition of PG synthesis blocked the preovulatory increase in collagenase mRNA without affecting the hCG-stimulated increase in collagenase IV (i.e., gelatinase) mRNA.

This chapter reports on the rat collagenase-3 (MMP-13) in contrast to the previous report (19) on the human interstitial collagenase (MMP-1), and a slightly different pattern of expression was observed for the two enzymes. At 8 hours after hCG we observed a peak in collagenase-3 mRNA expression that remained elevated at the 12-hour time point. Reich and co-workers (19) noted an increase in interstitial collagenase at 3 hours after hCG, which was diminished by 9 hours after gonadotropin treatment. In agreement with the inhibition of collagenase mRNA, several investigators have reported that indomethacin treatment attenuates collagenase protein production as indicated by a diminution of the preovulatory increase in collagenase activity (20,21). In previous findings from this laboratory, however, we noted that indomethacin did not inhibit the preovulatory increase in a latent (i.e., activatable) form of ovarian collagenase (22).

The possibility exists that the discrepancy in our present findings and our earlier observations reflects either the differences in mRNA levels versus enzyme activity, or the difficulty in measuring enzyme activity in tissue extracts. For example, enzyme activity may reflect "true" collagenase activity from either interstitial collagenase (MMP-1), collagenase-3 (MMP-13), or neutrophil collagenase (MMP-8). In this chapter indomethacin inhibited the increase in collagenase-3 mRNA, but neutrophil collagenase was not explored. There is an influx of white blood cells into the follicle following the LH surge (1) that may increase ovarian levels of neutrophil collagenase. The possibility exists that the increase in neutrophil collagenase may still take place in an environment where PGs remain at basal levels but the enzyme requires a PG-mediated step to become fully active. On the other hand, degradation of labeled collagen observed previously by ovarian extracts from rats treated with indomethacin may take place by enzymes other than collagenase. For example, gelatinases have been reported to have collagenolytic activity (23) and gelatinase mRNA increases after indomethacin treatment in the current study. Such postulates would, in part, explain the increased degradation of labeled collagen by ovarian extracts noted previously following indomethacin treatment.

MMP inhibitors are present in the ovaries of numerous species and have been postulated to maintain proteolytic homeostasis and provide localized control of extracellular degradation associated with follicular rupture (16,24). For example, TIMP-1 mRNA is abundant in periovulatory rat, ovine, and human ovaries (16,24–28). In concord with TIMP-1 mRNA expression, a TIMP-1-like protein has been identified in human follicular fluid (16), rat ovaries (26) and rat granulosa cell culture media (24). The levels of ovarian TIMP-1 mRNA and inhibitor activity increase following an LH/hCG stimulus (24–26). These findings collectively demonstrate that TIMP-1 is present in the ovary and is stimulated by the events associated with the preovulatory LH surge. In our study, there is differential regulation of the various TIMPs associated with the hormonal induction of follicular rupture by hCG; specifically, gonadotropin stimulation increases mRNA expression of TIMP-1, has no effect on TIMP-2 mRNA levels, but decreases the mRNA concentrations of the matrix-bound inhibitor TIMP-3. Such differential regulation of TIMP expression may reflect the varied physiological roles of the inhibitors during extracellular remodeling associated with follicular rupture. For example, the decline in TIMP-3 expression may decrease the inhibitor present in the apical extracellular matrix associated with the theca and surrounding fibroblasts, thereby allowing metalloproteinases to degrade the apical follicular wall. Stimulation of the secreted inhibitor TIMP-1 may ensure that any MMP activity not associated with follicular remodeling would be prevented. On the other hand, TIMP-1 may be in a different ovarian compartment (e.g., the granulosa cell layer) than the matrix-bound TIMP-3 and may act to protect the integrity of the granulosa cell basement membrane as progressive proliferation of the granulosa cells occurs.

In our study, TIMP-4 was not observed by Northern analysis using 45 µg of total RNA or 2–3 µg of poly A mRNA. Initial reports have demonstrated TIMP-4 in murine and human ovarian tissue (13,14). Our findings could be interpreted that TIMP-4 is not expressed at high levels during the ovulatory process but may display a hormonally induced pattern of expression at intermittent periods of ovarian function.

In summary, administration of hCG to induce ovulation results in an increase in the mRNA expression of collagenase-3, 72 kDa gelatinase, and TIMP-1 while decreasing the expression pattern of TIMP-3 mRNA. Inhibition of the periovulatory increase in prostaglandins by administration of indomethacin resulted in an inhibition of the hCG stimulated increase in collagenase-3 mRNA. These findings can be interpreted that the PG pathway is responsible for the regulation of collagenase associated with follicular rupture.

Acknowledgments. The authors would like to acknowledge the assistance of Ms. Sarah Wheeler in the preparation of the figures for this chapter. This work was supported by NIH HD23195 to T.E.C. Dr. Burns was supported by T32 NIH HD07436.

References

1. Espey LL, Lipner H. Ovulation. In: Knobil E, Neill JD, eds. The physiology of reproduction. New York: Raven Press; 1994:725.
2. Priddy AR, Killick SR. Eicosanoids and ovulation. Prostagland Leukot Essent Fat Acids 1993;49:827–31.

3. Kitai H, Yoshimura Y, Wright KH, Santulli R, Wallach EE. Microvasculature of preovulatory follicles: comparison of in situ and in vitro perfused rabbit ovaries following stimulation of ovulation. Am J Obstet Gynecol 1985;152:889–95.

4. Miyazaki T, Dharmarajan AM, Atlas SJ, Katz E, Wallach EE. Do prostaglandins lead to ovulation in the rabbit by stimulating proteolytic enzyme activity? Fertil Steril 1991;55:1183–88.

5. Yoshimura Y, Dharmarajan AM, Gips S, Adachi T, Hosoi Y, Atlas SJ, et al. Effects of prostacyclin on ovulation and microvasculature of the in vitro perfused rabbit ovary. Am J Obstet Gynecol 1988;159:977–82.

6. Hulboy DL, Rudolph LA, Matrisian LM. Matrix metalloproteinases as mediators of reproductive function. Mol Hum Reprod 1997;3:27–45.

7. McIntush EW, Smith MF. Matrix metalloproteinases and tissue inhibitors of metalloproteinases in ovarian function. Rev Reprod 1998;3:23–30.

8. Bjersing L, Cajander S. Ovulation and the mechanism of follicular rupture: V. Ultrastructure of tunica albuginea and theca externa of rabbit Graafian follicles prior to induced ovulation. Cell Tiss Res 1974;153:15–30.

9. Morales TI, Woessner JF, Marsh JM, LeMaire WJ. Collagen, collagenase and collagenolytic activity in rat Graafian follicles during follicular growth and ovulation. Biochim Biophys Acta 1983;756:119–22.

10. Brannstrom M, Woessner JF Jr, Koos RD, Sear CH, LeMaire WJ. Inhibitors of mammalian tissue collagenase and metalloproteinases suppress ovulation in the perfused rat ovary. Endocrinology 1988;122:1715–21.

11. Ichikawa S, Ohta M, Morioka H, Murao S. Blockage of ovulation in the explanted hamster ovary by a collagenase inhibitor. J Reprod Fert 1983;68:17–19.

12. Gomez DE, Alonso DF, Yoshiji H, Thorgeirsson UP. Tissue inhibitors of metalloproteinases: structure, regulation and biological functions. Eur J Cell Biol 1997;74: 111–22.

13. Leco KJ, Apte SS, Taniguchi GT, Hawkes SP, Khokha R, Schultz GA, et al. Murine tissue inhibitor of metalloproteinases-4 (Timp-4): cDNA isolation and expression in adult mouse tissues. FEBS Lett 1997;401:213–17.

14. Greene J, Wang M, Liu YE, Raymond LA, Rosen C, Shi YE. Molecular cloning and characterization of human tissue inhibitor of metalloproteinase 4. J Biol Chem 1996;271:30375–80.

15. Homanics GE, Silvia WJ. Effects of progesterone and estradiol-17 beta on uterine secretion of prostaglandin F2 alpha in response to oxytocin in ovariectomized ewes. Biol Reprod 1988;38:804–11.

16. Curry TE Jr, Sanders S, Pedigo NG, Estes SR, Wilson EA, Vernon M. Identification and characterization of metalloproteinase inhibitor activity in human ovarian follicular fluid. Endocrinology 1988;123:1611–18.

17. Chomoczynski P, Sacchi N. Single-step method of RNA isolation by acid guanidium thiocyanate-phenol-chloroform extraction. Anal Biochem 1987;162:156–59.

18. Nothnick WB, Edwards DR, Leco KJ, Curry TE Jr. Expression and activity of ovarian tissue inhibitors of metalloproteinases during pseudopregnancy in the rat. Biol Reprod 1995;53:684–91.

19. Reich R, Daphna-Iken D, Chun SY, Popliker M, Slager S, Adelmann-Grill BC, et al. Preovulatory changes in ovarian expression of collagenases and tissue metalloproteinase inhibitor messenger ribonucleic acid: role of eicosanoids. Endocrinology 1991;129:1869–975.

20. Reich R, Tsafriri A, Mechanic GL. The involvement of collagenolysis in ovulation in the rat. Endocrinology 1985;116:522–27.

21. Kawamura N, Himeno N, Okamura H, Mori T, Fukumoto M, Midorikawa O. Effect of indomethacin on collagenolytic enzyme activities in rabbit ovary. Nippon Sanka Fujinka Gakkai Zasshi 1984;36:2099.
22. Curry TE Jr, Clark MR, Dean DD, Woessner JF Jr, LeMaire WJ. The preovulatory increase in ovarian collagenase activity in the rat is independent of prostaglandin production. Endocrinology 1986;118:1823–28.
23. Aimes RT, Quigley JP. Matrix metalloproteinase-2 is an interstitial collagenase. Inhibitor-free enzyme catalyzes the cleavage of collagen fibrils and soluble native type I collagen generating the specific 3/4- and 1/4-length fragments. J Biol Chem 1995;270:5872–76.
24. Mann JS, Kindy MS, Hyde JF, Clark MR, Curry TE Jr. The role of prostaglandins, estrogen, and growth factors in rat ovarian metalloproteinase inhibitor production. Biol Reprod 1993;48:1006–13.
25. Smith GW, Goetz TL, Anthony RV, Smith MF. Molecular cloning of an ovine ovarian tissue inhibitor of metalloproteinases: ontogeny of messenger ribonucleic acid expression and in situ localization within preovulatory follicles and luteal tissue. Endocrinology 1994;134:344–51.
26. Zhu C, Woessner JF Jr. A tissue inhibitor of metalloproteinases and α-macroglobulins in the ovulating rat ovary: possible regulators of collagen matrix breakdown. Biol Reprod 1991;45:334–42.
27. Rapp G, Freudenstein J, Klaudiny J, Mucha J, Wempe F, Zimmer M, et al. Characterization of three abundant mRNAs from human ovarian granulosa cells. DNA Cell Biol 1990;9:479–85.
28. Satoh T, Kobayashi K, Yamashita S, Kikuchi M, Sendai Y, Hoshi H. Tissue inhibitor of metalloproteinases (TIMP-1) produced by granulosa and oviduct cells enhances in vitro development of bovine embryo. Biol Reprod 1994;50:835–44.

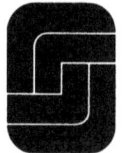

23

Expression and Function of CCAAT/ Enhancer Binding Proteins (C/EBPs) in the Ovary

Esta Sterneck and Peter F. Johnson

Introduction

Luteinizing hormone (LH) triggers a series of dramatic morphological and physiological changes in the ovarian follicle, that culminate in ovulation and subsequent differentiation into the corpus luteum. Underlying these events are alterations in the growth state and differentiation of the major follicular cell types, particularly the stratum granulosum and theca. These changes in cellular phenotype result from the expression of new genes, several of which are known, but the majority of which probably remain to be identified. The LH signal is relayed to the nucleus, where specific genes are activated through the actions of transcriptional regulatory proteins. Although the identities of these transcription factors are largely unknown, the cAMP-responsive element binding (CREB) protein has been implicated as an important nuclear target of LH signaling in granulosa cells (1). In addition, levels of c-Myc (2) and steroidogenic factor-1 (SF-1) (3) are modulated in granulosa cells during the ovulatory period. Members of the CCAAT/enhancer binding protein (C/EBP) family have also been identified as key transcriptional regulators in the ovarian follicle. These proteins play critical roles in ovulation as well as differentiation of granulosa cells into luteal cells. In this chapter we shall review the current information on the expression and functional roles of C/EBP family members in the mammalian ovary.

The C/EBP Protein Family

C/EBP, now designated C/EBPα, is a sequence-specific DNA-binding protein that was first isolated from rat liver nuclear extracts in a search for proteins that bind to *cis*-regulatory sequences of viral genes (4). DNase I footprinting studies led to the identification of a binding activity in liver extracts that protected certain viral CCAAT box elements as well as enhancer "core" sequences, hence the name *CCAAT/enhancer binding protein*. It was later recognized that CCAAT box and enhancer core elements represent weak C/EBP binding sites and are probably not true physiological targets of the C/EBPα protein. Nonetheless, the name *C/EBP* has been retained and is still used to refer to this family of proteins. Upon isolation of the gene encoding C/EBPα, Landschulz et al. (5) noted a motif of repeating leucine residues within the C-terminal portion of the DNA-binding domain. It was subsequently shown that this motif, termed the *leucine zipper*, mediates dimerization through a coiled-coil helical domain (5,6). An adjacent positively charged segment, the basic region, determines DNA sequence specificity (7) and makes base-specific contacts in the DNA major groove, as inferred from the crystallographic structure of the related yeast protein, GCN4 (8). Thus, C/EBPα is the prototype for a class of DNA-binding proteins defined by the basic region-leucine zipper (bZIP) structure. bZIP proteins in mammalian cells can be classified into several groups on the basis of their DNA-binding and dimerization specificities, and include the C/EBP, CREB/ATF, AP-1, and PAR families [(9) and references therein].

The C/EBP family consists of several members that were identified either by using functional screens to identify DNA-binding proteins with specificity for particular *cis*-regulatory sites or by cross-hybridization with the bZIP region of the C/EBPα gene [reviewed in (10)]. In addition to C/EBPα, three C/EBP-related proteins (C/EBPβ, C/EBPδ, and C/EBPε) have been characterized that function primarily as transcriptional activators (Fig. 23.1). Two more distantly related family members [Ig/EBP (C/EBPγ) and CHOP/gadd153] have been identified that may play inhibitory roles in regulating gene expression (11,12). With the exception of CHOP, all of the C/EBP proteins recognize the same DNA element and each protein, including CHOP, can form heterodimeric complexes with the other family members.

Four of the C/EBP proteins share an identical 17 amino acid segment spanning the basic region (Fig. 23.1). As a result, the C/EBP family members exhibit similar DNA binding properties, binding as dimers to the consensus palindromic sequence ATTGCGCAAT (9,13,14). An array of residues within the basic region known as the basic motif is shared by all bZIP proteins (13,15) (see Fig. 23.1B). The X-ray crystallographic structure of the yeast bZIP protein GCN4 bound to its cognate site revealed that five of the basic motif residues make all of the base-specific contacts to DNA (8). These amino acids are common to most bZIP proteins, which raises the question of how the distinct binding specificities of the various subfamilies are determined. Mutagenesis studies demonstrate that a major determinant of C/EBP specificity is a valine residue (arrow, Fig. 23.1B) located at an "invariant" position occupied by alanine in most other bZIP proteins (9,16,17).

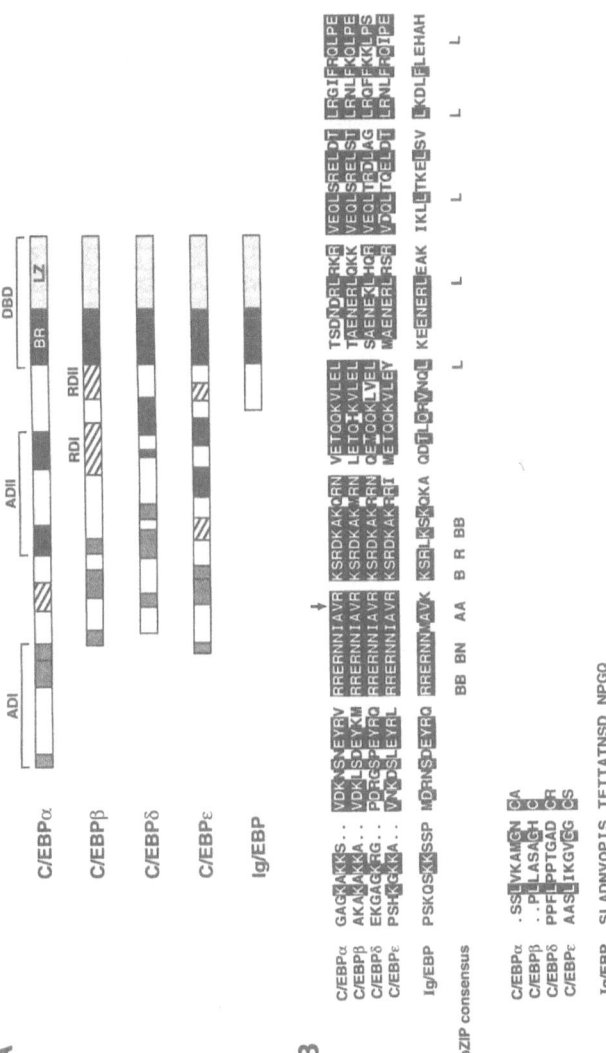

FIGURE 23.1. (A) Functional domains in the C/EBP proteins. Regions of sequence homology are shaded. AD, activation domain; RD, regulatory domain (hatched regions); BR, basic region; LZ, leucine zipper; DBD, DNA-binding domain. (B) Amino acid sequences of the basic/leucine zipper regions. Identical residues are shaded. The arrow denotes a valine residue that is an important determinant of C/EBP DNA-binding specificity. The bZIP consensus (13,15) shows conserved residues of the basic motif and the heptad leucine repeat (5). B, basic amino acid (R or K).

The C/EBPs are expressed in unique, cell-type restricted patterns that are partially overlapping. C/EBPα is found in differentiated hepatocytes and adipocytes, intestinal epithelial cells (18), skin (19), brain, lung, ovary, and myelomonocytic progenitor cells (20). C/EBPβ is the most widely distributed family member and its mRNA, protein, and/or DNA-binding activity can be detected in many cell types. Tissues with particularly high C/EBPβ levels include liver, skin (19), fat, and differentiated myelomonocytic cells (macrophages and neutrophils) (reviewed in Ref. 10). C/EBPδ expression is induced in several tissues, especially liver, by LPS and proinflammatory mediators (e.g., IL-6) (21–25). C/EBPδ transcripts are also present in several regions of the central and peripheral nervous systems (26). C/EBPε expression is the most restricted, occurring nearly exclusively in the myeloid lineage of the hematopoietic system (27–29).

C/EBP proteins have been implicated as important regulators of a large and growing number of target genes, many of which are markers of differentiated cells. In several cell lineages C/EBP proteins promote terminal phenotypes by activating differentiation-specific genes and causing cell growth arrest (30–32). Even though the detailed mechanism by which C/EBPs elicit cell growth arrest remains unclear, the current published data suggest the involvement of the cyclin-dependent kinase inhibitor p21, which has been identified as a target of both C/EBPα (33) and C/EBPβ (34).

The fact that the DNA-binding properties of the C/EBP proteins are highly related raises the question of whether the different members are functionally redundant or if each possesses the ability to activate a unique set of target genes. Work indicates that C/EBP proteins can exhibit either redundant (35) or isoform-specific (36,37) regulatory activities, depending on the target promoter analyzed. The underlying mechanism of differential transactivation of specific promoters by C/EBP family members has not been established, although cooperative interactions with other activator proteins such as Sp1 appear to play an important role in determining target specificity (36,38).

Expression of C/EBPs in the Ovary

Most, if not all, of the C/EBP family members are expressed in the ovary, which indicates a role for these proteins in female reproduction. C/EBPε (27) and C/EBPδ (the authors, unpublished) mRNA expression is detectable in human and mouse whole ovaries, respectively; however, no information is yet available on cell-type specificity of expression or regulation by hormones for these two genes. C/EBPα is widely and constitutively expressed in the rat ovary. Expression levels increase approximately twofold 24 hours after administration of pregnant mare serum gonadotropin (PMSG) and return to basal levels by 10 hours of subsequent treatment with human chorionic gonadotropin (hCG). Expression again increases with the formation of corpora lutea. Immunostaining localizes most expression to the granulosa cells and theca cells of preovulatory follicles, with the highest levels in cumulus cells (39). Sirois and Richards (40) analyzed expression in isolated rat granulosa cells and noted a decrease in mRNA at 1 hour hCG and specific downregulation of a low MW protein isoform. The same study reported hCG-inducible expression of C/EBPβ in granulosa cells, with mRNA levels increasing significantly at 30 minutes and protein levels at 2–10 hours hCG. Pall et al. (41) found that C/EBPβ protein expression was induced at 4 hours hCG in rat granulosa cells and, to a lesser extent, in theca cells. Expression was also high 1 day after hCG in CL, and low in residual ovarian tissue. We have reported induction of C/EBPβ mRNA expression between 4 and 7 hours hCG specifically in mouse granulosa cells of preovulatory follicles (42). The variations in the kinetics of C/EBPβ expression reported in these studies may be due to technical reasons (i.e., different species, timing and dose of injection, age of subjects and whether they were hypophysectomized). A clear picture emerges, however, showing that C/EBPβ expression is collectively dynamically regulated in the ovary, being highly inducible by hCG/LH in granulosa cells and also expressed to some extent in theca cells.

Functional Roles of C/EBP Proteins in the Ovary

The most powerful tool today for the analysis for gene function is provided by gene knockout technology. Mice deficient for C/EBPα, C/EBPβ, C/EBPδ, and C/EBPε have now been generated, and their reproductive phenotypes have been characterized to varying degrees. C/EBPε (43) and C/EBPδ (42) null mice are fertile, which indicates that these C/EBP proteins do not play vital roles in reproductive physiology. More thorough analyses in the future, however, may reveal subtle phenotypes that affect reproductive efficiency. C/EBPα null mice display perinatal lethality, which complicates the analysis of ovarian function in these animals (44). Piontkewitz et al. (45), however, were able to address the function of C/EBPα in the rat ovary by injecting specific antisense (AS) oligonucleotides, which diminish C/EBPα expression, into the ovarian bursa. When these oligonucleotides were applied 2 hours prior to PMSG treatment, ovulation in response to hCG was reduced by approximately 50%, whereas control (sense) oligonucleotides had no effect. Furthermore, the morphology of the ovaries was altered, with fewer corpora lutea than controls and large follicles containing entrapped oocytes remaining. In addition, c-myc expression was elevated in AS-treated ovaries compared with controls at 48 hours PMSG. In a subsequent study (41), C/EBPα AS oligonucleotides were applied by an ex vivo perfusion system just 30 minutes before addition of LH. In this experiment, the ovulation rate remained unaffected. In summary, these data demonstrate a role for C/EBPα in late follicular development from the antral to the preovulatory stage, with inhibition of C/EBPα expression during this phase having indirect effects on subsequent ovulation processes.

Two independent studies using different species and entirely different approaches established an important role for C/EBPβ in the ovulation mechanism. When Pall et al. (41) applied C/EBPβ AS oligonucleotides 2 hours before LH in the ex vivo perfusion experiments using rat ovaries, the ovulation rate was reduced to as little as 5% of control levels. This reduction occurred in an oligonucleotide dose-dependent manner. Estradiol and progesterone secretion remained normal at 7 and 20 hours LH, as well as induction of the PGS-2/COX-2 gene at 4 hour LH. As mentioned earlier, C/EBPα-specific AS had no effect on ovulation in these experiments. During differentiation of other cell types (e.g., adipocytes, hepatocytes and myeloid cells) consecutive expression of different C/EBP isoforms has been observed, which suggests that they may be involved in regulating each other. It is tempting to speculate that the reduced ovulation rate observed after inhibition of C/EBPα expression during late follicular development (45) may be due to impaired induction of C/EBPβ expression.

Using a targeted germline mutation in mice, we showed that C/EBPβ activity is important for ovulation and is essential for subsequent luteinization of the granulosa cells (42). C/EBPβ-deficient female mice are completely sterile, lack corpora lutea, and display a 90% reduction in ovulation rate in response to PMSG/hCG. Transplantation of ovaries between mutant and wild-type littermates demonstrated that the defect in luteinization is ovary intrinsic. Furthermore, the experiments showed that the granulosa cell defect does not affect oocyte maturation significantly because oocytes derived from unilateral mutant ovary transplants into wild-type host females could give rise to pups. Upon PMSG/hCG treatment mutant ovaries displayed large follicles, some hemorrhagic, with entrapped oocytes (42). Similar morphologies were observed in mutant ovaries transplanted into wild-type hosts. These observations are consistent with an impairment in ovulation.

A potential problem with both studies addressing C/EBPβ function in ovulation is the use of exogenous gonadotropins to assess ovulatory efficiency. When single mutant ovaries were implanted into wild-type hosts, approximately 20% of the progeny carried the mutant allele. Thus, the mutant ovaries were able to ovulate, albeit at a reduced rate (~40% of the expected amount). It is difficult to assess the ovulation rate quantitatively because transplants may not function as efficiently as resident host ovaries due to various degrees of regeneration and tissue scarring; however, the reduction in ovulation determined in ovarian transplantation studies is much less severe than the 90% decrease observed in PMSG/hCG stimulation experiments, which suggests that use of the superovulation protocol leads to an overestimate of the ovulatory defect. Nevertheless, it is fair to conclude that C/EBPβ is critically involved in the LH/hCG responsiveness of the ovary and is important for ovulation per se. To our knowledge, with the exception of nuclear hormone receptors, C/EBPβ is the first transcription factor shown by genetic analysis to be involved in the ovulation process. It is now important to identify C/EBPβ target genes in order to understand how this protein exerts its essential function in granulosa cells.

C/EBP-Regulated Genes in the Ovary

The induction of C/EBPβ by LH/hCG in granulosa cells suggested that it may regulate transcription of at least some LH-dependent genes in these cells. The PGS-2/COX-2 gene, which encodes prostaglandin endoperoxide synthase-2 and is upregulated by LH in granulosa cells, contains a C/EBP binding site in its promoter (40). Although initial studies indicated that C/EBPβ may activate transcription from the PGS-2 promoter (40), subsequent work suggested that the C/EBP element plays a negative role and counters positive regulation by an E-box element located nearby (46). Consistent with the latter interpretation, induction of PGS-2 transcripts by LH/hCG in ovaries of C/EBPβ-deficient mice or rats is comparable to that of control animals (41,42). It is interesting, however, that the rapid down regulation of PGS-2 expression that normally ensues upon luteinization does not occur in mutant ovaries (42), which implyies that C/EBPβ negatively influences PGS-2 gene expression. Whether this inhibitory effect is direct or indirect remains to be determined (see later).

Two other genes are also implicated as negative targets of C/EBPβ. The P450 aromatase (P450arom) gene is activated by FSH in granulosa cells and its expression is subsequently silenced in response to LH. P450arom transcripts, however, were maintained at high levels in C/EBPβ null ovaries (42). The gene encoding the α subunit of inhibin A and B, which are members of the transforming growth factor β (TGFβ) gene family, was similarly not efficiently repressed by LH/hCG in C/EBPβ null females in comparison to wild-type controls in which inhibin α expression was found to be downregulated (A. Mukherjee, E. Sterneck, P. Johnson, and K. Mayo, unpublished results). These effects on gene expression in mutant ovaries are depicted diagrammatically in Figure 23.2.

C/EBPβ typically stimulates expression of target promoter–reporter constructs in transient transactivation assays and therefore has been characterized as a transcriptional activator. It is surprising, however, that no genes have been identified to date that are positively regulated by C/EBPβ in the ovary, as determined by analysis of gene expression in knockout mice. Table 23.1 shows a compilation of genes whose expression has been compared in total RNA of ovaries from C/EBPβ null and control mice that had been subjected to a superovulation regimen. The data show two classes of genes— ones displaying defective shut-off in mutant ovaries, as described earlier, and another set whose expression is unaffected by the absence of C/EBPβ. Despite the failure to detect a class that is downregulated in C/EBPβ-deficient cells,

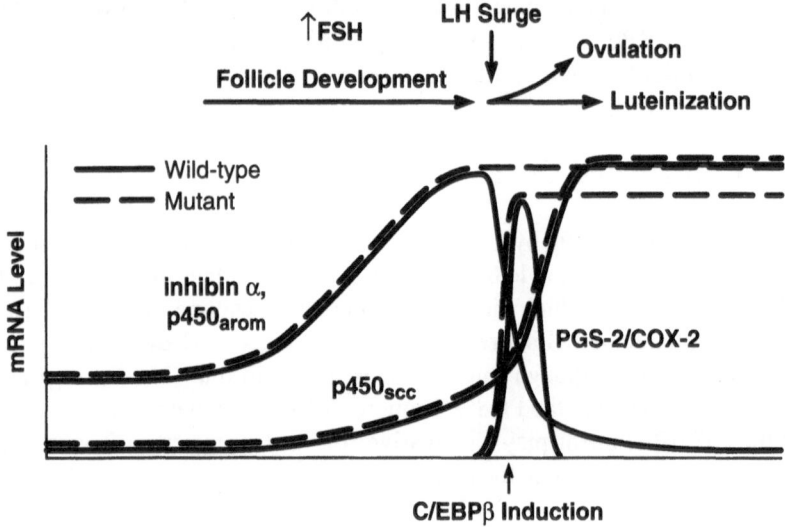

FIGURE 23.2. Temporal patterns of gene expression in wild-type and C/EBPβ-deficient ovaries. The diagram is an idealized representation of mRNA levels from several genes during late follicular development, ovulation, and luteinization. Expression in wild-type (solid lines) and C/EBPβ mutant mice (dashed lines) is shown. The approximate point at which C/EBPβ induction occurs is indicated. The data on mutant mice are from Sterneck et al. (42) and A. Mukherjee, E. Sterneck, P. Johnson, and K. Mayo (inhibin α; unpublished results). Adapted from Richards JS. Fitzpatrick SL, Clemens JW, et al. Ovarian cell differentiation: a cascade of multiple hormones, cellular signals, and regulated genes. Rec Prog Horm Res 1995;50:223–54. © The Endocrine Society, with permission.

TABLE 23.1. Expression of candidate target genes in C/EBPβ null ovaries.

Unchanged expression	Defective downregulation
P450scc	PGS-2/COX-2
angiotensinogen	P450 aromatase
estrogen receptor α	inhibin α
IL-1β	
prolactin receptor	
LH receptor	
StAR	
progesterone receptor	

Expression of each of the genes except inhibin α was determined by Northern blot analysis of total ovary RNA from superovulated control and C/EBPβ deficient mice at 4 and 7 hours after hCG injection. Inhibin α expression was analyzed by in situ hybridization of ovary sections 7 hours after hCG treatment.

it seems likely that ovarian genes exist whose expression is activated by C/EBPβ. We anticipate that future analyses (e.g., differential display or DNA microarray hybridization experiments comparing mRNA expression in normal and mutant tissue) will reveal genes that are induced by LH in a C/EBPβ-dependent manner.

How might C/EBPβ function as an inhibitor of gene expression? The C/EBPβ transcript contains an internal in-frame AUG codon that is proposed to function as an alternative translation startsite, generating a truncated protein known as liver-enriched inhibitory protein (LIP) (47). LIP lacks the transcriptional activation domain located in the C/EBPβ N-terminal region and can repress C/EBP-activated gene transcription (47). It is possible that LIP is expressed at high levels in granulosa cells and thereby inhibits expression of C/EBP-regulated genes. The notion that LIP is a translational product, however, has been called into question by studies showing that a protein identical in size to LIP can be generated by proteolysis during preparation of cell extracts (48,49). It is unclear, therefore, whether LIP-mediated repression is a plausible model. On the other hand, full-length C/EBPβ itself could serve as an inhibitor of specific genes. C/EBPβ contains a region termed *RD1* that is inhibitory to transactivation of a reporter gene (50). Thus, the RD1 element could be a repression domain that actively suppresses target gene transcription in a promoter-specific manner, thereby causing inhibition of selected genes in granulosa cells. Finally, it is possible that C/EBPβ functions indirectly to repress "target" genes in granulosa cells. Because differentiation of granulosa cells into luteal cells is defective in C/EBPβ null mice, C/EBPβ may act early in the differentiation pathway and activate genes encoding other regulatory proteins that directly repress genes such as PGS-2/COX-2, P450arom, and inhibin α. It has been reported that expression of inducible cAMP early repressor (ICER), a nuclear protein encoded by an alternative transcript from the CREM gene, is elicited in granulosa cells following the preovulatory surge (51). ICER binds to CREs, but, because it lacks a transcriptional activation domain, functions as an antagonist of CREB-activated transcription. Overexpression of ICER blocked basal and cAMP-induced expression from the inhibin α promoter in a granulosa cell line (51), suggesting that this factor is involved in attenuating inhibin α gene transcription. It is possible that C/EBPβ is required for the induction of ICER in response to LH, or, alternatively, that ICER and C/EBPβ cooperatively repress transcription from the inhibin α promoter. Further experimental studies will be necessary to test these hypotheses and to elucidate the mechanism by which C/EBPβ negatively regulates transcription of specific ovarian genes.

Conclusions, Speculations, and Future Directions

Studies examining C/EBP expression in the ovary, combined with gene ablation experiments and analysis of knockout mice to assess C/EBP protein function in vivo, have revealed that C/EBPα and C/EBPβ are key regulatory proteins involved in controlling late follicle development, ovulation, and luteinization. C/EBPα and C/EBPβ display reciprocal responses to gonadotropins because C/EBPα mRNA is increased by PMSG/FSH and declines in response to subsequent hCG/LH treatment, although C/EBPβ expression is not induced by PMSG and is dramatically upregulated by hCG/LH. Moreover, high C/EBPα levels are restored in corpora lutea, whereas C/EBPβ expression becomes nearly undetectable. These data raise the possibility that C/EBPα serves as a negative regulator of C/EBPβ gene transcription in granulosa cells. It is, however, also conceivable that C/EBPα is required for the *onset* (but not maintenance) of C/EBPβ expression in response to hCG/LH, as mentioned earlier. This notion would explain the observation that antisense ablation of C/EBPα causes abnormalities that are similar to, although not as severe as, those seen in C/EBPβ-deficient mice (see earlier). Additional work is necessary to establish the role of C/EBPα in maturation of follicles to the preovulatory stage, and to determine the possible interdependence between C/EBPα and C/EBPβ in granulosa cells. Future approaches to addressing these questions include using ovary transplants between wild-type and C/EBPα mutant mice or generating a conditional C/EBPα knockout (52) in the ovary or, more precisely, in granulosa cells. Experiments based on these strategies would allow an assessment of C/EBPα function during normal estrous cycles and might result in a definitive block to follicular maturation, if C/EBPα is indeed required for progression of follicles to the preovulatory stage.

The ovarian defects seen in C/EBPβ-deficient mice establish this transcription factor as an important nuclear effector of the LH signaling pathway in granulosa cells. Although the target genes whose deregulated expression cause ovarian dysfunction are not known, we can speculate about the nature of the signaling pathway leading to C/EBPβ from the LH receptor (Fig. 23.3). Ligand binding to the G-protein–coupled LH receptor elicits an increase in cAMP levels in the cell, leading to activation of protein kinase A (PKA) (53,54). PKA in turn phosphorylates and activates CREB, which is believed to regulate numerous target genes in granulosa cells, one of which may be C/EBPβ. The C/EBPβ gene promoter is stimulated by the PKA pathway and contains at least two CRE motifs that bind CREB and other members of the ATF/CREB protein family (55). These CREs were shown to be essential for mediating the stimulatory effects of PKA on the C/EBPβ promoter. Thus, we propose that the induction of C/EBPβ expression by LH involves the action of CREB or related cAMP-responsive family members. Additional signals may be required for translocation of C/EBPβ to the nucleus (56,57) or to induce posttranslational modifications that regulate C/EBPβ activity (58–61).

Although it is assumed that the complex processes of follicular maturation, ovulation, and luteinization are regulated by multiple transcription factors, few of these have been identified to date. The work summarized here

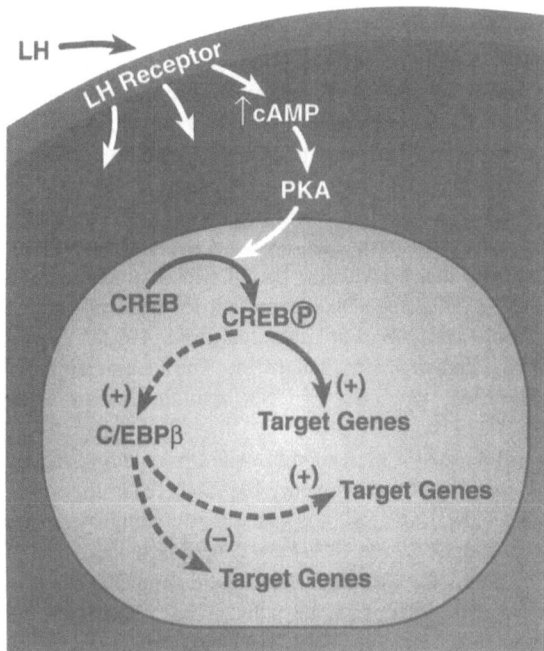

FIGURE 23.3. C/EBPβ is a nuclear effector of LH signaling in granulosa cells. LH binding to its receptor causes increased intracellular cAMP and activation of PKA. In this proposed pathway, PKA activates CREB, which stimulates transcription from the C/EBPβ promoter. CREB and C/EBPβ then activate or repress specific target genes.

from several laboratories shows that C/EBP proteins are key regulators of these events, although the precise molecular mechanisms (e.g., identification of critical target genes) have not yet been determined; however, we anticipate that the roles of C/EBP family members in ovarian development and physiology will become increasingly clear through continued studies of germline knockout mice and through the development of cell-specific knockout models. Such studies should significantly increase our understanding of gene regulation during the female reproductive cycle.

Acknowlegments. The authors are grateful to Kelly Mayo for providing unpublished data, Lars Hedin for critical reading of the chapter, and Madeline Wilson for expert secretarial assistance. The authors' research was sponsored by the National Cancer Institute, DHHS, under contract with ABL.

References

1. Mukherjee A, Park-Sarge OK, Mayo KE. Gonadotropins induce rapid phosphorylation of the 3',5'-cyclic adenosine monophosphate response element binding protein in ovarian granulosa cells. Endocrinology 1996;137:3234–45.

2. Piontkewitz Y, Sundfeldt K, Hedin L. The expression of c-myc during follicular growth and luteal formation in the rat ovary in vivo. J Endocrinol 1997;152:395–406.

3. Agarwal P, Peluso JJ, White BA. Steroidogenic factor-1 expression is transiently repressed and c-myc expression and deoxyribonucleic acid synthesis are induced in rat granulosa cells during the periovulatory period. Biol Reprod 1996;55:1271–75.

4. McKnight SL. CCAAT/enhancer binding protein. In: Transcriptional regulation. Cold Spring Harbor: Cold Spring Harbor Laboratory Press; 1992.

5. Landschulz WH, Johnson PF, McKnight SL. The leucine zipper: a hypothetical structure common to a new class of DNA binding proteins. Science 1988;240:1759–64.

6. Landschulz WH, Johnson PF, McKnight SL. The DNA binding domain of the rat liver nuclear protein C/EBP is bipartite. Science 1989;243:1681–88.

7. Agre P, Johnson PF, McKnight SL. Cognate DNA binding specificity retained after leucine zipper exchange between GCN4 and C/EBP. Science 1989;246:922–26.

8. Ellenberger TE, Brandl CJ, Struhl K, Harrison SC. The GCN4 basic region leucine zipper binds DNA as a dimer of uninterrupted alpha-helices: crystal structure of the protein-DNA complex. Cell 1992;71:1223–37.

9. Johnson PF. Identification of C/EBP basic region residues involved in DNA sequence recognition and half-site spacing preference. Mol Cell Biol 1993;13:6919–30.

10. Johnson P, Williams SC. CCAAT/enhancer binding (C/EBP) proteins. In: Yaniv M, Tronche F, eds. Liver gene expression. Austin, TX: R.G. Landes Company; 1994:231–58.

11. Ron D, Habener JF. CHOP, a novel developmentally regulated nuclear protein that dimerizes with transcription factors C/EBP and LAP and functions as a dominant-negative inhibitor of gene transcription. Genes Dev 1992;6:439–53.

12. Cooper C, Henderson A, Artandi S, Avitahl N, Calame K. Ig/EBP (C/EBPγ) is a transdominant negative inhibitor of C/EBP family transcriptional activators. Nucl Acids Res 1995;23:4371–77.

13. Vinson CR, Sigler PB, McKnight SL. Scissors-grip model for DNA recognition by a family of leucine zipper proteins. Science 1989;246:911–16.

14. Osada S, Yamamoto H, Nishihara T, Imagawa M. DNA binding specificity of the CCAAT/enhancer-binding protein transcription factor family. J Biol Chem 1996;271:3891–96.

15. Kouzarides T, Ziff E. The role of the leucine zipper in the fos-jun interaction. Nature 1988;336:646–51.

16. Suckow M, von Wilcken-Bergmann B, Muller-Hill B. The DNA binding specificity of the basic region of the yeast transcriptional activator GCN4 can be changed by substitution of a single amino acid. Nucl Acids Res 1993;21:2081–86.

17. Suckow M, von Wilcken-Bergmann B, Muller-Hill B. Identification of 3 residues in the basic regions of the bZIP proteins GCN4, C/EBP and TAF-1 that are involved in specific DNA binding. EMBO J 1993;12:1193–200.

18. Chandrasekaran C, Gordon JI. Cell lineage-specific and differentiation-dependent pat-

terns of CCAAT/enhancer binding protein α expression in the gut epithelium of normal and transgenic mice. Proc Natl Acad Sci USA 1993;90:8871–75.

19. Oh HS, Smart RC. Expression of CCAAT/enhancer binding proteins (C/EBP) is associated with squamous differentiation in epidermis and isolated primary keratinocytes and is altered in skin neoplasms. J Invest Dermatol 1998;110: 939–45.

20. Scott LM, Civin CI, Rorth P, Friedman AD. A novel temporal expression pattern of three C/EBP family members in differentiating myelomonocytic cells. Blood 1992;80:1725–35.

21. Alam T, An MR, Papaconstantinou J. Differential expression of three C/EBP isoforms in multiple tissues during the acute phase response. J Biol Chem 1992;267: 5021–24.

22. Ramji DP, Vitelli A, Tronche F, Cortese R, Ciliberto G. The two C/EBP isoforms, IL-6DBP/NF-IL6 and C/EBPδ/NF-IL6β, are induced by IL-6 to promote acute phase gene transcription via different mechanisms. Nucl Acids Res 1993;21:289–94.

23. Ray A, Ray BK. Serum amyloid A gene expression under acute-phase conditions involves participation of inducible C/EBPβ- and C/EBP-δ and their activation by phosphorylation. Mol Cell Biol 1994;14:4324–32.

24. Yamada T, Tobita K, Osada S, Nishihara T, Imagawa M. CCAAT/enhancer-binding protein δ gene expression is mediated by APRF/STAT3. J Biochem (Tokyo) 1997;121:731–38.

25. Cantwell CA, Sterneck E, Johnson PF. Interleukin-6-specific activation of the C/EBPδ gene in hepatocytes is mediated by Stat3 and Sp1. Mol Cell Biol 1998; 18:2108–17.

26. Sterneck E, Paylor R, Jackson-Lewis V, Libbey M, Przedborski S, Tessarollo L, et al. Selectively enhanced contextual fear conditioning in mice lacking the transcriptional regulator CCAAT/enhancer binding protein δ. Proc Natl Acad Sci USA 1998; 95:10908–13.

27. Antonson P, Stellan B, Yamanaka R, Xanthopoulos KG. A novel human CCAAT/enhancer binding protein gene, C/EBPε, is expressed in cells of lymphoid and myeloid lineages and is localized on chromosome 14q11.2 close to the T-cell receptor alpha/delta locus. Genomics 1996;35:30–8.

28. Chumakov AM, Grillier I, Chumakova E, Chih D, Slater J, Koeffler HP. Cloning of the novel human myeloid-cell-specific C/EBP-ε transcription factor. Mol Cell Biol 1997;17:1375–86.

29. Williams SC, Du Y, Schwartz RC, Weiler SR, Ortiz M, Keller JR, et al. C/EBPε is a myeloid-specific activator of cytokine, chemokine, and macrophage-colony-stimulating factor receptor genes. J Biol Chem 1998;273:13493–501.

30. Umek RM, Friedman AD, McKnight SL. CCAAT-enhancer binding protein: a component of a differentiation switch. Science 1991;251:288–92.

31. Buck M, Turler H, Chojkier M. LAP (NF-IL-6), a tissue-specific transcriptional activator, is an inhibitor of hepatoma cell proliferation. EMBO J 1994;13:851–60.

32. O'Rourke J, Yuan R, DeWille J. CCAAT/enhancer-binding protein-δ (C/EBP-δ) is induced in growth-arrested mouse mammary epithelial cells. J Biol Chem 1997;272: 6291–96.

33. Timchenko NA, Wilde M, Nakanishi M, Smith JR, Darlington GJ. CCAAT/enhancer-

binding protein α (C/EBPα) inhibits cell proliferation through the p21 (WAF-1/CIP-1/SDI-1) protein. Genes Dev 1996;10:804–15.

34. Chinery R, Brockman JA, Peeler MO, Shyr Y, Beauchamp RD, Coffey RJ. Antioxidants enhance the cytotoxicity of chemotherapeutic agents in colorectal cancer: a p53-independent induction of p21WAF1/CIP1 via C/EBPβ. Nat Med 1997; 3:1233–41.

35. Hu HM, Baer M, Williams SC, Johnson PF, Schwartz RC. Redundancy of C/EBP-α, -β, and -δ in supporting the lipopolysaccharide-induced transcription of IL-6 and monocyte chemoattractant protein-1. J Immunol 1998;160:2334–42.

36. Lee YH, Williams SC, Baer M, Sterneck E, Gonzalez FJ, Johnson PF. The ability of C/EBPβ but not C/EBPα to synergize with an Sp1 protein is specified by the leucine zipper and activation domain. Mol Cell Biol 1997;17:2038–47.

37. Colangelo AM, Johnson PF, Mocchetti I. Beta-adrenergic receptor-induced activation of nerve growth factor gene transcription in rat cerebral cortex involves CCAAT/enhancer-binding protein δ. Proc Natl Acad Sci USA 1998;95:10920–25.

38. Lee YH, Yano M, Liu SY, Matsunaga E, Johnson PF, Gonzalez FJ. A novel cis-acting element controlling the rat CYP2D5 gene and requiring cooperativity between C/EBPβ and an Sp1 factor. Mol Cell Biol 1994;14:1383–94.

39. Piontkewitz Y, Enerback S, Hedin L. Expression and hormonal regulation of the CCAAT enhancer binding protein-α during differentiation of rat ovarian follicles. Endocrinology 1993;133:2327–33.

40. Sirois J, Richards JS. Transcriptional regulation of the rat prostaglandin endoperoxide synthase 2 gene in granulosa cells. Evidence for the role of a cis-acting C/EBPβ promoter element. J Biol Chem 1993;268:21931–38.

41. Pall M, Hellberg P, Brannstrom M, Mikuni M, Peterson CM, Sundfeldt K, et al. The transcription factor C/EBP-β and its role in ovarian function; evidence for direct involvement in the ovulatory process. EMBO J 1997;16:5273–79.

42. Sterneck E, Tessarollo L, Johnson PF. An essential role for C/EBPβ in female reproduction. Genes Dev 1997;11:2153–62.

43. Yamanaka R, Kim GD, Radomska HS, Lekstrom-Himes J, Smith LT, Antonson P, et al. CCAAT/enhancer binding protein ε is preferentially up-regulated during granulocytic differentiation and its functional versatility is determined by alternative use of promoters and differential splicing. Proc Natl Acad Sci USA 1997;94:6462–67.

44. Wang ND, Finegold MJ, Bradley A, Ou CN, Abdelsayed SV, Wilde MD, et al. Impaired energy homeostasis in C/EBPα knockout mice. Science 1995;269:1108–12.

45. Piontkewitz Y, Enerback S, Hedin L. Expression of CCAAT enhancer binding protein-α (C/EBPα) in the rat ovary: Implications for follicular development and ovulation. Dev Biol 1996;179:288–96.

46. Morris JK, Richards JS. An E-box region within the prostaglandin endoperoxide synthase-2 (PGS-2) promoter is required for transcription in rat ovarian granulosa cells. J Biol Chem 1996;271:16633–43.

47. Descombes P, Schibler U. A liver-enriched transcriptional activator protein, LAP, and a transcriptional inhibitory protein, LIP, are translated from the same mRNA. Cell 1991;67:569–79.

48. Baer M, Williams SC, Dillner A, Schwartz RC, Johnson PF. Autocrine signals control CCAAT/enhancer binding protein β expression, localization, and activity in macrophages. Blood 1998;92:4353–65.

49. Lincoln AJ, Monczak Y, Williams SC, Johnson PF. Inhibition of CCAAT/enhancer-

binding protein α and β translation by upstream open reading frames. J Biol Chem 1998;273:9552–60.

50. Williams SC, Baer M, Dillner AJ, Johnson PF. CRP2 (C/EBPβ) contains a bipartite regulatory domain that controls transcriptional activation, DNA binding and cell specificity. EMBO J 1995;14:3170–83.

51. Mukherjee A, Urban J, Sassone-Corsi P, Mayo KE. Gonadotropins regulate inducible cyclic adenosine 3′,5′-monophosphate early repressor in the rat ovary: implications for inhibin alpha subunit gene expression. Mol Endocrinol 1998;12:785–800.

52. Lee Y-H, Sauer B, Johnson PF, Gonzalez FJ. Disruption of the *c/ebpα* gene in adult mouse liver. Mol Cell Biol 1997;17:6014–22.

53. Richards JS. Gonadotropin-regulated gene expression in the ovary. In: Adashi EY, Leung PCK, eds. The Ovary. New York: Raven Press; 1993:93–110.

54. Morris JK, Richards JS. Luteinizing hormone induces prostaglandin endoperoxide synthase-2 and luteinization in vitro by A-kinase and C-kinase pathways. Endocrinology 1995;136:1549–58.

55. Niehof M, Manns MP, Trautwein C. CREB controls LAP/C/EBPβ transcription. Mol Cell Biol 1997;17:3600–13.

56. Katz S, Kowenz-Leutz E, Muller C, Meese K, Ness SA, Leutz A. The NF-M transcription factor is related to C/EBP-β and plays a role in signal transduction, differentiation and leukemogenesis of avian myelomonocytic cells. EMBO J 1993;12:1321–32.

57. Chinery R, Brockman JA, Dransfield DT, Coffey RJ. Antioxidant-induced nuclear translocation of CCAAT/enhancer-binding protein β. A critical role for protein kinase A-mediated phosphorylation of Ser299. J Biol Chem 1997;272:30356–61.

58. Wegner M, Cao Z, Rosenfeld MG. Calcium-regulated phosphorylation within the leucine zipper of C/EBPβ. Science 1992;256:370–73.

59. Nakajima T, Kinoshita S, Sasagawa T, Sasaki K, Naruto M, Kishimoto T, et al. Phosphorylation at threonine-235 by a ras-dependent mitogen-activated protein kinase cascade is essential for transcription factor NF-IL6. Proc Natl Acad Sci USA 1993;90:2207–11.

60. Trautwein C, Caelles C, van dGP, Hunter T, Karin M, Chojkier M. Transactivation by NF-IL6/LAP is enhanced by phosphorylation of its activation domain. Nature 1993;364:544–47.

61. Engelman JA, Lisanti MP, Scherer PE. Specific inhibitors of p38 mitogen-activated protein kinase block 3T3-L1 adipogenesis. J Biol Chem 1998;273:32111–20.

62. Richards JS, Fitzpatrick SL, Clemens JW, Morris JK, Alliston T, Sirois J. Ovarian cell differentiation: a cascade of multiple hormones, cellular signals, and regulated genes. Rec Prog Horm Res 1995;50:223–54.

Part VI

Clinical Frontiers

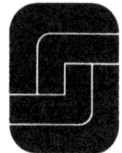

24

Designer Gonadotropins and Receptors: The Prospect of Recombinant Technology

David Puett and Prema Narayan

Introduction

Gonadotropins and Their Genes

The three human (h) gonadotropins, lutropin or luteinizing hormone (LH), follitropin or follicle stimulating hormone (FSH), and choriogonadotropin or chorionic gonadotropin (CG), are heterodimeric glycoproteins that contain a common α subunit and a hormone-specific β subunit (see in Refs. 1 and 2 for reviews on the chemical structures of the gonadotropins and the related glycoprotein hormone, thyrotropin). The α subunit contains 92 amino acid residues, has two sites of N-glycosylation at Asn-52 and Asn-78, and is encoded by a single copy gene ranging in length from 8 to 16.5 kbp, depending upon the species. In humans, the gene is 9.4 kbp and contains four exons and three introns, with a very large first intron of 6.4 kbp in length. It is mapped to chromosome 6p21.1-23. The α-subunit gene encodes an mRNA species of 730–800 nucleotides in all species and is expressed in both the pituitary and placenta (3–5).

hLHβ contains 121 amino acid residues and one site of N-glycosylation at Asn-30; the shortest of the human gonadotropin β subunits, hFSHβ contains 111 amino acid residues and two sites of N-glycosylation at Asn-7 and Asn-24. hLH and hFSH are expressed in gonadotrophs of the adenohypophysis and under the regulation of GnRH from the hypothalamus and of gonadal sex steroids and polypeptides.

hCG, originally believed to be expressed only by the syncytiotrophoblast in pregnancy and by certain neoplasms, is now known to be produced in the pituitary as well (6). The hCGβ subunit is the longest of the human glycoprotein hormone β subunits, containing 145 amino acid residues, with the C-terminal extension being referred to as the C-terminal peptide (CTP). Two sites of N-glycosylation occur in hCGβ at Asn-13 and Asn-30, although there are four sites of O-glycosylation at Ser-121,127,132, and 138 on the CTP.

The β-subunit genes are highly homologous with similar structures. The human LHβ and CGβ genes are organized in a large gene cluster spanning approximately 52 kbp that consists of six copies of the CGβ and a single copy of the LHβ gene (4,5). The LHβ gene is present at one end of the cluster, and the CGβ genes are arranged in tandem and inverted pairs. Both genes contain three exons and two introns. They are mapped in humans to locus q13.3 on chromosome 19. The LHβ gene is 1.1 kbp long and encodes an mRNA of 700 nucleotides, whereas the lengths of the CGβ genes are variable and are expressed to varying levels in the placenta. The highest level of expression, which results in an mRNA species 1000 nucleotides long, is observed from the CGβ5 gene (4,5). In contrast, FSHβ is encoded by a single copy gene in all species studied, and is present in humans on chromosome 11p13 (3,5). The FSHβ gene differs from the other glycoprotein hormone genes in that it contains a very long 3′ untranslated region and is about 4.2 kbp in length containing three exons and two introns. The bovine and rat genes encode a single mRNA 1800 nucleotides in length, whereas in humans four mRNA species are transcribed (3) due to alternate splicing and utilization of two polyadenylation sites.

In 1994 two laboratories reported the crystal structure of deglycosylated hCG (7,8). Despite little homology in the amino acid sequences of the α and β subunits, the conformations of the two chains were found to be quite similar. Each contained a cystine-knot motif, common in growth factor structures, and three extended loops. The elongated subunits are intertwined, and a portion of hCGβ, amino acid residues 90–110, wraps around α in a "seat belt" arrangement. A number of amino acid residues in the termini of both α and β, including the CTP, were not resolved, presumably due to flexibility of these regions in the crystal. Based upon the close homology of hLHβ and hFSHβ with hCGβ, it is inferred that the two other gonadotropins, hLH and hFSH, will have conformations very similar to that of hCG.

Gonadotropin Receptors and Their Genes

Excluding the CTP, the amino acid sequences of hCGβ and hLHβ are almost identical; not surprisingly, the two gonadotropins, hCG and hLH, bind to the same receptor, LHR, whereas FSH has its distinct receptor, FSHR. The two gonadotropin receptors, which are members of the G protein-coupled receptor superfamily, contain a relatively large N-terminal extracellular domain (ECD) and a membrane-imbedded C-terminal region consisting of seven transmembrane helixes (TMH), three extracellular loops, three cytoplasmic loops, and a C-terminal tail (9–11). The structure and organization of the LHR gene have been most extensively studied in the rat and to a lesser extent in the human and mouse (9,10,12). The single copy LHR gene, which is present at locus p21 on human chromosome 2, spans more than 70 kbp and consists of 11 exons separated by 10 introns. A striking feature of the LHR gene is that exons 1–10 encode the 5′ untranslated region and most of the ECD, with exons 2–8 encoding imperfect leucine-rich repeats, whereas exon 11 codes for 47 amino acid residues of the ECD adjacent to the plasma membrane, TMHs, connecting loops, and the C-terminal cytoplasmic tail. The FSHR gene is very similar to the LHR gene and is also a single copy gene, spanning a region of 54 kbp in the human and 84 kbp in the rat, and consisting of 10 exons and 9 introns (11). The first nine exons encode the majority of the ECD, which contains imperfect leucine-rich repeats as in LHR, whereas exon 10 encodes a portion of the ECD near TMH 1, the TMHs, connecting loops, and the C-terminal tail. The human FSHR gene is mapped to chromosome 2p21, the same chromosomal location as the LHR gene.

Although no structural data exist on the gonadotropin receptors, homology modeling of the ECD with porcine ribonuclease inhibitor, a leucine-rich protein (13), led to similar cusp-shaped structures (14–18). Results obtained on the arrangement of the seven TMHs of bacteriorhodopsin (19,20) and rhodopsin (21), as well as an analysis of heptahelical receptors by Baldwin (22), has been used to model the TMHs of LHR and FSHR (23,24).

The availability of detailed structural information of the gonadotropins and working models of the receptor have aided greatly in protein engineering of the gonadotropin subunits and receptors. Considerable work has been done on the nature of receptor activation, transmembrane and intracellular signaling, and ligand-mediated receptor uncoupling processes (e.g., desensitization and endocytosis), but these interesting aspects of gonadotropin-receptor function are not covered in this chapter; rather, our focus is on the use of recombinant technology to express wild-type and mutant forms of the gonadotropins and their receptors.

Protein Engineering

Site-Directed Mutagenesis

Early work on structure–function relationships of gonadotropins employed various techniques, including chemical modifications, limited proteolysis, immunochemistry, and synthetic peptides to elucidate the molecular nature of holoprotein formation and hormone-receptor binding. The availability of cDNAs and optimized expression systems have permitted a much more specific approach to studies of this type, and, when coupled with reliable structural information and working structural models, much more sophisticated questions can be asked. Numerous reports have appeared that characterize α and β mutants obtained by replacing one or more amino acid residues (see Refs. 2,25–36). Although there is controversy over direct and indirect effects of replacements on receptor binding, there is general agreement that both subunits contribute to high affinity binding.

As summarized in Table 24.1, a number of single and multiple amino acid residue replacements have been prepared in the human α and gonadotropin β subunits that lead to increased potency of the holoprotein; however, the increase in potency is not particularly high overall, with one possible exception being that of hCGβ-Arg-68 replacements (32). Thus, at this point, there is no evidence of a superagonist of any gonadotropin, in contrast to studies with hTSH (2,33). Numerous amino acid residue replacements on both subunits have been described that reduce receptor binding (cf. Ref. 26 for review). The holoprotein devoid of the N-linked oligosaccharide at position α-Asn-52 is the only derivative known that is a potent antagonist (37).

Protein Chimeras

In an effort to determine the important receptor specificity-determining regions on gonadotropin β subunits, a number of chimeras have been prepared in which segments of hCGβ and hFSHβ were switched via protein engineering. Heterodimers of the β chimeras were then prepared with human α and receptor specificity determined.

In a seminal study Moyle and co-workers (38) found that the substitution of limited regions of hCGβ with hFSHβ could change receptor specificity in the holoprotein from LHR-like to FSHR-like (Fig. 24.1). For example, with hCGβ subunits devoid of the CTP, replacement of amino acid residues 94–114 and of 94–117 with the homologous regions of hFSHβ (amino acid residues 88–108 and 88–111, respectively) yielded FSHR specificity and limited any LHR binding. Replacement with smaller segments of hFSHβ [e.g., in the region corresponding to hCGβ 108–114 (hFSHβ 102–108) in a CTP-deleted chain and hCGβ 94–97 (hFSHβ 88–91) in full length hCGβ] yielded LHR-specificity, although weak FSHR binding occurred with the former and the latter exhibited reduced LHR binding.

In a complementary study, Dias and colleagues (39) reported that a reciprocal replacement, amino acid residues of 94–97 from hCGβ in the homologous region of hFSHβ (amino acid residues 88–91) resulted in a gain of LHR-binding preference after combination with α, with the retention of some FSHR binding as well (Fig. 24.1). These are remarkable observations in that a limited number of amino acid residues can dictate receptor preferences. It is of considerable interest and a tribute to the insight of Dr. Darrell Ward that these regions are part of the determinant loop, a section of β influencing binding specificity originally proposed by Ward and Moore from a comparative analysis of the amino acid sequences of the β subunits of LH, CG, FSH, and TSH (40).

TABLE 24.1. Mutations in the α and β subunits of gonadotropins that increase in vitro potency.[a]

Replacements	Relative potency[b] (Ref.)	Replacements	Relative potency[b] (Ref.)
Mutant α + hCGβ		*Mutant α + hFSHβ*	
T11K[c]	2.5 (33)	F33A	2.2 (29)
Q13K[c]	2.8 (33)	R35A	1.9 (29)
P16K[c]	3.4 (33)	H90L	3.0 (31)
F18T	2.1 (34)	H90A	3.0 (31)
Q20K[c]	2.3 (33)	K91R	3.5 (31)
Q50P[c]	1.8 (33)	K91V	2.1 (31)
R67K[c]	1.5 (33)	K91H	2.0 (31)
H90L	3.3 (31)	RSK (42-44)→AAA	1.2 (29)
H90A	2.9 (31)		
H90S	1.3 (31)	*a + mutant hCGβ*	
K91R	2.6 (31)	R68A[c]	28.2(32)
K91E	1.7 (31)	R68K[c]	2.7 (32)
K91V	1.4 (31)	G71D	1.5 (30)
P16K+Q20K[c]	4.1 (33)	S81A	2.0 (30)
Q13K+P16K+Q20K[c]	4.4 (33)	S81R	1.3 (30)
Q13K+E14K+P16K+Q20K[c]	4.2 (33)	R94K[d]	1.4 (28)
		RLPG (68-71)→AAAA[c]	3.3 (32)
Mutant α + mutant hCGβ			
αF18T+βPRG (73-75)→AHH	2.9 (35)	*a + mutant hLHβ*	
αF18T+βGCPV (22-25)→ECRF	2.1 (35)	W8R[d]	1.7 (36)
αF74T+βPRG (73-75)→AHH	1.3 (35)	I15T[d]	1.3 (36)
		W8R+I15T[d]	1.6 (36)

[a]Unless indicated otherwise, the in vitro potency measurements were based on radioreceptor assays with ^{125}I-hCG or ^{125}I-hFSH and graded doses of hCG and hFSH, respectively, in a variety of cells [e.g., transfected COS-7 cells, transfected HEK 293 cells, and transformed Leydig (MA-10) cells, and membrane fractions from rat ovaries and testes].
[b]The potency was normalized to 1.0 for wild-type hCG (for comparison with mutant α+ hCGβ, mutant α + mutant hCGβ, and α + mutant hCGβ) and to 1.0 for wild-type hFSH (for comparison with mutant α + hFSHβ). In some cases, IC_{50}s were interpolated from dose-response curves and represent, at best, estimates of actual K_ds.
[c]Based on steroid production.
[d]Based on steroid production (K_d for mutant $\geq K_d$ wild-type hormone).

Protein engineering was also used to add one or two hCGβ CTPs to hFSHβ, followed by association with human α. The two modified FSHs exhibited an increase in in vivo potency compared with wild-type FSH; the heterodimer, hα·hFSHβ-CTP$_2$, was also shown to have a much longer circulatory half-life than did wild type hFSH (41).

In summary, it is possible to create recombinant gonadotropins with dual activities, to switch from one activity to another with minimal replacement of

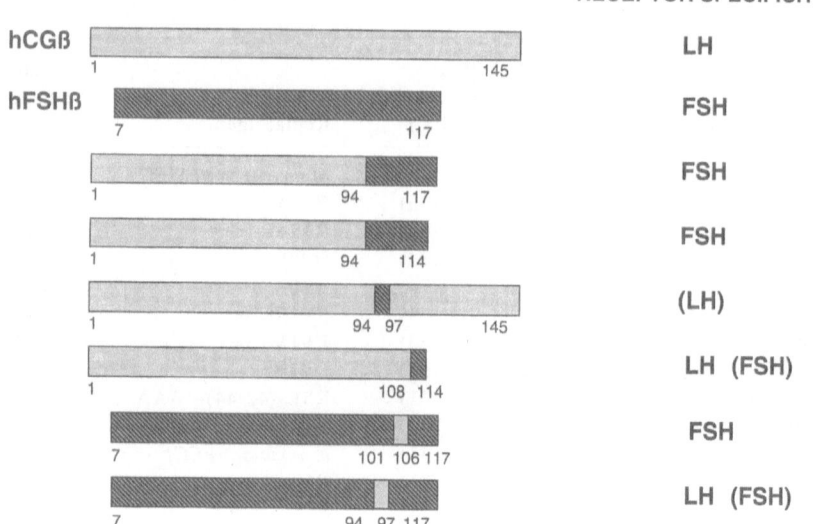

FIGURE 24.1. Summary of several chimeras of the hCG and hFSHβ subunits that have been prepared and characterized, along with the resulting receptor specificity of the resultant holoprotein (i.e., the α-chimeric β complex). Wild-type hCGβ and hFSHβ are shown at the top with the numbering for hFSHβ chosen to correspond to that of hCGβ following an amino acid sequence comparison to maximize homology. The four chimeras that are primarily from the hCGβ sequence are from Ref. 38; the two that are mainly from the FSHβ sequence are from Ref. 39. Receptor specificities are shown to the right; those in parentheses denote weak binding relative to wild-type hormone.

amino acid residues, and to enhance the circulatory half-life and in vivo potency of FSH greatly. It is clear that there will be many more examples showing the utility of protein engineering to achieve gonadotropins with desired properties.

Single Chain (Yoked/Tethered) Gonadotropins and Disulfide-Linked Heterodimers

The power of protein engineering in gonadotropin research was again demonstrated in 1995 with the publication of two papers showing that fusion products of the hα and hCGβ subunits could be expressed to yield bioactive single chain gonadotropins (42,43). Narayan et al. (42) expressed two constructs using the baculovirus system, one a full length β-α and the other a β-α with a shortened CTP; Boime, Hsueh, and co-workers (43) expressed a full length β-α construct in mammalian cells. Other reports demonstrated that single chains could be expressed of hCGβ-hα devoid of the CTP (44) and of hLHβ-hα (45) and hFSHβ-hα with and without a connecting CTP (44). It was also shown by Heikoop et al. (46) that biologically active fusion products of hCGβ and hα could be obtained with (Ser-Gly) linkers. Last, we have expressed an active hα-hCGβ fusion product (P. Narayan and D. Puett, unpublished results). These various single chain gonadotropins are summarized in Figure 24.2.

In a clever application of protein engineering, Heikoop et al. (47) used the crystal structure of hCG (7,8) to select certain amino acid residues on hα and the β subunits of hCG, hLH, and hFSH for replacement with Cys, thus leading to intermolecular disulfide cross-links. The following replacements yielded biologically active crosslinked α and β subunits: (hCG) α5-β8, α35-β35, and α37-β33; (hLH) α5-β8 and α35-β35; and (hFSH) α35-β29 and α37-β27.

Single Chain (Yoked/Tethered) Gonadotropin–Receptor Complexes

Our laboratory reported that yoked hCG could in turn be yoked to LHR with a [CTP-Factor Xa cleavage site] connector (48). This fusion product, hCGβ-hα-CTP-Factor Xa cleavage site-LHR (Fig. 24.3), was expressed in COS-7 cells and HEK 293 cells, as demonstrated by Western blots. It is interesting that the receptor is constitutively activated in both cell types, which indicates that the single chain gonadotropin–receptor complex folds correctly, undergoes proper trafficking within the cells to localize on the plasma membrane, and is capable of activating G_s as evidenced by a high basal production of cAMP (Fig. 24.3). Cells that express this yoked hormone–receptor complex bind exogenous hCG with an apparent K_d somewhat less than that of wild–type LHR and are only somewhat responsive to exogenous hCG in ligand-mediated cAMP production. These results suggest that the covalently attached yoked hCG is functionally bound to LHR, leading to persistent activation. Preliminary results show that yoked hα-LHR and yoked hCGβ-LHR are also active (Fig. 24.3), the fusion product of β and receptor much more so than that of α and receptor (49).

Clinical Use of Recombinant Gonadotropins

A number of clinical studies have appeared in which the three human recombinant gonadotropins have been used and, in some cases, compared with the natural forms purified from urine or pituitary (50–54). The recombinant forms have proven to be equipotent to, and in some cases more efficacious than, the natural gonadotropins. The purity is generally greater, and cross-contamination in hLH and hFSH preparations is avoided. Moreover, there is no evidence of adverse immunogenicity, and the potential exists for excellent batch-to-batch consistency and perhaps greater homogeneity. Last, by virtue of its shorter circulatory half-life compared with hCG, the availability of recombi-

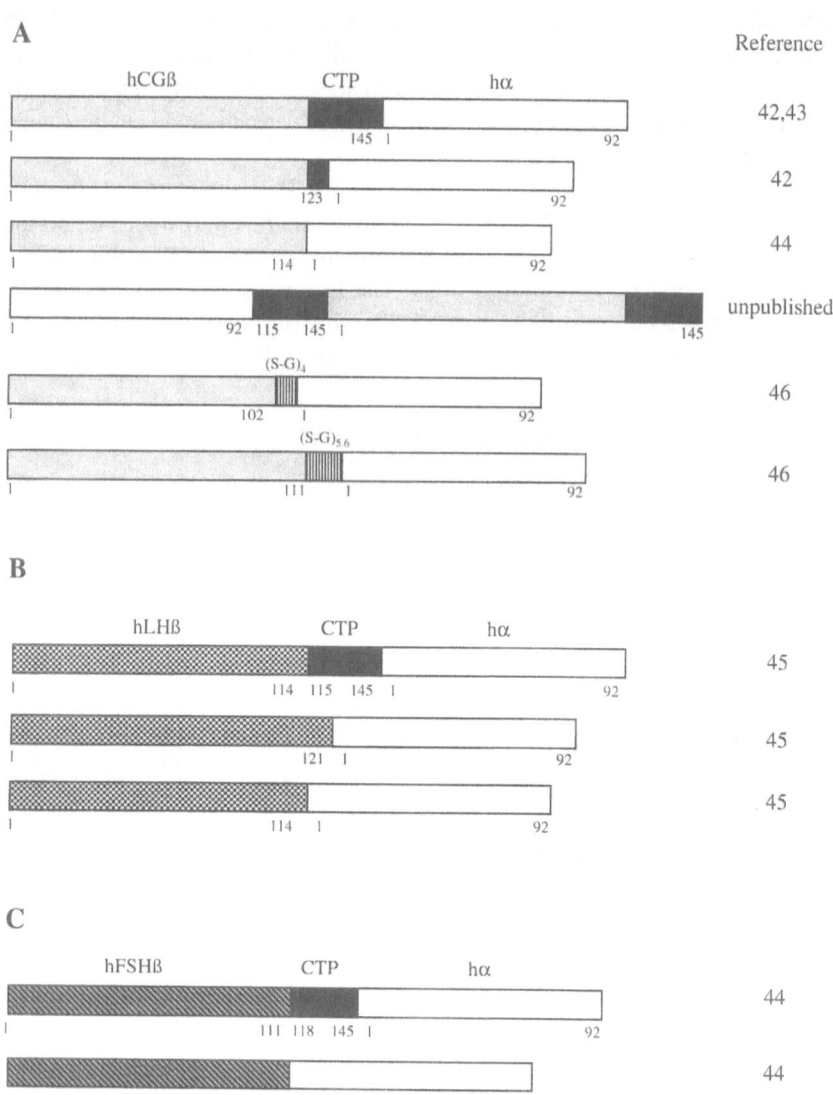

FIGURE 24.2. Summary of single chain (yoked/tethered) gonadotropins. Fusion products of hα and hCGβ (A), hα and hLHβ (B), and hα and hFSHβ (C). (S-G)₄ and (S-G)₅,₆ in panel (A) denote linkers of repeating Ser-Gly units; other linkers are CTP or a shortened version of CTP. Several single-chain gonadotropins are constructed with no linker between the subunits.

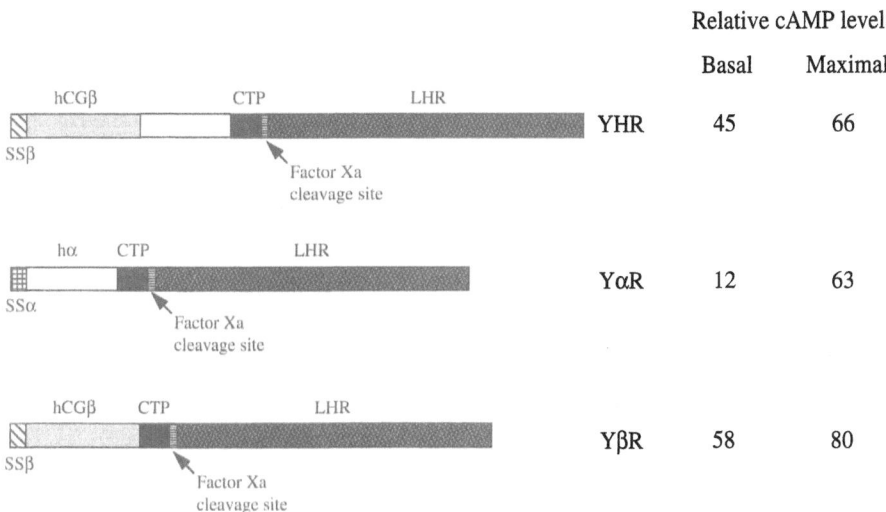

FIGURE 24.3. Single chain or yoked hCG and subunit LHR complexes. The basal and maximal cAMP levels were determined in the presence of 0 and 250 ng/ml hCG, respectively, and are expressed relative to the corresponding levels in mock transfected cells. SSβ and SSα denote the signal sequences of hCGβ and the hα subunits, respectively. YHR, yoked hCG-LHR; YαR, yoked hα-LHR; YβR, yoked hCGβ-LHR.

nant hLH may offer advantages in controlled ovarian stimulation cycles, particularly for women at risk of ovarian hyperstimulation syndrome.

Prospectus

The current status of protein engineering and recombinant technology offers the promise of many new gonadotropin and receptor derivatives for research and clinical use in the coming years. In addition to the advantages of recombinant gonadotropins mentioned earlier, one can expect the availability of gonadotropins with superagonist and superantagonist properties, of increased stability, with greater receptor specificity, and, if desired, with mixed activities. Moreover, it should be possible to prepare mini-gonadotropins using linked α and β fragments, as well as soluble receptor ligand-binding domains. A variety of yoked or single chain gonadotropin-receptor complexes should be available for cell models of male-limited precocious puberty, hormone-mediated transformation, and other disorders. Last, in view of the similarities in the conformation of the hCG subunits with various growth factors (7,8), it may be possible to prepare αα and ββ homodimers, as well as many other forms, that act on receptors different from LHR and FSHR.

Acknowledgments. This work was supported by NIH Research Grant DK33973. We are most appreciative of the many graduate students and research associates who have contributed to our studies on hCG and LHR.

References

1. Ryan RJ, Charlesworth MC, McCormick DJ, Milius RP, Keutmann HT. The glycoprotein hormones: recent studies of structure-function relationships. FASEB J 1988;2:2661–69.

2. Grossman M, Weintraub BD, Szkudlinski MW. Novel insights into the molecular mechanisms of human thyrotropin action: structural, physiological, and therapeutic implications for the glycoprotein hormone family. Endocrine Rev 1997;18:476–501.

3. Gharib SD, Wierman ME, Shupnik MA, Chin WW. Molecular biology of the pituitary gonadotropins. Endocrine Rev 1990;11:177–99.

4. Jameson JL, Hollenberg AN. Regulation of chorionic gonadotropin gene expression. Endocrine Rev 1993;14:203–21.

5. Albanese C, Colin IM, Crowley WF, Ito M, Pestell RG, Weiss J, et al. The gonadotropin genes: evolution of distinct mechanisms for hormonal control. Recent Prog Horm Res 1996;51:23–61.

6. Birken S, Maydelman Y, Gawinowicz MA, Pound A, Liu Y, Hartree AS. Isolation and characterization of human pituitary chorionic gonadotropin. Endocrinology 1996;137:1402–11.

7. Lapthorn AJ, Harris DC, Littlejohn A, Lustbader JW, Canfield RE, Machin KJ, et al. Crystal structure of human chorionic gonadotropin. Nature 1994;369:455–61.

8. Wu H, Lustbader JW, Liu Y, Canfield RE, Hendrickson WA. Structure of human chorionic gonadotropin at 2.6 Å resolution from MAD analysis of the selenomethionyl protein. Structure 1994;2:545–58.

9. Segaloff DL, Ascoli M. The lutropin/choriogondotropin receptor . . . 4 years later. Endocrine Rev 1993;14:324–47.

10. Dufau M. The luteinizing hormone receptor. Annu Rev Physiol 1998;60:461–96.

11. Simoni M, Gromoll J, Nieschlag E. The follicle-stimulating hormone receptor: biochemistry, molecular biology, physiology, and pathophysiology. Endocrine Rev 1997;18:739–73.

12. Koo YB, Ji I, Slaughter RG, Ji TH. Structure of the luteinizing hormone receptor gene and multiple exons of the coding sequence. Endocrinology 1991;128:2297–308.

13. Kobe B, Deisenhofer J. Crystal structure of porcine ribonuclease inhibitor, a protein with leucine-rich repeats. Nature 1993;366:751–56.

14. Moyle WR, Campbell RK, Venkateswara Rao SN, Ayad NG, Bernard MP, Han Y, et al. Model of human chorionic gonadotropin and lutropin receptor interaction that explains signal transduction of the glycoprotein hormones. J Biol Chem 1995;270:20020–31.

15. Kajava AV, Vassart G, Wodak SJ. Modeling of the three-dimensional structure of proteins with the typical leucine-rich repeats. Structure 1995;3:867–77.

16. Jiang X, Dreano M, Buckler DR, Cheng S, Ythier A, Wu H, et al. Structural predictions for the ligand-binding region of glycoprotein hormone receptors and the nature of hormone-receptor interactions. Structure 1995;3:1341–53.

17. Couture L, Naharisoa H, Grebert D, Remy J-J, Pajot-Augy E, Bozon V, et al. Peptide and immunochemical mapping of the ectodomain of the porcine LH receptor. J Mol Endocrinol 1996;16:15–25.

18. Bhowmick N, Huang J, Puett D, Isaacs NW, Lapthorn AJ. Determination of residues

important in hormone binding to the extracellular domain of the luteinizing hormone/ chorionic gonadotropin receptor by site-directed mutagenesis and modeling. Mol Endocrinol 1996;10:1147–59.

19. Pebay-Peyroula E, Rummel G, Rosenbusch JP, Landau EM. X-ray structure of bacteriorhodopsin at 2.5 Angstroms from microcrystals grown in lipidic cubic phases. Science 1997;277:1676–80.

20. Kimura Y, Vassytyev DG, Miyazawa A, Kidera A, Matsushima M, Mitsuoka K, et al. Surface of bacteriorhodopsin by high-resolution electron crystallography. Nature 1997;389:206–11.

21. Unger VM, Hargrave PA, Baldwin JM, Schertier GFX. Arrangement of rhodopsin transmembrane helices. Nature 1997;389:203–6.

22. Baldwin JM. The probable arrangement of the helices in G protein-coupled receptors. EMBO J 1993;12:1693–703.

23. Hoflack J, Hibert MF, Trumpp-Kallmeyer S, Bidart J-M. Three-dimensional models of gonado-thyrotropin hormone receptor transmembrane domain. Drug Design Disc 1993;10:157–71.

24. Lin Z, Shenker A, Pearlstein R. A model of the lutropin/choriogonadotropin receptor: insights into the structural and functional effects of constitutively activating mutations. Protein Engr 1997;10:501–10.

25. Dias JA. Human follitropin heterodimerization and receptor binding structural motifs: identification and analysis by a combination of synthetic peptide and mutagenesis approaches. Mol Cell Endocrinol 1996;125:45–54.

26. Puett D, Bhowmick N, Fernandez LM, Huang J, Wu, C, Narayan P. hCG-receptor binding and transmembrane signaling. Mol Cell Endocrinol 1996;125:55–64.

27. Ji TH, Ryu K-S, Gilchrist R, Ji I. Interaction, signal generation, signal divergence, and signal transduction of LH/CG and the receptor. Rec Progr Horm Res 1997;52:431–54.

28. Chen F, Puett D. Contributions of Arginines-43 and -94 of human choriogonadotropin β to receptor binding and activation as determined by oligonucleotide-based mutagenesis. Biochemistry 1991;30:10171–75.

29. Liu CL, Roth KE, Lindau Shepard BA, Shaffer JB, Dias JA. Site-directed alanine mutagenesis of Phe[33], Arg[35], Arg[42]-Ser[43]-Lys[44] in the human gonadotropin α-subunit. J Biol Chem 1993;268:21613–17.

30. Xia H, Puett D. Identification of conserved amino acid residues in the β subunit of human choriogonadotropin important in holoprotein formation. J Biol Chem 1994;269:17944–53.

31. Zeng H, Ji I, Ji TH. Lys[91] and His[90] of the α-subunit are crucial for receptor binding and hormone activation of follicle-stimulating hormone (FSH) and play hormone-specific roles in FSH and human chorionic gonadotropin. Endocrinology 1995;136:2948–53.

32. Shen L, Xia H, Bhowmick N, Narayan P, Puett D. Mutations of Arg[68] of the human chorionic gonadotropin β subunit lead to reduced secretion. J Mol Endocrinol 1996;17:257–62.

33. Szkudlinski MW, Teh NG, Grossman M, Tropea JE, Weintraub BD. Engineering human glycoprotein hormone superactive analogues. Nat Biotech 1996;14:1257–63.

34. Shao K, Purohit S, Bahl OP. Effect of modification of all loop regions in the α- and β-subunits of human choriogonadotropin on its signal transduction activity. Mol Cell Endocrinol 1996;122:173–82.

35. Shao K, Bahl OP. Effect of modification of the β-hairpin and long loops simultaneously in both α- and β-subunits on the function of human choriogonadotropin: part II. Mol Cell Endocrinol 1997;127:179–87.

36. Suganuma N, Furui K, Kikkawa F, Tomoda Y, Furuhashi M. Effects of the mutations (Trp^8→Arg and Ile^{15}→Thr) in human luteinizing hormone (LH) β-subunit on LH bioactivity in vitro and in vivo. Endocrinology 1996;137:831–38.

37. Matzuk MM, Keene JL, Boime I. Site specificity of the chorionic gonadotropin N-linked oligosaccharides in signal transduction. J Biol Chem 1989;264:2409–14.

38. Campbell RK, Dean-Emig DM, Moyle WR. Conversion of human choriogonadotropin into a follitropin by protein engineering. Proc Natl Acad Sci USA 1991;88:760–64.

39. Dias JA, Zhang Y, Liu X. Receptor binding and functional properties of chimeric human follitropin prepared by an exchange between a small hydrophilic intercysteine loop of human follitropin and human lutropin. J Biol Chem 1994;269:25289–94.

40. Ward DN, Moore WT. In: Alexander NJ, ed. Animal models for research on contraception and fertility. Baltimore: Harper & Row; 1979:151–64.

41. Fares FA, Suganuma W, Nishimori K, LaPolt PS, Hsueh AJW, Boime I. Design of a long-acting follitropin agonist by fusing the C-terminal sequence of the chorionic gonadotropin β subunit to the follitropin β subunit. Proc Natl Acad Sci USA 1992;89:4304–8.

42. Narayan P, Wu C, Puett D. Functional expression of yoked human chorionic gonadotropin in baculovirus-infected insect cells. Mol Endocrinol 1995;9:1720–26.

43. Sugahara T, Pixley MR, Minami S, Perlas E, Ben-Menahem D, Hsueh AJW, et al. Biosynthesis of a biologically active single peptide chain containing the human common α and chorionic gonadotropin β subunits in tandem. Proc Natl Acad Sci USA 1995;92:2041–45.

44. Sugahara T, Sato A, Kudo M, Ben-Menahem D, Pixley MR, Hsueh AJW, et al. Expression of biologically active fusion genes encoding the common α subunit and the follicle-stimulating hormone β subunit. J Biol Chem 1996;271:10445–48.

45. Garcia-Campayo V, Sato A, Hirsch B, Sugahara T, Muyan M, Hsueh AJW, et al. Design of stable biologically active recombinant hormones. Nature Biotech 1997;15:663–67.

46. Heikoop JC, van Beuningen-de Vaan MMJACM, van den Boogaart P, Grootenhuis PDJ. Evaluation of subunit truncation and the nature of the spacer for single chain human gonadotropins. Eur J Biochem 1997;245:656–62.

47. Heikoop JC, van der Boogaart P, Mulders JWM, Grootenhuis PDJ. Structure-based design and protein engineering of intersubunit disulfide bonds in gonadotropins. Nat Biotech 1997;15:658–62.

48. Wu C, Narayan P, Puett D. Protein engineering of a novel constitutively active hormone-receptor complex. J Biol Chem 1996;271:31638–42.

49. Puett D, Wu C, Narayan P. The tie that binds: design of biologically active single-chain chorionic gonadotropins and a gonadotropin-receptor complex using protein engineering. Biol Reprod 1998;58:1337–42.

50. Shoham Z, Insler V. Recombinant technique and gonadotropin production: new era in reproductive medicine. Fertil Steril 1996;66:187–201.

51. Geurts TBP, Peters MJH, van Bruggen JGC, de Boer W, Out HJ. Puregon (ORG 32489)-recombinant human follicle-stimulating hormone. Drugs Today 1996;32:239–58.

52. Eshkol A. Recombinant gonadotropins: an introduction. Hum Reprod 1996;11 (suppl. 1):89–94.

53. Loumaye E, Martineau I, Piazzi A, O'Dea L, Ince S, Howles C, et al. Clinical assessment of human gonadotropins produced by recombinant DNA technology. Hum Reprod 1996;11(suppl. 1):95–107.

54. Hull ML, Livesey JH, Evans JJ, Benny PS. The effect of recombinant follicle stimulating hormone (Gonal-F) on endogenons luteinizing hormone secretion in women. Hum Reprod 1998;13:1139–43.

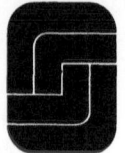

25

Triggering Ovulation
with GnRH Analogs

Shahar Kol and Joseph Itskovitz-Eldor

Introduction

Since their introduction in the early 1960s, human menopausal gonadotropins (hMG) have been used in millions of ovulation induction cycles, particularly since 1980 in the context of in vitro fertilization (IVF). In these cycles human chorionic gonadotropin (hCG) is typically used as a surrogate to luteinizing hormone (LH) for the purpose of oocyte maturation and induction and ovuation. Given its significantly longer half-life [>24 hours. 60 minutes for LH (1,2)], hCG administration results in a prolonged luteotrophic effect, characterized by the development of multiple corpora lutea and supraphysiologic levels of estradiol (E_2) and progesterone (P). This sustained luteotrophic effect may result in the development of ovarian hyperstimulation syndrome (OHSS), which is the most frequent and severe complication of hMG trearment (3). The treat of OHSS often leads to cycle cancellation.

An alterative to hCG-driven ovulation is the use of gonadotropin-releasing hormone analogs (GnRHa). These compounds induce a sustained release of LH (and FSH) from the pituitary (also known as the "flare effect") that effectively induces oocyte maturation and ovulation. It is of note that they also provide a means by which OHSS is completely and effectively eliminated (4–11). The endocrine basis for the use of GnRHa for ovulation triggering, and its clinical application in assisted reproductive technology (ART), are reviewed herein.

The Spontaneous LH/FSH Surge

The midcycle spontaneous LH surge is characterized by three phases: a rapidly ascending limb of 14-hour duration, a plateau of 14 hours, and a descendibng phase of 20 hours (12). The parallel follicle stimulating hormone (FSH) surge is

308

of lower amplitude. Serum E_2 levels reach a peak at the time of the onset of LH surge and then decline rapidly. Serum levels of P begin to rise 12 hours before LH surge, continue to rise for additional 12 hour, and then plateau until follicular rupture (36 hours after LH surge onset). Follicular rupture is associated with a second rise in P and a fall in E_2, as luteal pattern of ovarian steroidogenesis is attained.

The threshold duration of LH surge required for the final stage of follicular and oocyte maturation has been studied in primates. Based on these studies (13,14), 14–18 hours of LH surge are required to reinitiate oocyte meiosis, whereas metaphase II oocytes are obtained after a 28-hour exposure to LH.

The GnRHa-Induced LH/FSH Surge

GnRHa elicits pituitary secretion of gonadotropins, which can be utilized for triggering oocyte maturation and ovulation, if given at the right time of the cycle. Numerous compounds, administered in different regimens, have been successfully used for that purpose (3–11). Based on these studies it appears that a single administration of a GnRHa in a dose of 200–500 µg effectively and reliably triggers the required gonadotropin surge (10,11); however, the minimal effective dose of GnRHa required to trigger an endogenous midcycle LH surge sufficient to induce oocyte maturation and ovulation remain to be established. Preliminary experience (15) suggests that a single dose of 50 µg intranasal buserelin is the most effective minimal dose consistently to trigger ovulation.

The pituitary and ovarian responses to midcycle GnRHa injections in stimulated cycles are displayed in Figure 25.1. The injection of GnRHa results in an acute release of LH and FSH. The serum LH and FSH levels rise 4 and 12 hours, respectively, and are elevated for 24–36 hours. The amplitude of the surge is similar to that seen in the normal menstrual cycle, but, by contrast with the natural cycle, the surge consists of only two phases: a short ascending limb (>4 hours) and a long descending limb (>20 hours). This has no bearing on ovarian hormones secretion pattern, which is qualitatively similar to the pattern observed in a natural cycle. As depicted in Figure 25.1, the LH surge is associated with a rapid rise of P and the attainment of peak E_2 levels during the first 12 hours after GnRHa administration. This followed by a transient suppression of P biosynthesis and a gradual decline in E_2 levels during the 24 hours preceding follicle aspiration. After oocyte retrieval, a second rapid rise in P and continuous fall in E_2 are observed, which reflects normal transition from follicular to luteal phase in ovarian steroidgenesis.

The Luteal Phase

Although the endogenous LH surge triggered by GnRHa is associated with a normal folliclar–luteal shift in ovarian steroidogensis, serum levels of E_2 and P during the luteal phase are lower compared with those achieved after hGC

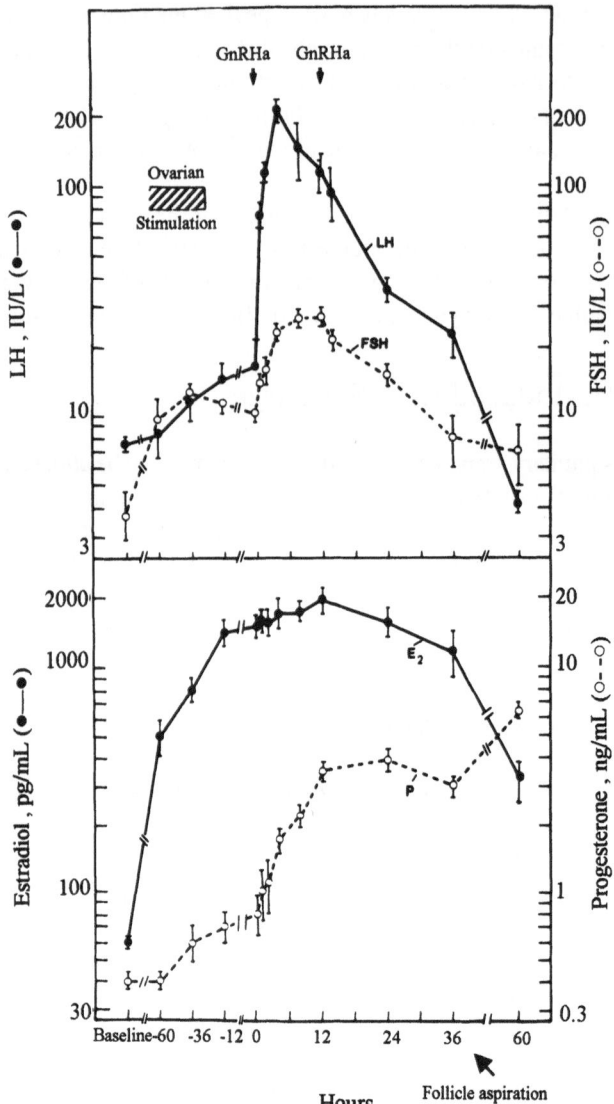

FIGURE 25.1. Hormonal levels (mean ± standard error of the mean) before and afer the injection of two dose of buserelin acetate, 500 µg, in six IVF patients. Mean serum E_2 level: before GnRHa injection was 1494 ± 422 pg/ml (± standard deviation). The baseline is Day 3 of the menstrual cycle. Reprinted by permission from the American Society for Reproductive Medicine, Fertil Steril 1991;56:213–20.

administration (Fig. 25.2). This may be related to the longer duration of plasma hCG activity compared with the shorter GnRHa-induced LH elevation. Normal function of the corpus luteum is dependent on pituitary LH (16). It is possible, therefore, that the prolonged down regulation of pituitary GnRH receptors after a midcycle injection of a GnRHa results in reduced LH support for the development corpora lutea, reduced steroidogenesis, and early luteolysis. Based on these considerations, it is prudent to support the luteal phase with P (and possibly E_2) in patients treated with midcycle GnRHa. Whether continued support during early pregnancy (i.e., until the luteal–placental shift) is required, has yet to be determined.

Prevention of OHSS

The most important benefit emerging from the use of GnRHa, rather than hCG, for ovulation induction, is the ability of this regimen to eliminate the threat of clinically significant OHSS completely. It should be emphasized that the clinical findings attributable to mild (17) OHSS (e.g., ovarian enlargement, abdominal discomfort, excessive steroid production) are an integral part of most cases of ovulation induction in IVF; hence, they are meaningless in this context. As mentioned earlier, the clinical experience with midcycle administration of GnRHa in the context of OHSS prevention is very encouraging. Effective ovulation is triggered effectively with no risk of OHSS, even in patients with extremely high E_2 levels during the late follicular phase (9). We are aware of three reports detailing cases in which OHSS developed despite the use of GnRHa to induce ovulation. Three cases were reported by van der Meer et al. (18). The clinical details of the three cases are in line with a mild-to-moderate OHSS. Severe ascites, hypovolemia, or electrolyte imbalance did not occur, nor were the patients hospitalized. Note was made of the fact that three patients received nasal GnRH-a preparations (buserelin; Superfact; Hoechst, Germany). In one of them, a very weak response to GnRH-a was noted, with an LH surge peak of 15.9 mIU/ml, which suggests that the dosage used or the route of administration were less than optimal. The possibility of incomplete absorption using nasal administration clearly cannot be ignored. It is of note that the three patients were stimulated in preparation for intrauterine insemination (IUI). Gerris et al. (19) have also reported OHSS following this approach; however, in this case, use was made of *native* GnRH (and not *GnRH-a*), which resulted in successful ovulation triggering, but without the critcal gonadotropin suppression, which is the key element in preventing OHSS. Last, Shoham et al. (20) reported a personal communication in which two cases of OHSS were described; however, the complete details of the treatment protocols, symptoms and signs leading to the diagnosis of OHSS, severity of the syndrome, and clinical outcome were not available.

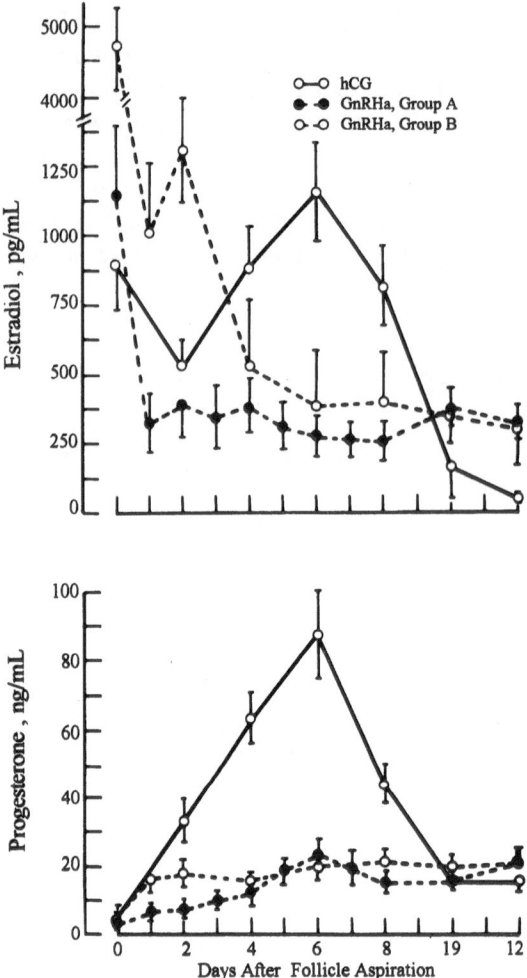

FIGURE 25.2. Serum E$_2$ and P levels (mean ± standard error of the mean) throughout the luteal phase in "normal responders" injected with either hCG (O—O), $n = 14$, E$_2$ on the day of hCG=1182 ± 562 pg/ml (± standard deviation) or GnRHa (group A, ●—●, $n =$ 6, E$_2$ on the day of GnRHa=1494 ± 422 pg/ml) and in "high responders" injected with GnRHa (group B, O- - -O, $n = 8$, E$_2$ on the day of GnRHa=7673 ± 3028 pg/ml). Control normal responders treated with hGC were supplemented with progesterone in oil 25–50 mg/day from Day 2 to Day 12. Normal and high responders injected with GnRHa were supplemented with estradiol valerate and progesterone in oil to maintain serum E$_2$ and P levels at approximately 200–400 pg/ml and 15–20 ng/ml, respectively. Reprinted by permission from the American Society for Reproductive Medicine, Fertil Steril 1991;56:213–20.

For more than 10 years of utilizing GnRHa to trigger ovulation in both IVF and ovulation induction high risk patients, we have not seen a single case of severe OHSS.

Benefits and Limitations

As discussed earlier, GnRHa is an effective alternative to hCG in ART, particularly, when the threat of OHSS is imminent. In addition, it offers a more physiological stimulus for ovulation, combining both LH and FSH surges. The presence of a midcycle FSH is apparently not obligatory for successful ovulation given the widespread use of hGC; hence, it is not known whether the FSH surge associated with GnRHa is of any advantage.

The major limitation of GnRHa-induced ovulation is that it could not be effective in woman with low gonadotropin reserve. It is not applicable, therefore, in IVF stimulation cycles during which use is made of pituitary downregulation with a GnRH agonist that renders the pituitary unresponsive for induction of endogenous LH surge. Because GnRH agonist-based protocols are used routinely by most IVF programs, GnRHa-induced ovulation for OHSS prevention has not gained much popularity.

Eye to the Future

The introduction of GnRH antagonists in COH protocols (21,22), and their anticipated debut in the clinical arena have opened new opportunities in the context of OHSS prevention. One possibility is to prevent spontaneous LH in high risk patients with high dose GnRH antagonist safely, waiting patiently for follicular demise and ovarian quiescence (23). In order to prevent OHSS effectively and to rescue the cycle at the same time, the quick reversibility of the antagonist-induced pituitary suppression can be of advantage by allowing the use of a GnRHa for the purpose of ovulation triggering. This possibility was assessed thus far in small-scale studies (24,25). It can be deduced from these preliminary reports that the pituitary response to GnRH or GnRHa is preserved folling GnRH antagonist-based follicular stimulation protocols. The extent of pituitary gonadotrophs suppression depends on the dose used. Under the minimal effective dose of GnRH antagonists it is most probable that ovulation could be safely and effectively triggered with a GnRH agonist. This may become a significant potential advantage of GnRH antagonist-based COH protocols for IVF because it lets the clinician choose the agent that will trigger ovulation. If OHSS is imminent, ovulation may be triggered with a GnRHa, eliminating any threat for significant OHSS. In fact, we feel it is safe to speculate that OHSS will become a very rare clinical condition once the approach described is widely adopted, even in cases at low risk for OHSS.

The responsiveness of the pituitary gonadotrophs to GnRHa may be blunted by pretreatment with a GnRH antagonist. The relatively short half-life of the GnRH antagonists that will become available soon (ganirelix and certrorelix), and the fact that the agonist will be given 12–30 hours after the last dose of the antagonist, set the stage for an adequate endogenous LH (and FSH) rise.

The effects of the proposed approach needs to be further studied; however, it gives clinicians a powerful and safe tool to prevent OHSS without the need to abort the cycle. Under current protocols, for reasons of safety, it is considered mandatory to cancel ovarian stimulation in the face of clear signs of imminent OHSS. The main reason for this attitude is that proposed prophylactic treatments (i.e., intravenous albumin) have not proved to be effective (26).

Last, the development of recombinant LH, and the current research for attenuated (in terms of biological half-life) recombinant gonadotropins, will offer further possibilities for ovulation induction in different clinical situations.

Summary

The physiologic basis and clinical applications of the use of GnRHa, rather than hCG, to induce the final stage of oocyte maturation and ovalation in gonadotrpin-treated cycles were reviewed. A single midcycle dose of GnRHa is able to trigger a preovlatory LH/FSH surge, leading to oocyte maturation in women undergoing ovarian stimulation for IVF, or induction of ovulation in vivo. The main advantage of this approach is the elimination of clinically significant OHSS. We speculate that the popularity of this approach will increase as GnRH antagonists become clinically available.

References

1. Yen SSC, Lenera G, Little B, Pearson OH. Disappearance rate of endogenous luteinizing hormone and chorionic gonadotropin in man. J Clin Endocrinol Metab 1968;28:1763–67.
2. Damewood MD, Shen W, Zacur HA, Schaff WD, Rock JA, Wallach EE. Disappearance of exogenously administered human chorionic gonadotropin. Fertil Steril 1989,52.398–400.
3. Golan A, Ron-El R, Herman A, Soffer Y, Weinraub Z, Caspi E. Ovarian hyperstimulation syndrome: an update review. Obstet Gynecol Surv 1989;44:430–40.
4. Emperaire JC, Ruffie A. Triggering ovulation with endogenous luteinizing hormone may prevent the ovarian hyperstimulation syndrome. Hum Reprod 1991;6:506–10.
5. Imoedemhe DAG, Chan RCW, Sigue AB, Pacpaco ELA, Olazo AB. A new approach to the management of patients at risk of ovarian hyperstimulation in an in-vitro ferilization programme. Hum Reprod 1991;6:1088–91
6. Itskovitz J, Boldes R, Barlev A. Erlik Y, Kahana L, Brandes JM. The induction of LH surge and oocyte maturation by GnRH analogue (buserelin) in woman undergoing ovarian stimulation for in vitro ferilization. Gynecol Endocrinol 1988;2(suppl. 2):165.
7. Itskovitz J, Boldes R, Levron J, Erlik Y, Kahana L, Brandes JM. Induction of preovu-

latory luteinizing hormone surge and prevention of ovarian hyperstimulation syndrome by gonadotropin-releasing hormone agonist. Fertil Steril 1991;56:213–20.

8. Lanzone A, Fulghesu AM, Villa P, Guida C, Guido M, Nicoletti MC, et al. Gonadotropin-releasing hormone agonist versus human chorionic gonadotropin as a trigger of ovulation in polycystic ovarian disease gonadotropin hyperstimulated cycles. Fertil Steril 1994;62:35–41.

9. Lewit N, Kol S, Manor D, Itskovitz-Eldor J. The use of GnRH analongs for induction of the preovulatory gonadotropin surge in assisted reproduction and prevention of the ovarian hyperstimulation syndrome. Gynecol Endocrinol 1995;4(suppl.):13–17.

10. Segal S, Casper RF. Gonadotropin-releasing hormone agoinst versus human chorionic gonadotropin for triggering folliclar maturation in in vitro fertilization. Fertil Steril 1992;57:1254–58.

11. Lewit N, Kol S, Manor D, Itskovitz-Eldor J. Comparison of GnRH analogs and hCG for the induction of ovulation and prevention of ovarian hyperstimulation syndrome (OHSS): a case-control study. Hum Reprod 1996;11:1399–402.

12. Hoff JD, Quingley ME, Yen SSC. Hormonal dynamics at midcycle: a reevaluation. J Clin Endocrinol Metab 1983;57:792–96.

13. Seibel MM, Smith DM, Levesque L, Borten M, Taymor ML. The temporal relationship between the luteinizing hormone surge and human oocyte maturation. Am J Obstet Gynecol 1982;142:568–72.

14. Zelinski-Wooten MB, Lanzendorf SE, Wolf DP, Chandrasekher YA, Stouffer RL. Titrating luteinizing hormone surge requirements for ovulatory changes in primate follicles, I: oocyte maturation and corpus luteum function. J Clin Endocrinol Metab 1991;73:577–83.

15. Buckett WM, Bentick B, Shaw RW. Induction of the endogenous gonadotrophin sugre for oocyte mauration with intra-nasal gonadotrophin-releasing hormone analogue (buserelin): effective minimal dose. Hum Reprod 1998;13:811–14.

16. Mais V, Kazar RR, Cetel NS, Rivier J, Vale W, Yen SSC. The dependency of folliculogenesis and corpus luteum function on pulsatile gonadotropin secretion in cycling women using a gonadotropin-releasing hormone antagonist as a probe. J Clin Endocrinol Metab 1986;62:1250–55.

17. Schenker JG, Weinstein D. Ovarian hyperstimulation syndrome: a current survey. Fertil Steril 1978;30:255–68.

18. van der Meer S, Gerris J, Joostens M, Tas B. Triggering of ovulation using a gonadotropin-releasing hormone agonist does not prevent ovarian hyperstimulation syndrome. Hum Reprod 1993;8:1628–31.

19. Gerris J, De Vits A, Joostens M, Van Royen E. Triggering of ovulation in human menopausal gonadotropin-stimulated cycles: comparison between intravenous administered gonadotrophin-releasing homone (100 and 500 µg), GnRH agonist (buserelin, 500 µg) and human chorionic gonadotrophin (10000 IU). Hum Reprod 1995;10:56–62.

20. Shoham Z, Schachter M, Loumaye E, Weissman A, MacNamee M, Insler V. The luteinizing hormone surge—the final stag in ovulation induction: modern aspects of ovulation triggering. Fertil Steril 1995;64:237–51.

21. Albano C, Smitz J, Camus M, Riethmuller-Winzen H, Van Steirteghem A, Devroey P. Comparison of different doses of gonadotropin-releasing hormone antagoist Cetrorelix during controlled ovarian hyperstimulation. Fertil Steril 1997;67:917–22

22. Itskovitz-Eldor J, Kol S, Mannaerts B, Coelingh Bennink H. Case report: first estab-

lished pregnancy after controlled ovarian hyperstimulation with recombinant follicle stimulating hormone and gonadotrophin-releasing hormone antagonist ganirelix (Org 37462). Hum Reprod 1998;13:294–95.

23. de Jong D, Macklon NS, Mannaerts BMJL, et al. High dose gonadotrophin-releasing hormone antagonist (ganirelix) may prevent ovarian hyperstimulation syndrome caused by ovarian stimulation for in-vitro ferilization. Hum Reprod 1998;13:573–75.

24. Felberbaum RE, Raissmann T, Kupker W, Bauer O, al Hasani S, Diedrich C, et al. Preserved pituitary response under ovarian stimulation with HMG and GnRH antagonists (Cetrorelix) in women with tubal infertility. Eur J Obstet Gynecol Reprod Biol 1995;61:151–55.

25. Olivennes F, Fanchin R, Bouchard P, Taieb J, Frydman R. Triggering of ovulation by a gonadotropin-releasing hormone (GnRH) agonist in patients pretreated with a GnRH antagonist. Fertil Steril 1996;66:151–53.

26. Lewit N, Kol S, Ronen N, Itskovitz-Eldor J. Does intravenous administration of human albumin prevent severe ovarian hyperstimulation syndrome? Fertil Steril 1996; 66:654.

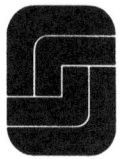

26

Closing Comments:
Ovulation from 1672 to 1998

GILBERT S. GREENWALD

In a classic study, "A New Treatise Concerning the Generative Organs of Women," Regnier de Graaf in 1672 described the effects of coitus on the rabbit ovary (1). Twenty-four hours after coitus, the egg follicles were transformed into new structures: the corpora lutea. Thus, de Graaf is one of the founding fathers of reproductive research and the first in the quest to understand ovulation.

Fast forwarding to the twentieth century, the first major international meeting—the Singer-Polignac Colloquium—was held in Paris in 1937, followed by a major conference in Syracuse, NY, in 1958. The closing remarks by Sir Zolly Zuckerman stressed that the major advances since 1980 were mainly attributable to the chemists unraveling the nature of the steroid nucleus and establishing the basis for hormonal reactions. He was less sanguine about the progress of reproductive biology: "I ask whether the area of our ignorance today is really smaller than it appeared in the '30s." He felt that endocrinologists tend to generalize too much with relatively little new concrete data to work with. Is this still true today?

I doubt that Sir Zolly's verdict was correct even then. The past half century has certainly witnessed an unprecedented increase in knowledge of reproductive physiology, attributable to several factors: remarkable advances in technology culminating in molecular techniques; the interlocking nature of the life sciences and the rapidity with which breakthrough findings are transferred between them; the recognition that analysis of homologous gene sequences in yeast, *Drosophila, C. elegans, Xenopus*, and so on, can be extrapolated to mammals. Finally, the exponential increase in the number of workers in the field is also an important factor accelerating the growth of our discipline. These advances are all blended together in this book.

The stage for Salt Lake City was set by key findings in the mid-1950s to early 1970s; for example, time-lapse photography of ovulation in the rat (2); studies on the mechanism of ovulation (3); ultrastructure of ovulation in the rabbit (4); biophysical aspects of ovulation (5). The following are some of the major themes that have been discussed.

Ovulation as an Inflammatory Process

For many years, Larry Espey was a voice in the wilderness in establishing the role of inflammation as a key factor in ovulation. There is no doubt about the significance of this concept. The problem is the increasing complexity of the system involving, among others, prostanoids, eicosanoids, reactive oxygen species, leukocytic release of inflammatory factors, and vasoactive agents, makes it difficult to assess what are primary or secondary steps. The good old days when LH entered the black box and ovulation exited is no longer feasible to explain a multifactorial system. Several authors explored this theme.

The rennin–angiotensin system, studied in vivo, and in vitro shows a connection between angiotensin II and prostaglandin production (Mikuni et al.). In *COX-2 knockout mice* (a key rate-limiting enzyme in prostanoid synthesis), the animals are infertile because of impaired ovulation (Sirois). When *prostaglandin synthesis is blocked by indomethacin,* after hCG injection, gelatinase and TIMP-1 increase independent of an increase in prostanoids; the characteristic rise in progesterone (P_4) and decline of estradiol are also unaffected. Although $PGF_{2\alpha}$ mRNA does not increase in the indomethacin treated rats, ovulation still occurred at 24 hours, albeit at a reduced rate (Curry et al.). *Depletion of neutrophils or macrophages* from the ovary of the prepubertal rat decreases the ovulation rate, but adding a crude leukocytic fraction to the perfused prepubertal ovary restores ovulation to the normal rate (Brännström et al.). In vivo *follicular vascular changes* were studied by intravital microscopy. Blood flow is intermittently interrupted in apical vessels of the enlarging preovulatory follicle, and microemboli concomitantly block apical but not lateral vessels (Zackrisson et al.). The *angiopoetins* (ANG) are a newly characterized family involved in angiogenesis along with VEGF. In the immature rat model, VEGF is initially restricted to the cumulus oophorus; however, after PMS the reaction spreads to the membrana granulosa (Wiegand et al.). On the other hand, before PMS Ang-1 is localized in thecal blood vessels, whereas Ang-2 (an antagonist of Ang-1) is not expressed. By the afternoon of proestrus, Ang-2 is now intensely present in the theca. Ang-1 and -2 are normally limited to endothelial cells but in *atretic* antral follicles, Ang-2 is found in the granulosa compartment—a nonvascular tissue.

Preantral Follicles: The Last Frontier

We are all grateful to Dr. Alain Gougeon for his herculean task of sectioning 107 human ovaries, but more importantly for providing a detailed analysis of follicular kinetics. This stresses the still-significant role of morphometric analysis that provides answers that are not always met by molecular techniques. I recommend a review by Dr. Gougeon (6). Gougeon classifies resting follicles into three categories: primordial, intermediate, primary (surrounded by one layer of cuboidal granulosa cells). At present, we know absolutely nothing about what factors recruit primordial follicles into the growing pool. The best species to explore this problem is perhaps the pig, where through simple enzymatic dissociation (7) it is possible to recover 400,000 primordials per ovary (8).

A topic that has excited considerable interest reveals that an mRNA to a growth factor differentiation factor-9 (GDF-9) is present in mouse oocytes of all stages except primordial follicles. GDF-9 persists until 1 day postovulation (9). Moreover, GDF-9 knockout mice are infertile with follicular development limited to primary follicles; PMS fails to overcome the block to further follicular development (10). In prepubertal rats stimulated by PMS, primary follicles similarly are the only stage not affected (Kishi and Greenwald, unpublished).

Our knowledge of preantral follicles is fragmentary and controversial. For example, preantral follicles isolated by enzymatic dissociation (7) or manually dissected respond in vitro to FSH by growth and differentiation in cow, hamster, human, mouse, and rat and FSH receptors are present in preantral follicles of all five species plus ovine and porcine follicles. Thus, the dogma that preantral follicles are gonadotropin independent may have to be modified.

Another issue to be resolved is the extent of atresia in preantral follicles. One of the problems is the diverse criteria used in defining atresia in various species. Atresia in rat preantral follicles is purportedly very low, but clear morphometric analyses are unavailable. Atresia occurs, however, at appreciable rates in various species (e.g., human [30%], mouse [18%], hamster [19%], sheep [40% in follicles <1 mm], rabbit [61%], and pig [58% based on zona pellucida staining]). Thus, there are considerable species differences in the rate of atresia of preantral follicles.

Still another apparent example of species differences is the effect of estrogens in recruiting preantral follicles. It is certainly true in the rat and mouse, but not in the hypophysectomized hamster or in some rat, guinea pig, and macaque models (11). Thus, the problem has not been tested in enough species to determine whether the direct effect of estrogens on follicular numbers is the rule or the exception.

The Fate of the Graafian Follicle: Atresia or Ovulation

As soon as the antral cavity develops, the majority of follicles are destined to become atretic; only a minority go on to ovulate. As Erickson pointed out, the deciding factor in survival is the concentration of follicular stimulating hormone (FSH), as elegantly demonstrated by McNatty (12). FSH is therefore critical, acting as a growth factor in preventing apoptosis in cultured early antral follicles and preantral follicles. It is capable of inducing ovulation as a substitute for human chorionic gonadotropin (hCG) (Hsueh et al.). Still another function of FSH is to stimulate DNA synthesis in the smallest preantral follicles in the hamster ovary—follicles with one to four layers of granulosa cells, but no theca. This reinforces Gougeon's hypothesis that the preovulatory peak in gonadotropin levels may stimulate DNA replication even in small follicles. These "privileged" follicles may develop over several cycles, boosted by gonadotropin surges before they either ovulate or become atretic.

Erickson gave an excellent summary of the heterogeneity of the healthy antral follicle with three distinct regional zones of the granulosal compartment: cumulus oophorus, basal cells of the membrana granulosa, and peripheral cells bordering on the antral cavity. These regions differ in structure and function, responding differently to luteinizing hormone (LH) and FSH (and possibly steroids?).

Erickson raised the question: What is the role of follicular fluid (FF)? Some investigators have speculated that FF is not of physiological consequence, representing only a sink for steroids produced by thecal–granulosal interactions and that the only functionally significant steroids are exported to the periphery via thecal blood vessels. Some light is provided by studies involving follicular growth supported only by FSH and minimal or completely absent LH.

The story begins in 1942 when Greep and associates (13) showed that porcine FSH administered to hypophysectomized rats produced large antral follicles, but no evidence of estrogen secretion. In women with 17α-hydroxylase deficiency, treatment with a GnRH agonist and prednisone suppressed gonadotropin secretion (14). Subsequent injection of pure FSH matured large follicles, but plasma estradiol was undetectable. Cynomologus monkeys injected with a GnRH antagonist for 20 days followed by rFSH, similarly, developed multiple follicles, but there were minimal levels of estradiol in serum and FF (15). Another study by Zelinski-Wooten and colleagues (16) used an aromatase inhibitor injected on Days 8–10 to reduce serum estradiol drastically by 84%. In the monkey studies, estradiol was not completely suppressed, but the same year the Zelinski-Wooten results were published we found even greater reduction in estradiol in a model involving hypophysectomized mice: The animals were untreated for 12 days before injecting FSH for 4 days (see Ref. 17). Preovulatory follicles were incubated on Day 4 of FSH treatment and estradiol was undetectable in the medium. When the animals were injected with hCG and mated, the fertilized eggs only progressed to the two-celled stage in vivo. When two-celled embryos were grown in vitro only 22% developed into blastocysts by 96 hours of culture compared with 80% forming blastocysts by 72 hours by embryos of normal mice (17).

Similar results were obtained when rabbit ovaries were perfused with clomiphene citrate (CC), an antiestrogen, and the contralateral ovary perfused with CC plus estradiol (18). The addition of hCG induced similar rates of ovulation and fertilization in both ovaries, but whereas 87.5% of recipients were pregnant from the CC plus E_2 ovary, only 25.0% were pregnant from the CC-treated ovary. The latter papers (17,18) therefore suggest that the lack of estrogen affected postovulatory embryogenesis. In this connection, estrogen receptor mRNA is detectable in human and mouse oocytes (19).

To return to the initial question: Is follicular fluid of physiological importance? The somewhat devious line of evidence I have mustered suggests that follicular steroids, especially estrogens, may function as autocrine and paracrine factors in maintaining the membrana granulosa and *maturation of the oocyte*, respectively. A final point is that we showed in 1985 that binding sites for FSH and hCG are demonstrable, by autoradiography, in oocytes stripped of zonae in rodents and rabbits (20). The availability now of RT-PCR makes this a worthwhile area to pursue.

The Midcycle Gonadotropin Surge

After *pulsatile administration of GnRH* (at a greatly reduced rate) to women with a GnRH deficiency, ovulation occurred in seven women, which suggests that the amount of GnRH does not increase at midcycle, which in turn suggests that the pituitary is the site where positive feedback of LH is elicited (Taylor, et al.). In animals with intact and functional hypothalamic axes, however, a preovulatory surge of GnRH exists in rat, rabbit, monkey, and sheep. For ethical reasons the question whether a similar temporal sequence is operative in women will obviously never be answered. A rhesus model of *preovulatory follicular development* was tested by dose–response administration of GnRH, or hCG, or LH (Zelinski-Wooten et al.). The conclusion was that the duration of gonadotropin surges determines whether oocyte maturation will occur with longer periods required for sustained luteal function.

FSH induces ovulation in hypophysectomized rats and reinstates oocyte meiosis (Hsueh et al.). Furthermore, in Trilostane-treated monkeys a bolus of rFSH initiates oocyte meiosis, fertilization, and P_4 production by granulosa cells (Zelinski-Wooten et al.). Ovarian hyperstimulation syndrome (OHSS) is a major problem in ovulation induction and is attributable to increased levels of the rennin–angiotensin system, endothelin, VEGF, and cytokines (Jones). These complications are related to the long half-life of hCG used to induce ovulation. An alternative is to *substitute GnRH*, which completely eliminates OHSS as a problem (Kol and Itskovitz-Eldor). Finally, recombinant technology has created *designer gonadotropins and receptors* of yoked single chain gonadotropins of greater stability than wild-type hormones with the prospect of future superagonists and antagonists (Puett and Narayan).

The Oocyte as the "Soul" of the Follicle

A 1970 paper from Nalbandov's lab (21) showed that "ovectomizing" rabbit follicles led 3 days later to luteinization and elevated concentration of progesterone in ovarian venous effluent. Thus, removal of the oocyte took away a restraining influence that prevented luteinization. Nalbandov told me that the oocyte was therefore the "soul" of the follicle. Several chapters herein stressed the pivotal role of the oocyte in regulating follicular function.

In previous work, Dr. Salustri showed that before the LH surge *hyaluronic acid* is located in the cumulus cells and then spreads to engulf the membrana granulosa after the gonadotropin surges on proestrus. In this volume she shows that the oocyte is responsible for producing a soluble factor that interacts with two matrix proteins in cumulus cells. In vitro, absence of the oocyte hinders the increase of "hyaluron" synthase in cumulus cells in response to FSH. Two hours after LH, ascorbic acid (AA) decreases in granulosa cells and germinal vesicle breakdown begins at 4h (Behrman et al.). Thus AA depletion precedes oocyte meiosis. Direct intraoocyte injection of AA significantly delays the onset of GVBD. It has been suggested that oxygen radicals induce GVBD after depletion of antioxidants. An isoform of endothelial synthase (ENOS) is localized in follicular somatic cells and oocytes and the levels increase substantially before and after ovulation (Olson et al.). In ENOS knockout mice fewer oocytes advance to MII, and ovulation is reduced by 61% in a superovulation model. *Ovarian teratomas* are quite common in LT strain mice in which MI arrest is frequently observed (Eppig et al.). This is associated with oocyte failure to degrade Cyclin G; concurrently, a cytostatic factor (MOS) persists.

Progesterone: A Key Player in Ovulation

An intriguing paper from Greep's lab (22) dealt with rats hypophysectomized at 1550 hours on proestrus (when the LH surge was initiated) but the animals did not ovulate; however, massive injections of P_4 restored ovulation. In the perfused rat ovary that has been treated with LH, addition of a 3β-hydroxysteroid steroid inhibitor similarly decreases the number of ovulations that are restored by addition of P_4 (23).

P_4 knockout mice have normal preovulatory follicular development, but they fail to ovulate (Robker and Richards). This is associated with normal numbers of macrophages, but deficient neutrophils and evidence for a possible deficiency of a specific protease that prevents cleavage of MMP-13 to a smaller active form. In Trilostane-treated monkeys injected with hCG, simultaneous administration of a progestin restores luteinization, P_4 levels, and mRNAs for MMP-1 and TIMP-1 (Stouffer et al.). In normal mice and rats, P_4 receptors localize in granulosa cells.

Paracrine and Autocrine Factors in the Preovulatory Follicle

One of the revelations of the past few decades is the universal distribution of peptide hormones in "aberrant" locations where they function in paracrine and autocrine roles in gut, placenta, and the ovary. In antral follicles, the majority are restricted to granulosa cells, but notable exceptions are found in thecal cells. Several of the peptides do not reach peak levels until shortly before ovulation, which suggests that their presence is possibly related more to luteal than follicular function.

Thus, *oxytocin* in the bovine follicle is synthesized and secreted by granulosa cells (GC) and is induced by the LH surge; it increases P_4 production, which reciprocates by stimulating oxytocin (Fortune et al.). The *inhibin related peptides* are also restricted to GCs (Findlay et al.). In vitro experiments suggest that inhibin stimulates LH-induced androgen production by rat and human thecal cells. This may be important in selecting the dominant follicle(s) by providing the C-19 precursors for estrogen synthesis. Immunizing sheep with the N-terminal portion of the inhibin-a subunit leads to atresia of all follicles > 1 mm. Contrary to oxytocin and inhibin, *nerve growth factor* is found in theca and interstitial cells with peak activity after the LH surge (Dissen and Ojeda). Intrabursal administration of an NRF antiserum blocks ovulation. To my knowledge, renin is restricted to the theca (rabbit) and angiotensin-II to granulosa cells (rat). Hence, interaction of both follicular compartments may be needed for functional activity. With the distribution of peptides in theca and granulosa, one wonders whether LH is the sole stimulus or whether FSH might also be involved.

Unraveling the Puzzle: Targeted Gene Deletions

The ability to dissect intricate systems by knockout mice is one of the most significant advances, but whether the findings in mice can be extrapolated to all species remains to be proven. The value of gene deletions has been shown by knockouts for cyclin D2 (Richards and Robker), C/EBP (Johnson and Sterneck), prostaglandin synthase (Sirois), NO synthase (Olson et al.), P_4 receptor (Robker and Richards), and NGF (Dissen and Ojeda). An obvious word of caution is that with so much redundancy built into any system the possibility of compensation by other factors must be considered if a function is not lost (e.g., FSH —> cAMP —> EGF in the hamster follicle).

References

1. De Graaf R. A new treatise concerning the generative organs of women, 1672. Jocelyn HD, Setchell BPJ, eds. J Reprod Fert 1972(suppl. 17).

2. Blandau RJ. Ovulation in the living albino rat. Fertil Steril 1955;6:391–404.

3. Zachariae F. Studies on the mechanism of ovulation: permeability of the blood–liquor barrier. Acta Endocrinol 1958;27:339–42.

4. Espey LL. Ultrastructure of the apex of the rabbit Graafian follicle. Endocrinology 1967;81:267–76.

5. Rondell P. Biophysical aspects of ovulation. Biol Reprod 1970;2(suppl. 2):64–89.

6. Gougeon A. Regulation of ovarian follicular development in primates: facts and hypotheses. Endocrine Rev 1996;17:121–55.

7. Roy SK, Greenwald GS. An enzymatic method for dissociation of intact follicles from the hamster ovary: histological and quantitative aspects. Biol Reprod 1985;32:203–15.

8. Greenwald GS, Moor RM. Isolation and preliminary characterization of porcine primordial follicles. J Reprod Fert 1989;87:561–71.

9. McGrath SA, Esquela AF, Lee S-J. Oocyte-specific expression of growth/differentiation factor-9. Mol Endocrinol 1995;9:131–36.

10. Dong J, Albertini DF, Nishimori K, Kumar TR, Lu N, Matzuk MM. Growth differentiation factor-9 is required during early ovarian folliculogenesis. Nature 1996;383:531–35.

11. Hutz RJ. Disparate effects of estrogens on in vitro steroidogenesis by mammalian and avian granulosa cells. Biol Reprod 1989;40:709–13.

12. McNatty KP, Hunter WM, McNeilly AS, Sawers RS. Changes in the concentration of pituitary and steroid hormones in the follicular fluid of human Graafian follicles throughout the menstrual cycle. J Endocrinol 1975;64:555–71.

13. Greep RO, van Dyke HB, Chow BF. Gonadotropins of the swine pituitary. Endocrinology 1942;30:635–49.

14. Rabinovici A, Blankenstein J, Goldman B, Rudak E, Dor Y, Pariente C, et al. In vitro fertilization and primary embryonic cleavage are possible in 17α-hydroxylase deficiency despite extremely low intrafollicular 17β-estradiol. J Clin Endocrinol Metab 1989;68:693–97.

15. Karnitis VJ, Townson DH, Friedman CI, Danforth DR. Recombinant human follicle-stimulating hormone stimulates multiple follicular growth, but minimal estrogen production in gonadotropin-releasing hormone antagonist-treated monkeys: examining the role of luteinizing hormone in follicular development and steroidogenesis. J Clin Endocrinol Metab 1994;79:91–97.

16. Zelinski-Wooten MB, Hess DL, Baughman WL, Molskness TA, Wolf DP, Stouffer RL. Administration of an aromatase inhibitor during the late follicular phase of gonadotropin-treated cycles in rhesus monkeys: effects on follicle development, oocyte maturation, and subsequent luteal function. J Clin Endocrinol Metab 1993;76:988–95.

17. Wang X-N, Greenwald GS. Human chorionic gonadotropin or human recombinant follicle-stimulating hormone (FSH)-induced ovulation and subsequent fertilization and early embryo development in hypophysectomized FSH-primed mice. Endocrinology 1993;132:2009–16.

18. Yoshimura Y, Hosoi Y, Atlas SJ, Dharmarajan AM, Adachi T, Wallach EE. Effect of the exposure of intrafollicular oocytes to clomiphene citrate on pregnancy outcome in the rabbit. Fertil Steril 1988;50:153–58.

19. Wu T-CJ, Wang L, Wan Y-JY. Detection of estrogen receptor messenger ribonucleic acid in human oocytes and cumulus-oocyte complexes using reverse transcriptase-polymerase chain reaction. Fertil Steril 1993;59:54–59.

20. Roy SK, Greenwald GS. Evidence for binding sites for FSH and hCG in mammalian

oocytes. Proceedings of the fifth Ovarian Workshop. In: Toft D, Ryan R, eds. Champaign, IL; Ovarian Workshop Inc., 1985:143–47.

21. El-Fouly MA, Cook B, Nekola M, Nalbandov AV. Role of the ovum in follicular luteinization. Endocrinology 1970;87:288–93.

22. Takahashi M, Ford JJ, Yoshinaga K, Greep RO. Induction of ovulation in hypophysec-tomized rats by progesterone. Endocrinology 1974; 95:1322–26.

23. Brännström M, Janson PO. Progesterone is a mediator in the ovulatory process of the in vitro-perfused rat ovary. Biol Reprod 1989;40:1170–78.

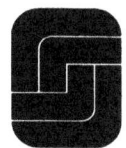

Author Index

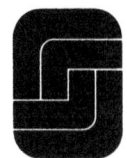

Subject Index

PROCEEDINGS IN THE SERONO SYMPOSIA USA SERIES

(Continued)

FOLLICLE STIMULATING HORMONE: Regulation of Secretion and Molecular Mechanisms of Action
Edited by Mary Hunzicker-Dunn and Neena B. Schwartz

SIGNALING MECHANISMS AND GENE EXPRESSION IN THE OVARY
Edited by Geula Gibori

GROWTH FACTORS IN REPRODUCTION
Edited by David W. Schomberg

UTERINE CONTRACTILITY: Mechanisms of Control
Edited by Robert E. Garfield

NEUROENDOCRINE REGULATION OF REPRODUCTION
Edited by Samuel S.C. Yen and Wylie W. Vale

FERTILIZATION IN MAMMALS
Edited by Barry D. Bavister, Jim Cummins, and Eduardo R.S. Roldan

GAMETE PHYSIOLOGY
Edited by Ricardo H. Asch, Jose P. Balmaceda, and Ian Johnston

GLYCOPROTEIN HORMONES: Structure, Synthesis, and Biologic Function
Edited by William W. Chin and Irving Boime

THE MENOPAUSE: Biological and Clinical Consequences of Ovarian Failure: Evaluation and Management
Edited by Stanley G. Korenman